Chlamydia - Secret Enemy From Past to Present

Edited by Mehmet Sarier

Published in London, United Kingdom

Chlamydia - Secret Enemy From Past to Present
http://dx.doi.org/10.5772/intechopen.106108
Edited by Mehmet Sarier

Contributors
Ibrahim Duman, Saurabh Krishna Misra, Ankita Pundir, Panagiota Xaplanteri, Charalampos Potsios, Nikiforos Rodis, Mehmet Besir Akpinar, Elçin Yenidünya Konuk, Erhan Alkan, Gül Banu Çiçek Bideci, Özlem Koca, Atakan Yanikoglu, Ramón Scharbaai-Vázquez, Francisco J. J. López Font, Félix Zayas Rodriguez, Hande Berk Cam, Anna Fedorova, Seçil Özdemir Şahin, Walter C Millanzi, Nurgül Uzun, Gül Aydın Tığlı, Esin Kasap, Alev Özlem Özdemir-Karabağ, Hayriye Daloglu, Sibel Surmen Usta

First published in London, United Kingdom, 2023 by IntechOpen
IntechOpen is the global imprint of INTECHOPEN LIMITED, registered in England and Wales, registration number: 11086078, 5 Princes Gate Court, London, SW7 2QJ, United Kingdom
Printed in Croatia

British Library Cataloguing-in-Publication Data
A catalogue record for this book is available from the British Library

Additional hard and PDF copies can be obtained from orders@intechopen.com

Chlamydia - Secret Enemy From Past to Present
Edited by Mehmet Sarier
p. cm.

This title is part of the Infectious Diseases Book Series, Volume 23
Topic: Bacterial Infectious Diseases
Series Editor: Alfonso J. Rodriguez-Morales
Topic Editors: Tomas Jarzembowski and Katarzyna Garbacz

Print ISBN 978-1-83768-760-2
Online ISBN 978-1-83768-761-9
eBook (PDF) ISBN 978-1-83768-762-6
ISSN 2631-6188

For EU product safety concerns:
IN TECH d.o.o., Prolaz Marije Krucifikse Kozulić 3, 51000 Rijeka, Croatia,
info@intechopen.com or visit our website at intechopen.com.

IntechOpen Book Series

Infectious Diseases

Volume 23

Aims and Scope of the Series

This series will provide a comprehensive overview of recent research trends in various Infectious Diseases (as per the most recent Baltimore classification). Topics will include general overviews of infections, immunopathology, diagnosis, treatment, epidemiology, etiology, and current clinical recommendations for managing infectious diseases. Ongoing issues, recent advances, and future diagnostic approaches and therapeutic strategies will also be discussed. This book series will focus on various aspects and properties of infectious diseases whose deep understanding is essential for safeguarding the human race from losing resources and economies due to pathogens.

Meet the Series Editor

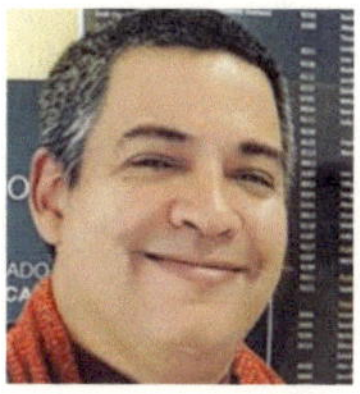

Dr. Rodriguez-Morales is an expert in tropical and emerging diseases, particularly zoonotic and vector-borne diseases (notably arboviral diseases), and more recently COVID-19 and Monkeypox. He is the president of the Publications and Research Committee of the Pan-American Infectious Diseases Association (API), as well as the president of the Colombian Association of Infectious Diseases (ACIN). He is a member of the Committee on Tropical Medicine, Zoonoses, and Travel Medicine of ACIN. Dr. Rodriguez-Morales is a vice-president of the Latin American Society for Travel Medicine (SLAMVI) and a member of the Council of the International Society for Infectious Diseases (ISID). Since 2014, he has been recognized as a senior researcher at the Ministry of Science of Colombia. He is a professor at the Faculty of Medicine of the Fundacion Universitaria Autonoma de las Americas, in Pereira, Risaralda, Colombia, and a professor, Master in Clinical Epidemiology and Biostatistics, at Universidad Científica del Sur, Lima, Peru. He is also a non-resident adjunct faculty member at the Gilbert and Rose-Marie Chagoury School of Medicine, Lebanese American University, Beirut, Lebanon, and an external professor, Master in Research on Tropical Medicine and International Health, at Universitat de Barcelona, Spain. Additionally, an invited professor, Master in Biomedicine, at Universidad Internacional SEK, Quito, Ecuador, and a visiting professor, Master Program of Epidemiology, at Diponegoro University, Indonesia. In 2021 he was awarded the "Raul Isturiz Award" Medal of the API and, the same year, the "Jose Felix Patiño" Asclepius Staff Medal of the Colombian Medical College due to his scientific contributions to the topic of COVID-19 during the pandemic. He is currently the Editor in Chief of the journal Travel Medicine and Infectious Diseases. His Scopus H index is 55 (Google Scholar H index 77) with a total of 725 publications indexed in Scopus.

Meet the Volume Editor

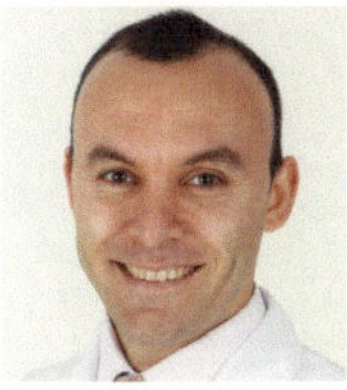

Mehmet Sarier, MD, is an associate professor in the Department of Urology, Faculty of Medicine, Istinye University, Turkey. He has published nearly fifty articles in national and international journals and presented more than fifty oral and written abstracts at congresses. He has also written three book chapters, edited one book, and served as a reviewer for more than 400 articles indexed in Publons. His research interests include endourology, andrology, sexually transmitted diseases, and urological complications following renal transplantation. He is a member of the Turkish Urologic Association and Society of Urological Surgery.

Contents

Preface

Chlamydia – Secret Enemy from Past to Present is written by a group of distinguished clinicians, scientists, and educators from different countries. The book examines chlamydial infections using a comprehensive multidisciplinary approach. The microbiology, clinical presentation, and current approaches in the diagnosis and treatment management of chlamydial infection are presented from the viewpoint of different clinics, accompanied by recent literature. We believe this book will be a useful resource for researchers and clinicians.

The book consists of twenty-one chapters organized into five sections: “Chlamydia as a Bacterium and Current Approaches in Diagnosis”, “Chlamydia as a Zoonosis and the Treatment of Chlamydial Infection”, “Multidisciplinary Approach to Chlamydial Infection”, “Chlamydia as a Sexually Transmitted Disease”, and “Pediatric and Adolescent Chlamydial Infection”.

Section 1 describes the characteristics of chlamydial bacteria, the laboratory tests that play an important role in infection management, molecular developments in the diagnosis of chlamydial infection, and the latest innovations in chlamydia immunology.

Section 2 presents chlamydia as a zoonosis and discusses treatment approaches and antibiotic resistance in chlamydial infection.

Section 3 examines the clinical presentations of human chlamydial infection in different disciplines and explains the broad range of treatment approaches to chlamydial infection. This section updates the management of chlamydial infection from the perspectives of cardiology, neurology, gastroenterology, cardiovascular surgery, and ophthalmology.

Section 4 presents chlamydial infection from the andrological and gynecological perspective as a sexually transmitted disease (STD) and discusses the effect of chlamydial infection on fertility. It also explains the importance of chlamydial infection as an STD in terms of public health.

Section 5 evaluates chlamydial infection in the pediatric and adolescent period, its association with pediatric asthma, and its social impact on adolescents.

I would like to thank my wife Pınar Sarıer and my children Nil and Alp, who have added meaning to my life and were always supportive during the preparation of this book.

I also extend my condolences to everyone affected by the devastating earthquake that occurred earlier this year in Turkey and Syria. I wish a speedy recovery to all those injured. Thanks as well to our publisher IntechOpen, who contacted us after the earthquake and offered their sympathies.

Mehmet Sarier M.D.
Assistant Professor,
Department of Urology,
Medical School of Istinye University,
Istanbul, Turkey

Section 1

Chlamydia as a Bacterium and Current Approaches in Diagnosis

Chapter 1

Chlamydia: The Secret Enemy from the Past to Present, and Future

Saurabh Krishna Misra and Ankita Pundir

Abstract

Chlamydia was discovered in 1907 by Halberstaedter and Von Prowazek in conjunctival scrapings from an experimentally infected orangutan. Once being thought of as symbiont in plant like unicellular amoebae to intracellular parasites of vertebrates to viruses to currently as obligate intracellular bacteriae. Chlamydia is able to survive indefinitely as viable but non cultivable altered forms being a bacteria. It's a supremely adaptable microorganism as seen with the emergence of it's Swedish New variant (nvCT) in 2006, which was not a product of mutation or recombination but due to losing a short segment of DNA from it's plasmid. The disease expression of Chlamydia is due to the interplay between the differences in the plasticity zone of it's genome and the host factors. Despite the recombination of genes and emergence of new variants there is no evidence of circulating genomic resistance in *Chlamydia trachomatis*. The 'seek and treat' Chlamydia control strategy shortens the genital infection yet it's rising sequelae of tubal infertility, the evidence of neoplastic change in cervix via modulation of caveolin-1 and c-myc RNA expression and it's under investigated role in pathogenesis of atherosclerosis and ischemic heart disease is a sign of how exponentially this organism is evolving.

Keywords: evolution, future, diagnostics, treatment, vaccine

1. Introduction

Humans have bravely faced this magically cloaked organism since the past till present; and their efforts to deal with it in the future are still going on strong. They are dwelling worldwide among livestock, humans and free-living animals. The true color of Chlamydia will be discussed as how secretively it has spread its roots among humans playing constant hide and seek with us without our suspicion. One chapter is never enough to talk about Chlamydia and how it might soon get the status of being omnipresent. Our hope is not only to touch upon its journey from past to present as concisely as possible, but also to express our views about conjoined future with us. Before talking about the present scenarios, we need to understand about the organism first.

2. Chlamydia: the organism

The phylum of Chlamydiae has obligate intracellular, Gram-negative bacteria. They consist of the following four groups (Simkania, Waddila, Chlamydiaceae and

Parachlamydia family) with five added Candidatus families (Parilichlamydiaceae, Clavichlamydiaceae, Rhabdochlamydiaceae, Criblamydiaceae, and Piscichlamydiaceae) [1]. Literature search tells us that chlamydia like caused diseases in the eye have occurred in ancient Egyptian papyri (1555–1553 BC) and Chinese writings (2700 BC). The associates of Albert Neisser, von Prowazek and Halberstaedter, noticed inclusions within the cytoplasm of cells in the scrapings of conjunctiva, from patients with trachoma in 1907. Chlamydiae was isolated by Levinthal, Cole and Lillie between 1929 and 1930 while they were studying psittacosis. It was described as a virus by Bedson an Bland in 1932 [2]. Earlier chlamydiae were considered to be protozoa in 1997 as chlamydia-like microorganisms were first found in single-celled, free-living environmental acanthamoebae [3]. Then as they passed through filters of 0.45 μm diameter and had a biphasic intracellular development cycle, they were thought of as viruses. However, as it had- both RNA and DNA, the ability to synthesize nucleic acids, proteins and lipids, the susceptibility to antibiotics; hence they were concluded as bacteria. However, as they are obligate intracellular pathogens, they are cultivated only within living cells, unlike free living bacteria [2].

At present there are 16 species put forward in the *Chlamydiaceae* family, which infect a broad range of hosts and different anatomical sites. Out of which humans are primarily infected by *C. trachomatis* and *C. pneumoniae*, with *C. psittaci* having proven zoonotic potential in humans [4].

C. trachomatis remains an elusive human infecting species constantly under focus. It consists of four ocular serovars A, B, Ba, and C that cause endemic trachoma, with at least eight serovars, D to K, that cause infections of the genital tract. In addition three L serovars are also included that cause lymphogranuloma venerum. Genome sequencing helped in knowing this enigmatic organism more. An early study on genomic phylogeny described the "trachoma clade" in which *C. trachomatis* is divided into two distinct clades of LGV and the ocular and genital tract isolates [5]. This clade has two lineages (T1 and T2). Clade T1 includes more common urogenital isolates, whereas T2 contains rarer urogenital isolates and ocular strains, that makes this cluster, making one suspect that these ocular isolates could have emerged from a urogenital ancestor. It is suspected that chlamydiae spread further from a urogenital niche to infect the eye, resulting in trachoma [6]. This notion evolves from the ability of urogenital isolates to utilize indole and synthesize tryptophan that is abundant in the vagina due to it's microbiome, but ocular strains lack this ability. Hence, urogenital strains can flourish both in the eye and genital tract, whereas ocular strains fail to thrive in the genital tract [7]. Myths like, *C. trachomatis* is a parasite as it derives energy from the eukaryotic host cell have been quashed with the help of genome sequencing with the discovery of all the required genes for the biosynthesis of ATP [8].

Over the years Chlamydiacae family evolved to give rise to new variants, serovars and species and humans have discovered new species as well while studying this organism over the years. The process of Lateral gene transfer (LGT) influences bacterial ecology and pathogenesis of diseases, evolution of Chlamydia and the propagation of antibiotic resistance across different species. Also known as Horizontal gene transfer, it involves genetic material (DNA) transfer between the cells followed by it's integration into the recipient cell's genome. Mutation is not the only adaptive strategy of *C. trachomatis* to evolve. High recombination rates among the strains seen using phylogenetic analysis of genomes, tell us otherwise. The overall average recombination rate seen has been around 26% (5–32%) [9]. The phenomenon of intrastrain recombination among *C. trachomatis* was first reported in literature, in the 1990s. It was based on gene-specific sequence analysis of gene *ompA*, that is responsible for synthesis of major outer membrane protein (MOMP). A wide range of such regions with high recombination rates are present in *C. trachomatis* and *C. pneumonia* like *ompA*, *tarp* (the translocated actin-recruiting phosphoprotein encoding gene), the polymorphic membrane protein-encoding genes (*pmps*), and *incA*, as well as the plasticity zone (PZ). Studies show that recombination events keep occurring across the complete genome leading to evolution of *C. trachomatis* as well as other chlamydial species such as *C. pneumoniae*, *C. suis and C. psittaci*. Cross-species and intraspecies genetic transfer vary. Intraspecies LGT maintains wild-type genomes within the cell, that otherwise might be considered stressful and mutagenic [10]. Whereas interspecies recombination leads to replication termination. It is now possible to genetically modify the organism, as evident in knockout mutants where the genes that are involved in LGT are inactivated [11].

The more we write about it and understand this organism, more is the number of doors we see that take us forward to amazement.

3. Chlamydia and it's rainbow spectrum of diseases

Chlamydia was recognized as STI in the 1970s, became notifiable in the year 1988. New cases were reported routinely in the STI statistics 1990 onwards. After 1995 the noted cases then began to rise steeply [12]. More number of couples started seeking infertility treatment. It became a disease which was turning into a direct threat for the propagation of life on earth. How could the human attention not go towards this gram-negative bacterium then, that has made humans err a lot in its identification as a bacteria. Gradually, more research has unveiled a lot of diseases where intensity of the role of chlamydia is still under constant scrutiny.

Table 1 is known hosts and their corresponding infective species of the Chlamydiaceae family.

The information in **Table 1** is an established limited knowledge. Multiple reports and research are continuing to highlight the involvement of Chlamydia.

Chlamydia has not spared the newborns. Many infants infected with *C. trachomatis* at birth have remained so for long period of time without appropriate antimicrobial therapy. This may misdirect us to sexual abuse. The cumulative infected proportion of infants at 1 year of age has been noted to be 35% [13]. The account of longest persistence of infection in one child, in the conjunctiva, nasopharynx, and oropharynx, has been around 866 days (28.5 months), until treatment cured it. Same serovars of *C. trachomatis* were reported in specimens from infants and their respective mothers and the serological tests in all infants pointed to the acquisition of infection during birth only [13].

Genital Chlamydia infection: In women it encompasses mucopurulent cervicitis, urethritis, and endometritis. Mucopurulent cervicitis can complicate into—salpingitis, pelvic inflammatory disease (PID), tubal pregnancy, chronic pelvic pain, Fitz Hugh Curtis Syndrome; premature rupture of membrane during pregnancy, chorioamnionitis, premature delivery, puerperal and neonatal infections (like conjunctivitis and interstitial pneumonia) and recurrent spontaneous abortions due to its immune reactions in human body. It's considered to be the leading cause of infertility. Around 20–30% of PID cases have been accredited to *C. trachomatis* in USA [14]. A study from India reported the prevalence of *C. trachomatis* infection around 23% in gynecology OPD (outpatient

Primary host	Species	Disease site
Human	*C. trachomatis*	Urogenital, ocular
Bird	*C. psittaci*	Respiratory and placenta
Human	*C. pneumonia*	Respiratory
Pig	*C. suis*	Urogenital, ocular
Cat	*C. felis*	Urogenital, ocular and respiratory
Livestock	*C. abortus*	Placenta
Mice	*C. muridarum*	Urogenital
Guinea pig	*C. caviae*	Urogenital, ocular and respiratory
Bird (pigeon)	*C. avium*	Respiratory
Marsupials, livestock	*C. pecorum*	Urogenital and conjunctiva
	C. ibidis	
	C. gallinacean	
Snake	*C. serpentis*	Cloacal, choanal
	C. poikilothermis	
	C. corallus	

Table 1.
Host, Chlamydia infective species & their disease sites.

department) [15] and around 19.9% of total STD patients [16]. In a systematic literature review from India, the rate of prevalence among infertile women was reported as 9–68% based on PCR results which took into account mostly the urban metro cities with only two studies from rural settings [17]. The reason that Chlamydia is an intense threat because, a large reservoir of unknown infected transmitting sources exist while leaving everlasting sequelae. Around 70–80% of females and up to 50% males carry asymptomatic infection [18]. Urethritis and epididymitis is on the male spectrum of genital chlamydia. An uncommon complication of untreated chlamydial infection is Reiter's syndrome, that is more common in females. Intra-articular *C. trachomatis* infection has been found in seronegative spondyloarthropathies using PCR [19].

In the past there has been a huge buzz around female infertility caused due to it, continuing till present. What about male infertility? *C. trachomatis* can lead to male infertility because it causes epididymitis and, consequently prostatitis and orchitis in them. According to Sonnenberg et al., Chlamydia infection can directly damage the sperms as well [20]. It can also cause testicular atrophy and obstructive azoospermia.

STIs are generally known to have good camaraderie with each other. Chlamydia is no exception here to our dismay. *C. trachomatis* infection increases risk of acquiring Human Immunodeficiency Virus infection, it's transmission by 3 to 4 fold and flourishes as co-infection with human papillomavirus (HPV) as well [21, 22]. But this is not a synergistic association. In study done by Martinelli et al., no association was observed between presence of *C. trachomatis* and abnormal Pap smear. In the study, *C. trachomatis* and HPV co-infections were seen in 4.9% and 9.3% of patients with and without cervical cytology abnormalities respectively [23]. This prevalence figure is in line with the rates previously reported in the literature. The prevalence of chlamydia was more in the normal cytology ones. But one cannot deny that, the co-existence of the *C. trachomatis* and HPV 16 might increase the risk of cervical carcinoma [24]. The carcinomatous changes are more profound with co-infection as compared to mono-infection in various studies. It's intriguing that, the load of *C. trachomatis* DNA has been found to be significabtly higher in cases of co infection as compared to mono infection. This points out to how the relationship between Chlamydia infection and the host immune response makes the foundation to understanding the disease process.

Chlamydia has been implicated in the causation of diseases where its role is still under question and research. Extragenital manifestations of chlamydia have come up with changing societal behavior and acceptance, as compared to the limited data and prevalence in the past. Most extragenital infections in women remain asymptomatic, estimated at—100% of pharyngeal chlamydia, 36–100% of rectal chlamydia, 93% of pharyngeal gonorrhea and 53–100% of rectal gonorrhea [25]. Rectal gonorrhea or chlamydia without history of anal sex has been reported in a significant number of women. Extragenital infections are higher among MSM. The prevalence in MSM (Men who have Sex with Men) ranged from 2.1 to 23% for rectal chlamydia (median 8.9%), 0.2 to 24% for rectal gonorrhea (median 5.9%), 0 to 3.6% for pharyngeal chlamydia (median 1.7%) and 0.5 to 16.5% for pharyngeal gonorrhea (median 4.6%) [26]. The prevalence of extragenital infections among MSW (HIV positive Heterosexual Men) in the studies reviewed ranged from 0 to 11.8% for rectal chlamydia (median 7.7%), 0 to 5.7% for rectal gonorrhea (median 3.4%), 0 to 22.0% for pharyngeal chlamydia (median 1.6%) and 0.4 to 15.5% for pharyngeal gonorrhea (median 2.2%) [26]. *C. pneumoniae* has been shown to have synergistic association with development of Coronary Artery Disease, with higher rate of positivity for *C. pneumoniae* IgA than IgG in positive PCR of CAD patients [27]. *C. pneumoniae* antibody positivity has been found to be independently associated with ischemic stroke in elderly patients without altering stroke outcome [28]. *Chlamydia pneumoniae* also has role in childhood asthma. In a study, anti-*C. pneumoniae* IgM was positive in 25% of patients with uncontrolled and partly controlled bronchial asthma [29]. Also duration of hospital stay was found to be longer in patients of uncontrolled asthma who had anti-Cp IgM positive [29]. *C. pneumoniae* IgG antibody has been found to be independently associated with migraine in Indian patients [30]. *C. trachomatis* has been proposed to play a role in photosensitive dermatoses and melasma, with variable positivity for IgA, IgM and IgG antibodies to *C. trachomatis* [31, 32].

Chlamydia has risen like a huge eagle from past to the present and humans are yet counting the feathers. Mankind does not know the extent but indeed it will be and it has to gear up to face chlamydia.

4. The journey of diagnostics for chlamydia

The diagnostic methodology of chlamydia has undergone a transformative change over the last two decades spanning from the traditional culture to high throughput NAAT (nucleic acid amplification test)/NGS (next generation gene sequencing). Testing for chlamydia infection is indicated for patients having ocular, urogenital and anorectal symptoms. Close contacts of such patients should also be tested for chlamydia and other sexually transmitted infections along with medico legal cases destined for such testing.

Laboratory investigations include both direct and indirect methods. Direct methods depend on detection of the antigen or nucleic acid. It includes culture, antigen tests (Enzyme Immune Assay, direct fluorescent antibody (DFA), and immune chromatographic RDTs), nucleic acid hybridization and amplification tests. Indirect methods detect antibodies against CT and have a role in diagnosing chronic and invasive infection like pelvic inflammatory disease (PID), lymphogranuloma venerum (LGV) and post infectious complications, like sexually acquired reactive arthritis (SARA) [33]. As *C. trachomatis* crosses the epithelial barrier and may no longer be detectable in swabs in these chronic/invasive infections. However, serology is not recommended for diagnosis of acute genitourinary infections, as the antibody response comes into play only after weeks to months of infection and the titers are usually insignificant.

4.1 Individual methods

4.1.1 Cell culture

"Cell lines for isolation of *C. trachomatis* include Mc Coy, HeLa 229 or Buffalo Green Monkey Kidney cells" [33]. Swabs are taken from different anatomical sites (endocervix, urethra, anal canal, conjunctivae) and inoculated. However, swab collection requires special collection device and transport media as culture can detect only viable organisms. "The detection rate is around 60–80%, in reference laboratories with experienced technicians" [33]. Limiting factors for culture include extended turn-around time, intensive labor requirement and difficulties in standardization. Hence cell culture is remotely used nowadays, however it has an important niche in reference laboratories and in few conditions like to monitor antibiotic susceptibility and change in virulence.

4.1.2 Nucleic acids amplification tests (NAATs)

NAATs have replaced culture as the diagnostic gold standard as they have high sensitivity and specificity and are currently the standard of care in diagnosing CT infections. With introduction of dual-target assays which incorporates a 2nd target region in NAATs the detection of new variants with deletions or recombination in one of the target regions is possible. Use of coated magnetic beads for nucleic acids isolation in the pre analytical steps also enhances the diagnostic sensitivity [34]. "These bead-based extractions systems allow simultaneous testing of chlamydia and gonococci with high sensitivity and specificity, can be automated and are used in several high-output systems" [33].

4.1.3 Clinical specimens required for CT testing

NAAT can analyze any clinical material like vulvo-vaginal, anorectal, urethral, cervical, ocular swabs, first void urine (FVU), sperms or living tissues. FDA approved NAAT's are available for first void urine, urethral, vaginal and cervical swabs. For screening asymptomatic individual's noninvasive specimen like first void urine is preferred. In contrast to collection of urine for routine culture sensitivity for other organisms where mid-stream sample is preferred, for chlamydia detection first void urine is recommended as the concentration of chlamydia sharply decreases during urination. Genital swabs are preferred in women as the CT concentration is comparatively higher when compared to urine. "A study analyzing urine, vaginal and cervical swabs taken simultaneously from asymptomatic women showed that the NAAT detection rate was highest in self-collected vaginal swabs. Hence, vaginal swabs (self-collected or clinician-collected) are the recommended sample type for women. Endocervical swabs may also be used, especially when a pelvic examination is indicated" [33].

For detection of extra genital infection like conjunctivitis, pharyngeal or anorectal infections, testing of corresponding swabs or tissue samples is recommended.

4.1.4 Recent developments

Proteomics are also being deployed in CT detection with encouraging results. These results might be used to characterize antibodies specific to detect different stages of infection.

> *"The Management of Chlamydia Cases in Australia (MoCCA) study is a new initiative to address gaps in chlamydia management in Australian general practice through implementing interventions shown to improve chlamydia management in specialist services. MoCCA will focus on improving retesting, partner management including patient-delivered partner therapy) and PID diagnosis" [35].*

> *"Accelerated partner therapy contact tracing for people with chlamydia (LUSTRUM): a crossover cluster-randomised controlled trial results suggest that accelerated partner therapy can be safely offered as a contact tracing option and is also likely to be cost saving" [36].*

5. Treatment and control: how far have we come?

Well we have come far in understanding Chlamydia. Once surprised humans by its lack of peptidoglycan in its structure yet being sensitive to penicillin [37]. Years later research revealed that unlike other bacterial species, members of the Chlamydiacae do not synthesize Peptidoglycan (PG) in their cell wall or "sacculus" but their PG is maintained in a narrow band that corresponds to the plane of septal division [38]. This PG "ring" has an active role in cell division of Chlamydia [39]. It is therefore included in the group of 'peptidoglycan-intermediate' organisms. Other such organisms are the Wolbachia, *Orientia tsutsugamushi* and *Anaplasma marginale* [40]. Peptidoglycan is a potent stimulator of the immune system and Chlamydia has perfectly cloaked it once to be a mystery for quite some time.

Treatment was targeted using the initial available antibiotics such as penicillin, amoxicillin in 1970s. Penicillin did not eradicate *C. trachomatis* but did inhibt its inclusion formation in in vitro studies when added within 1 h [41]. Amoxicillin 10 day course did eradicate it (unpublished observations of W. R. Bowie, E. R. Alexander, and K. K. Holmes). Gentamicin, Streptomycin, metronidazole and nalidixic acid were inactive against *C. trachomatis*. Tetracycline and erythromycin exhibited poor effects clinically, with good in vitro activity. In vitro under all tested conditions, doxycycline, minocycline and rifampin were more efficacious than tetracycline. The emerging most effective antimicrobial agent was turning out to be doxycycline [42].

In 1990s a new azalide antibiotic azithromycin was found effective both in vitro and in vivo; with ability to block formation of elementary bodies [43]. Azithromycin and doxycycline were then extensively investigated various studies and experiments.

Studies reported Single dose azithromycin superior to 3 days course of doxycycline for various species of chlamydia [44]. Mass drug administration (MDA) of single dose of Azithromycin began to be employed widely for trachoma as part of its elimination strategy. Later studies emerged which reported that single round of MDA brought down the overall active trachoma prevalence but had no influence on ocular *C. trachomatis* infection [45]. MDA of azithromycin has shown to be inadequate when encountered with heavy infection load, and this leads to persistence of infection post MDA. There is concern that MDA can lead to development of resistance in other organisms, notably *Streptococcus pneumoniae.* This is not after single round of MDA, but multiple rounds [46]. The first report of persistent or relapsing infection due to multidrug-resistant *C. trachomatis* came forward in year 2000. All 3 isolates in the report demonstrated resistance to azithromycin, ofloxacin and doxycycline at concentrations >4.0 μg/mL [47].

Azithromycin rapidly rose as the choice of treatment because of its less frequent dosing and high efficacy, was incorporated in trachoma elimination strategy. In 1998 Centers for Disease Control recommended Azithromycin as the first-line therapeutic regimen to treat genital infections in women and men. But then came growing emergence of resistance to it in urogenital and rectal isolates. Its detailed pharmacokinetics study unearthed the reasons for its new challenges. The action of azithromycin being pH dependant, unionized at high pH and only unionized form can go intracellular. It needs polymorphonuclear cells to be transported to the site of inflammation. More bacterial load is reported in rectoanal samples than endocervical. Higher MIC values have been found for Azithromycin in these samples, almost 2 fold higher.

A double blind RCT (2021) in 177 participants reported a "1-week course of doxycycline was significantly more effective than a single dose of azithromycin for the treatment of rectal CT in MSM" [48]. It is a conundrum that a significant proportion of women, with no history of anal intercourse, have asymptomatic rectal chlamydia infection. In what way this will influence the treatment in women is still unfolding. There is a theory that this rectal infection might be a "reservoir for reinfection of the vagina and sexual transmission" [49]. Hence antibiotic that tackles the rectal *Chlamydia trachomatis* is the need of the hour [50]. For the same STI, same antimicrobial or same regimen of dosing might not be the answer for different sites of infection in the body.

More research and trials, and the limitations with azithromycin are taking us back to Doxycycline when it comes to *C. trachomatis*. Doxycycline is promising even when used as a prophylaxis to prevent bacterial STIs as seen in short term RCTs and clinical studies, but robust evidence is still in need for this [51]. The target population for this need of prophylaxis is MSM, which would also help in less transmission of HIV by maintaining the mucosal integrity that gets broken which allows easy transmission of HIV and vice versa.

But the challenges are increasing each day when it comes to fight with CT. In a study from India that investigated isolates from females with recurrent chlamydial infection, decreased susceptibility to the present first line antibiotics (doxycycline and azithromycin) was noticed [52].

There is indeed a compelling need to research more about the antimicrobial resistance mechanism. There are two types of resistance that have been seen in Chlamydia species-homotypic and heterotypic. In homotypic resistance the organisms mostly survive above MIC (Minimal Inhibitory Concentration) of the antibiotic, whereas in heterotypic less than 1% of the organisms can survive above MIC [53]. "Azithromycin resistance of *C. trachomatis* is often a result of the mutations in the peptidyl transferase region of 23S rRNA genes, tetracycline resistance is usually linked to the presence of foreign genomic islands integrated in chlamydial chromosome, a predominant mechanism of fluoroquinolone resistance is a point mutation in the gyrA quinolone-resistance-determining region. A nucleotide substitution in rpoB gene is responsible for rifampin resistance" [54].

As we have no effective new antimicrobials for STI on the horizon, there is a dire need to optimize the use of available antibiotics with respect to their dose, regimen of dosing and their simultaneous use with other antibiotics.

Humans have been devising new control strategies continuously. SAFE has been able to decrease the load of trachoma very well. But when it comes to urogenital and rectal Chlamydia, the screening approaches have their pros and cons. It's still a debate whether universal screening or targeted screening is the solution. Universal screening is indeed obviously more effective, but the question is- is it cost effective?

Who to screen and how is still being subjected to multiple studies and reviews in order to frame the best pronged guidelines. Among 18–31 years old women, Mehta et al. observed that a greater number of PID cases were prevented by screening (universal and selective) using Ligase Chain Reaction (LCR) in urine for chlamydia and gonorrhea as compared to the usual practice of treating only self-reported or symptomatic cases [55]. Combining both standard procedure and screening turned out to be more cost effective in women, as the sequelae affect them for their future lives. Whereas in men the standard method of treating detected cases was better with respect to the cost involved, when compared to enhanced screening [55].

Mass Drug Administration has proven quite useful in control of trachoma, but the frequency of it depends on the prevalence and transmission rates in the area targeted. In high prevalence areas with trachoma annual MDA is not enough, quarterly MDA has been thought as a better control strategy. When it comes to urogenital and rectal Chlamydia control, the acceptability of MDA is not established. Pre-exposure prophylaxis in population at risk e.g. MSM has reduced transmission in pilot studies [56]. Also the impending threat of antibiotic resistance always prevails.

While talking of control practices one thing that should never be missed is safe sexual practices and stress over sex education from early adolescent life can be the best cost effective strategy.

6. The future of chlamydia

The past had unfolded to become the present and the present will continue to unfold into the future. Hence looking at the evolution of different aspects related to chlamydia from past to present, let us see what we might see at the forefront in future.

With rapid discoveries of new chlamydial species, there is definitely increasing risk of zoonoses in humans. *Chlamydia psittaci*—the causative microorganism of ornithosis, is the most well-known zoonotic pathogen. Chlamydiae are quite prevalent microorganisms in the animal kingdom. Constant human exposure via research keeps us always on the verge of contracting zoonoses.

Despite more than 20 years of screening programme and chlamydia testing in many countries and regions, chlamydia control strategies still rely on assumptions rather than robust evidence. The trend is shifting from the approach of diagnose and treat to more focused management of patients and their partners [57]. The focus is on management of disease rather than management of infection. A wide array of approaches are being proposed and tested for chlamydia control.

On one hand there's this notion developing regarding early antibiotic intervention programme and pre exposure prophylaxis in at risk population. A randomized study under "Ipergay trial" done in the MSM group used doxycycline prophylaxis that consisted of two doses of the drug administered after the sexual encounter within a period of 72 h. It reported that Doxycycline Post Exposure Prophylaxis decreases the incidence of a first symptomatic bacterial STI in at risk MSM [58]. Yet on other hand early antibiotic intervention strategy may have undesirable impact of reducing the herd immunity as it eliminates "bottlenecks to *Chlamydia* transmission" among humans [59].

Macrolides, quinolones and tetracyclines are the usual antimicrobials used to treat acute Chlamydial infections. However, Chlamydiae can develop "persistent forms (atypical reticular bodies)" that remain uninfluenced by usual available therapies [60]. This is not genetic resistance, but actually is phenotypic resistance. Persistent infections can turn to have clinically chronic courses.

So many questions and doubts revolve around antibiotics. One answer is leading us to the next new question. Hence there was a need to look at other options to battle with chlamydia. The focus is around a vaccine, alternative therapies for chlamydia and educating humans for being responsible for their sexual behavior. A vaccine for chlamydia carries the hope of an ideal protective strategy. Why is there an evolving urgent need of vaccine against chlamydial infection? An infection that has accessible antibiotic treatment but behaves exactly like its name—a cloaked organism. A magical cloak that allows it to spread rapidly, create new variants, have high rates of re-infection, be asymptomatic so often yet lead to drastic sequelae that has potential to change the nature's human anatomy and physiology by rendering it infertile or play a probable role in carcinogenesis! Accessible treatment, screening programmes and awareness programmes leading with—"Chlamydia is not a flower" have not been enough! The quest for an effective vaccine has utilized multiple chlamydial species and their different antigens. The trajectory of different antigens has included whole cell and subunit vaccines—utilizing Major Outer Membrane Proteins, Polymorphic Membrane Proteins, Plasmid antigens etc. MOMP has shown promising results. The challenge in the vaccine development has been it's mucosal protective immunity and robust immune response. After more than 70 years of several vaccine trials, first in human vaccine trial via both intramuscular and intranasal routes, has reported good immunogenicity with good tolerability. "Antigen CTH522 with either CAF01 liposomes or aluminium hydroxide (AH)" as adjuvants were studied, where liposomal adjuvant formulation had a better profile [61]. A variety of alternative therapies are also being utilized to derive whatever benefit they might provide. Non antibiotic approaches include synthetic drugs like "Broad-Spectrum Antiviral Compound ST-669", a "small-molecule inhibitor of type III secretion INP0400", "Lipopolysaccharide-Binding Alkylpolyamine DS-96"; polyphenols like "Baicalin, luteolin and catechins". Peptides like "Transferrin", "WLBU2 Peptide", "Cecrotin peptides", "Cathelicidin peptides", "Spider venom peptides" etc. have also shown slow therapeutic effect. The hurdle with these alternative therapies is that they are needed in high concentrations where they have unpredictable efficacy [62]. Vitamin E supplementation has shown increased humoral response towards chlamydia [63]. Interferon and interferon inducers have shown reduced growth of chlamydiae in vitro, when subjected to it six or eighteen hours prior to infection, and when treated early (within four hours) after infection reduced yield was detected in the cell cultures [64].

Recently the interest has spiked in anti-infective drugs that disarm the organism and help the host immunity in clearing infection. This surpasses the hurdle of antimicrobial resistance. For example—small-molecule LpxC inhibitors blocks the synthesis of lipopolysaccharide in Chlamydia due to which it replicates within vacuoles intracellularly, but cannot transition into the invasive form—"the elementary body". Yet there is time for further development of such drugs and whether they can be commercially viable therapeutics [59].

Single measures or a few combined measures are not what will help control Chlamydia. Impeccable efforts to develop a plan with designed steps, is the need for any major success. An "Integrated Care Model with Implementation Roadmap to Improve *C. trachomatis* Management and Control" has been developed in India [65]. It focuses on 4 key areas- Awareness, timely and effective management, aggressive follow up, and prevention. In developing countries the barriers to Chlamydia control narrow down to two main categories—Logistics & Resources and Culture & Education.

It is seen that younger age has higher association with *C. trachomatis* infection prevalence, due to more risky sexual behavior. Hence the role of timely sex education in pre-adolescence or adolescence with sufficient information about such STIs and the protection measures could lead to a more responsible and informed young adult population. This could culminate into a healthier thriving young population over the years [66].

7. Conclusions

Humans have come forward extensively from past to the future; when it comes to knowing the organism Chlamydia as discussed in the chapter, the range of diseases it causes, the development of diagnostic techniques we have to detect it and understand it further, the journey of finding the best treatment options to tackle it, the realization of the need of a preventive strategy before treatment strategy, the celebrated steps towards developing a vaccine, the development of comprehensive plans to instill an inclusive programme that aims to control the spread of chlamydia and hence to stop the further sequelae and it's impact on human race with a little peek window into the expected future of chlamydia and humans.

Acknowledgements

I Dr. Saurabh Krishna Misra would like to express my special thanks to my wife Dr. Richa Dokania Pedodontist for her constant encouragement thought the journey and Dr. Ankita (co Author) for her support and valuable suggestions in the preparation of this chapter.

Dr. Ankita Pundir, would like to express my humble gratitude to Dr. Saurabh K Misra (the author) for giving me the opportunity to work on this chapter and for investing his belief in me. I hope I have done my part as per his expectations. I would also like to thank my beloved husband, Dr. Aakash Kumar Singh who is a budding rheumatologist, for his inputs and help in developing this chapter.

we also thank Marica Novakovic for being empathetic towards our personal aspects affecting the submission deadline of this chapter and for offering help all along.

Conflict of interest

"The authors declare no conflict of interest."

Author details

Saurabh Krishna Misra[1*] and Ankita Pundir[2]

1 Govt Medical College, Kaushambi, UP, India

2 B.R.D. Medical College, Gorakhpur, India

*Address all correspondence to: drsaurabhkmishra@gmail.com

References

[1] Kim H, Kwak W, Yoon SH, Kang DK, Kim H. Horizontal gene transfer of chlamydia: Novel insights from tree reconciliation. PLoS One. 2018;**13**(4):e0195139. DOI: 10.1371/journal.pone.0195139

[2] Zaręba-Marchewka K, Szymańska-Czerwińska M, Niemczuk K. Chlamydiae—What's new? Journal of Veterinary Research. 2020;**64**(4):461-467. DOI: 10.2478/jvetres-2020-0077

[3] Amann R et al. Obligate intracellular bacterial parasites of Acanthamoebae related to chlamydia spp. Applied and Environmental Microbiology. 1997;**63**(1):115-121

[4] Phillips S, Quigley BL, Timms P. Seventy years of *chlamydia* vaccine research - limitations of the past and directions for the future. Frontiers in Microbiology. 2019;**10**:70. DOI: 10.3389/fmicb.2019.00070

[5] Seth-Smith et al. Co-evolution of Genomes.

[6] Shaw A et al. Genetic differences in the chlamydia trachomatis tryptophan synthase alpha-subunit can explain variations in serovar pathogenesis. Microbes and Infection. 2000;**2**(6):581-592

[7] Fehlner-Gardiner C et al. Molecular basis defining human Chlamydia trachomatis tissue tropism: A possible role for tryptophan synthase. Journal of Biological Chemistry;**277**(3)

[8] Iliffe-Lee E, McClarty G. Glucose metabolism in chlamydia trachomatis: The 'energy parasite' hypothesis revisited. Molecular Microbiology. 1999;**33**(1):177-187

[9] Rodríguez-Domínguez M, González-Alba JM, Puerta T, Martínez-García L, Menéndez B, Cantón R, et al. Spread of a new chlamydia trachomatis variant from men who have sex with men to the heterosexual population after replacement and recombination in ompA and pmpH genes. Clinical Microbiology and Infection. 2017;**23**(10):761-766. DOI: 10.1016/j.cmi.2017.03.009. Epub 2017 Mar 18

[10] Maharjan RP, Ferenci T. A shifting mutational landscape in 6 nutritional states: Stress-induced mutagenesis as a series of distinct stress input–mutation output relationships. PLoS Biology. 2017;**15**:e2001477. DOI: 10.1371/journal.pbio.2001477

[11] Marti H, Suchland RJ, Rockey DD. The impact of lateral gene transfer in *chlamydia*. Frontiers in Cellular and Infection Microbiology. 2022;**12**:861899. DOI: 10.3389/fcimb.2022.861899

[12] Worboys M. Chlamydia: A disease without a history. In: Szreter S, editor. The Hidden Affliction: Sexually Transmitted Infections and Infertility in History. Rochester (NY): University of Rochester Press; 2019. Chapter Five

[13] Bell TA. Chronic chlamydia trachomatis infections in infants. JAMA: The Journal of the American Medical Association. 1992;**267**(3):400

[14] Soper DE. Pelvic inflammatory disease. Obstetrics & Gynecology. 2010;**116**:419-428

[15] Patel LA, Sachdev D, Nagpal P, Chaudary U, Sonkar AS, Mendiratta LS, et al. Prevalence of Chlamydial infection among women visiting a gynaecology outpatient department: Evaluation of

an in-house PCR assay for detection of *Chlamydia trachomatis*. Annals of Clinical Microbiology and Antimicrobials. 2010;**9**:24-33

[16] Malhotra M, Bala M, Muralidhar S, Khunger N, Puri P. Prevalence of sexually transmitted infections in patients attending a tertiary care hospital in North India—A retrospective study. Indian Journal of Sexually Transmitted Diseases. 2008;**29**:82-85

[17] Thomas P, Spaargaren J, Kant R, Lawrence R, Dayal A, Lal JA, et al. Burden of chlamydia trachomatis in India: A systematic literature review. Pathogens and Disease. 2017;**75**(5):1-10. DOI: 10.1093/femspd/ftx055

[18] Stamm WE. *Chlamydia trachomatis*: Progress and problems. The Journal of Infectious Diseases. 1999;**179**:S380-S383

[19] Kumar P, Bhakuni DS, Rastogi S. Diagnosis of *Chlamydia trachomatis* in patients with reactive arthritis and undifferentiated spondyloarthropathy. Journal of Infection in Developing Countries. 2014;**8**(5):648-654. DOI: 10.3855/jidc.3644

[20] Sonnenberg P, Clifton S, Beddows S, Field N, Soldan K, Tanton C, et al. Prevalence, risk factors, and uptake of interventions for sexually transmitted infections in Britain: Findings from the National Surveys of Sexual Attitudes and Lifestyles (Natsal). Lancet. 2013;**382**:1795-1806. DOI: 10.1016/s0140-6736(13)61947-9

[21] Reda S, Gonçalves FA, Mazepa MM, de Carvalho NS. Women infected with HIV and the impact of associated sexually transmitted infections. International Journal of Gynecology & Obstetrics. 2018;**142**:143-147. DOI: 10.1002/ijgo.12507

[22] Kumari S, Bhor VM. A literature review on correlation between HPV coinfection with *C. trachomatis* and cervical neoplasia-coinfection mediated cellular transformation. Microbial Pathogenesis. 2022;**168**:105587. DOI: 10.1016/j.micpath.2022.105587

[23] Martinelli M, Musumeci R, Rizzo A, Muresu N, Piana A, Sotgiu G, et al. Prevalence of *Chlamydia trachomatis* infection, serovar distribution and co-infections with seven high-risk HPV types among Italian women with a recent history of abnormal cervical cytology. International Journal of Environmental Research and Public Health. 2019;**16**(18):3354. DOI: 10.3390/ijerph16183354

[24] Challagundla N, Chrisophe-Bourdon J, Agrawal-Rajput R. Chlamydia trachomatis infection co-operatively enhances HPV E6-E7 oncogenes mediated tumorigenesis and immunosuppression. Microbial Pathogenesis. 2022 Dec;**22**(175):105929. DOI: 10.1016/j.micpath.2022.105929

[25] Peters RPH, Nijsten N, Mutsaers J, Jansen CL, Morré SA, van Leeuwen AP. Screening of oropharynx and anorectum increases prevalence of *Chlamydia trachomatis* and *Neisseria gonorrhoeae* infection in female STD clinic visitors. Sexually Transmitted Diseases. 2011;**38**(9):783-787. DOI: 10.1097/olq.0b013e31821890e9

[26] Chan PA, Robinette A, Montgomery M, Almonte A, Cu-Uvin S, Lonks JR, et al. Extragenital infections caused by *Chlamydia trachomatis* and *Neisseria gonorrhoeae*: A review of the literature. Infectious Diseases in Obstetrics and Gynecology. 2016;**2016**:5758387. DOI: 10.1155/2016/5758387

[27] Jha HC, Vardhan H, Gupta R, Varma R, Prasad J, Mittal A. Higher incidence of persistent chronic infection of *Chlamydia pneumoniae* among

coronary artery disease patients in India is a cause of concern. BMC Infectious Diseases. 2007;7:48. DOI: 10.1186/1471-2334-7-48

[28] Bandaru VC, Boddu DB, Mridula KR, Akhila B, Alladi S, Laxmi V, et al. Outcome of *Chlamydia pneumoniae* associated acute ischemic stroke in elderly patients: A case-control study. Clinical Neurology and Neurosurgery. 2012;**114**(2):120-123. DOI: 10.1016/j.clineuro.2011.09.016

[29] Awasthi S, Yadav KK, Agarwal J. *Chlamydia pneumoniae* infection associated with uncontrolled asthma: A hospital based cross sectional study. Indian Journal of Pediatrics. 2012;**79, 10**:1318-1322. DOI: 10.1007/s12098-012-0809-6

[30] Chaudhuri JR, Mridula KR, Keerthi AS, Prakasham PS, Balaraju B, Bandaru VC. Association between *Chlamydia pneumoniae* and migraine: A study from a tertiary Center in India. Journal of Oral & Facial Pain and Headache. 2016;**30**(2):150-155. DOI: 10.11607/ofph.1570

[31] Sawhney M, Arora S, Khetrapal A. Chlamydia trachomatis infection and photosensitive dermatoses. Medical Journal Armed Forces India. 2008;**64**(4):340-342. DOI: 10.1016/S0377-1237(08)80016-0. Epub 2011 Jul 21

[32] Sawhney M, Batra RB. IgM *Chlamydia trachomatis* antibodies in cases of melasma. Medical Journal, Armed Forces India. 2005;**61**(4):351-352. DOI: 10.1016/S0377-1237(05)80063-2

[33] Meyer T. Diagnostic procedures to detect *Chlamydia trachomatis* infections. Microorganisms. 2016;**4**:25

[34] Xu L, Zhao Z, Mai H, Tan X, Du Y, Fang C. Clinical and chest computed tomography features associated with severe *Chlamydia psittaci* pneumonia diagnosed by metagenomic next-generation sequencing: A multicenter, retrospective, observational study. Medicine (Baltimore). 2022;**101**:1-7

[35] Goller JL, Coombe J, Temple-Smith M, Bittleston H, Sanci L, Guy R, et al. Management of chlamydia cases in Australia (MoCCA): Protocol for a non-randomised implementation and feasibility trial. BMJ Open. 2022;**12**:e067488

[36] Estcourt CS, Stirrup O, Copas A, Low N, Mapp F, Saunders J, et al. Accelerated partner therapy contact tracing for people with chlamydia (LUSTRUM): A crossover cluster-randomised controlled trial. The Lancet Public Health. 2022;7:e853-e865

[37] Moulder JW. Why is chlamydia sensitive to penicillin in the absence of peptidoglycan? Infectious Agents and Disease. 1993;**2**(2):87-99

[38] Liechti GW, Kuru E, Hall E, Kalinda A, Brun YV, VanNieuwenhze M, et al. A new metabolic cell-wall labelling method reveals peptidoglycan in *Chlamydia trachomatis*. Nature. 2014;**506**:507-510. DOI: 10.1038/nature12892

[39] Liechti G, Kuru E, Packiam M, Hsu YP, Tekkam S, Hall E, et al. Pathogenic *Chlamydia* lack a classical sacculus but synthesize a narrow, mid-cell peptidoglycan ring, regulated by MreB, for cell division. PLoS Pathogens. 2016;**12**:e1005590. DOI: 10.1371/journal.ppat.1005590

[40] Otten C, Brilli M, Vollmer W, Viollier PH, Salje J. Peptidoglycan in obligate intracellular bacteria. Molecular Microbiology. 2018;**107**(2):142-163. DOI: 10.1111/mmi.13880

[41] Lee CK, Bowie WR, Alexander ER. In vitro as says of the efficacy of antimicrobial agents in controlling *Chlamydia trachomatis* propagation. Antimicrobial Agents and Chemotherapy. 1978;**13**:441-445

[42] Bowie WR, Lee CK, Alexander ER. Prediction of Efficacy of Antimicrobial Agents in Treatment of Infections Due to Chlamydia trachomatis1978. DOI: 10.1093/infdis/138.5.655

[43] Engel JN. Azithromycin-induced block of elementary body formation in *Chlamydia trachomatis*. Antimicrobial Agents and Chemotherapy. 1992;**36**(10):2304-2309. DOI: 10.1128/AAC.36.10.2304

[44] Malinverni R, Kuo CC, Campbell LA, Lee A, Grayston JT. Effects of two antibiotic regimens on course and persistence of experimental *Chlamydia pneumoniae* TWAR pneumonitis. Antimicrobial Agents and Chemotherapy. 1995;**39**(1):45-49. DOI: 10.1128/AAC.39.1.45

[45] Harding-Esch EM, Holland MJ, Schémann JF, Sillah A, Sarr B, Christerson L, et al. Impact of a single round of mass drug administration with azithromycin on active trachoma and ocular *Chlamydia trachomatis* prevalence and circulating strains in the Gambia and Senegal. Parasites & Vectors. 2019;**12**(1):497. DOI: 10.1186/s13071-019-3743-x

[46] Coles CL, Mabula K, Seidman JC, Levens J, Mkocha H, Munoz B, et al. Mass distribution of azithromycin for trachoma control is associated with increased risk of azithromycin-resistance *S. pneumoniae* carriage in young children 6 months after treatment. Clinical Infectious Diseases: An Official Publication of the Infectious Diseases Society of America. 2013. Epub 2013/03/15. DOI: 10.1093/cid/cit137

[47] Somani J, Bhullar VB, Workowski KA, Farshy CE, Black CM. Multiple drug-resistant *Chlamydia trachomatis* associated with clinical treatment failure. The Journal of Infectious Diseases. 2000;**181**(4):1421-1427. DOI: 10.1086/315372

[48] Dombrowski JC, Wierzbicki MR, Newman LM, Powell JA, Miller A, Dithmer D, et al. Doxycycline versus azithromycin for the treatment of rectal chlamydia in men who have sex with men: A randomized controlled trial. Clinical Infectious Diseases. 2021;**73**(5):824-831. DOI: 10.1093/cid/ciab153

[49] Llata E, Braxton J, Asbel L, Chow J, Jenkins L, Murphy R, et al. Rectal *Chlamydia trachomatis* and *Neisseria gonorrhoeae* infections among women reporting anal intercourse. Obstetrics and Gynecology. 2018;**132**(3):692-697. DOI: 10.1097/AOG.0000000000002804

[50] Hammerschlag MR, Sharma R. Azithromycin in the treatment of rectogenital *Chlamydia trachomatis* infections: End of an era? Expert Review of Anti-Infective Therapy. 2021;**19**(4):487-493. DOI: 10.1080/14787210.2021.1834850

[51] Grant JS, Stafylis C, Celum C, Grennan T, Haire B, Kaldor J, et al. Doxycycline prophylaxis for bacterial sexually transmitted infections. Clinical Infectious Diseases. 2020;**70**(6):1247-1253. DOI: 10.1093/cid/ciz866

[52] Bhengraj AR, Vardhan H, Srivastava P, Salhan S, Mittal A. Decreased susceptibility to azithromycin and doxycycline in clinical isolates of chlamydia trachomatis obtained from recurrently infected female patients in India. Chemotherapy. 2010;**56**(5):371-377. DOI: 10.1159/000314998

[53] Suchland RJ, Geisler WM, Stamm WE. Methodologies and cell lines

used for antimicrobial susceptibility testing of Chlamydia spp. Antimicrobial Agents and Chemotherapy. 2003;**47**:636-642. DOI: 10.1128/AAC.47.2.636-642.2003

[54] Mestrovic T, Ljubin-Sternak S. Molecular mechanisms of *Chlamydia trachomatis* resistance to antimicrobial drugs. Frontiers in Bioscience-Landmark. 2018;**23**(4):656-670. DOI: 10.2741/4611

[55] Mehta SD, Bishai D, Howell MR, Rothman RE, Quinn TC, Zenilman JM. Cost-effectiveness of five strategies for gonorrhea and chlamydia control among female and male emergency department patients. Sexually Transmitted Diseases. 2002;**29**(2):83-91. DOI: 10.1097/00007435-200202000-00004

[56] Dubourg G, Raoult D. The challenges of preexposure prophylaxis for bacterial sexually transmitted infections. Clinical Microbiology and Infection. 2016;**22**(9):753-756. DOI: 10.1016/j.cmi.2016.08.022

[57] Dukers-Muijrers NHTM, Evers YJ, Hoebe CJPA, Wolffs PFG, de Vries HJC, Hoenderboom B, et al. Controversies and evidence on Chlamydia testing and treatment in asymptomatic women and men who have sex with men: A narrative review. BMC Infectious Diseases. 2022;**22**(1):255. DOI: 10.1186/s12879-022-07171-2

[58] Doxycycline PEP reduced the occurrence of a first episode of bacterial STI in high-risk men who have sex with men

[59] Valdivia RH. Thinking outside the box: New strategies for antichlamydial control. Future Microbiology. 2012;**7**(4):427-429. DOI: 10.2217/fmb.12.25

[60] Rohde G, Straube E, Essig A, Reinhold P, Sachse K. Chlamydial zoonoses. Deutsches Ärzteblatt International. 2010;**107**(10):174-180. DOI: 10.3238/arztebl.2010.0174

[61] Thoma C. First chlamydia vaccine trial in humans. Nature Reviews Urology. 2019;**16**:566

[62] Hou C, Jin Y, Wu H, Li P, Liu L, Zheng K, et al. Alternative strategies for *Chlamydia* treatment: Promising non-antibiotic approaches. Frontiers in Microbiology. 2022;**13**:1-13. DOI: 10.3389/fmicb.2022.987662

[63] Nockels CF. Protective effects of supplemental vitamin E against infection. Federation Proceedings. 1979;**38**(7):2134-2138

[64] Kazar J, Gillmore JD, Gordon FB. Effect of interferon and interferon inducers on infections with a nonviral intracellular microorganism, *Chlamydia trachomatis*. Infection and Immunity. 1971;**3**(6):825-832. DOI: 10.1128/iai.3.6.825-832.1971

[65] Thomas PPM, Allam RR, Ambrosino E, Malogajski J, Lal JA, Morré SA, et al. An integrated care model with implementation roadmap to improve *Chlamydia trachomatis* management and control in India. Frontiers in Public Health. 2018;**6**:321. DOI: 10.3389/fpubh.2018.00321

[66] Saurabh et al. Knowledge and attitude about sexually transmitted infections among paramedical 1st year students in a tertiary care teaching institute in Pondicherry. IJOD. DOI: 10.18203/issn.2455-4529.IntJResDermatol20193225

Chapter 2

Virulence Factors of *Chlamydia* Spp. Involving Human Infections

Panagiota Xaplanteri, Nikiforos Rodis and Charalampos Potsios

Abstract

Chlamydia spp. are the culprit of many human infections with severe complications, especially involving human eye, reproductive system, and lungs. The scope of the project is to delineate the virulence factors of the bacterium that facilitate invasion in human tissues, their mechanism of action, the ability to hide from immune system and the complications of infection. *Chlamydia* spp. are obligate intracellular pathogens that in their evolution, they use multiple mechanisms to enter host cell, to form the inclusion body, and to promote intracellular replication and survival. The T3SS effectors, the inclusion membrane proteins (Incs), are not only structural components of the membrane but also interfere with the host cell pathways. They also have an atypical mechanism of cell division. Description of the mechanisms of pathogenicity may lead to the development of new ways to face this major pathogen.

Keywords: *Clamydia* spp., virulence factors, human infections, chlamydial proteins, virulence factors

1. Introduction

The order Chlamydiales, family Chlamydiaceae comprises obligate intracellular bacteria, classified as Gram-negative bacteria due to the cell wall structure but are difficult to stain. The cell wall has no peptidoglycan but contains an outer lipopolysaccharide membrane. Instead of peptidoglycan it contains proteins which confer the same functional properties as peptidoglycan. Those proteins are rich in cysteine. Due to this unique cell wall structure, the microorganism can divide intracellularly and survive extracellularly. The shape is coccoid or rod-shaped. Both survive intracellularly in aerobic conditions and are not able to synthesize its own ATP or grow on an artificial medium [1, 2].

Chlamydiae are not metabolically active outside the host cell. This is a unique characteristic of *Chlamydiae* and in contrast with other intracellular bacteria [3]. The life cycle of *Chlamydia* is biphasic and is characterized by a succession between the infectious inactive elementary body which does not replicate and represents the dispersal form of the microorganism, and the noninfectious reticulate body which can replicate [1]. Upon contact with the host cell, the bacterium provokes endocytosis by injecting chlamydial proteins into the epithelial cell it attacks. Those injected proteins force the epithelial cells to endocytose particles they would never do otherwise [4].

Once inside the host cell, the interaction with glycogen drives the elementary body to germinate and take its reticulate form [4]. The microorganism survives intracellularly into a protective parasitophorous vacuole [1]. To do so, the microorganisms act on host cell cytoskeletal structures and endocytic pathways so as not to fuse the parasitophorous vacuole with the infected cell lysosomes [4]. In those vacuoles, the microbe uptake nutrients and energy and simultaneously alter host cell transcriptional pathways to prevent apoptosis and hide from host defense mechanisms [4]. Some proteins of the bacterium are secreted into the inclusion membrane. Those proteins are called inclusion membrane proteins and their role as virulence factors still needs to be elucidated [4]. The reticulate form has an incubation period of about 7–21 days in its host as it divides every 2–3 hours. When division is complete, in about 48 hours, it takes the elementary form and is released from the host cell via exocytosis to infect new cells [1].

Chlamydophila (Chlamydia) pneumoniae is a main culprit of community-acquired pneumonia, bronchitis, and adult-onset asthma. They are also linked in the literature to atherosclerosis and multiple sclerosis [2, 5]. *Chlamydia psittaci* causes infection in birds and can cause severe pneumonia in humans who inhale the feces of those birds [1].

Chlamydia trachomatis, depending on the disease they induce and different tissue tropisms, are divided into biovars. Depending on the humoral response they provoke are divided into serovars (genovars) [1, 4, 6]. Based on antigenic variation of the major outer membrane protein (MOMP), *C. trachomatis* is classified into 15 serovars [6]. The genital strains of *C. trachomatis* serovars D through K cause the sexually transmitted disease chlamydia (cervicitis in women and urethritis in men) [1, 6]. The microbe infects squamocolumnar or transitional epithelial cells. Ascending infection causes Pelvic Inflammatory Disease in women and epididymitis and reactive arthritis in men. In women, infection may lead to infertility, ectopic pregnancy, and chronic pelvic pain [6]. Serovars L1–L3 cause the invasive lymphoma granuloma venereum (LGV), also sexually transmitted infection [1, 6]. The ocular biovar that causes Trachoma includes the serovars A through C [1]. Trachoma is a state directly linked with blindness. The disease is transmitted via infected secretions of the genital urinary tract or through ocular discharge or contact with eye-seeking flies. The microorganism binds to the mucosal membranes of the cervix, rectum, urethra, throat, and conjunctiva [1].

Chlamydia gallinacea is an obligate intracellular bacterium and an opportunistic human pathogen. In human, it is known to cause pneumonia in poultry slaughterhouse workers [7].

The genome of *Chlamydial* microorganisms has significant similarities that make it difficult to comprehend the way they provoke so diverse diseases [1]. Comparing the genome structure of *C. trachomatis* to *Chlamydia pneumoniae* may lead to better understanding of the ways those microorganisms act. The genome of *C. trachomatis* is described to be 1,042,519, while the respective of *C. pneumoniae* is 1,230,230 base pairs long. There are clear differences between the two: 186 genes on the *C. pneumoniae* genome are not present on the *C. trachomatis* genome, and seventy genes on the *C. trachomatis* genome are not represented on the *C. pneumoniae* genome [8]. The *C. trachomatis* genome is considered small. Nonetheless, there have been specified 900 coding sequences on the chromosome and the plasmid of the microbe. The over 200 open reading frames encode proteins their function still needs to be elucidated and are all responsible for the virulence, intracellular survival, and replication of the bacterium [9].

2. Virulence factors

Chlamydia can evade both intra- and extracellular host defense [1]. Further understanding of the virulence factors they possess, and elucidation of the mechanisms of action can provide essential tools for prevention and treatment.

2.1 The cell wall structure

The *C. trachomatis* LPS is a genus-specific antigen. It is a "rough" type molecule provoking weak macrophage activation. Lipid A portion is pentaacylated with more than C14 fatty acids. The cell wall of *C. trachomatis* inhibits phagolysosome fusion in phagocytes [10].

2.2 Type III secretion systems

Intracellular pathogens secrete contact-dependent protein products of conserved secretory genes [3]. Those proteins promote the viability and multiplication of the microbe within the host cell and are well-described virulence factors. Their role is to intercept host signaling pathways in favor of the intruder [3]. Type III secretion systems serve as a conduit to promote the delivery of pathogen-effector proteins into the cytoplasm of the host cell. Via this apparatus, the microorganism can inject proteins directly into the host cell and avoid lysosomes [10]. *Chlamydiae* have a unique life cycle where the elementary body is metabolically dormant and therefore expresses no contact secretion. This contrasts with other intracellular pathogens, where contact-dependent secretion begins before they have been internalized in the host cell [3]. In *Chlamydiae* contact secretion is triggered from within by the intracellular metabolically active reticulate body. Therefore, characterization and description of *Chlamydiae* contact-dependent secretion mechanisms are of great interest [3]. The product of *scc1* gene has homology to chaperone proteins of other intracellular pathogens. *Cds1 and cds2* locuses are acquired by horizontal transfer and thus are included in a classical pathogenicity island. They are expressed during the intracellular life cycle of the bacterium and are related to the translocation of the pathogen across the cytoplasmic membrane [3]. Effector protein IncA of *C. trachomatis* mediates inclusion fusion and is related to strain-dependent disease severity [10]. Another chlamydial phosphoprotein is delivered into host cell cytoplasm and promotes actin recruitment in favor of the pathogen. This so-called Translocated Actin Recruiting Phosphoprotein causes internalization of the microbe and is related to disease severity [10, 11].

2.3 Chlamydial proteins present in the cytosol of infected cells

Many chlamydial proteins have been described in literature to be present in the cytosol of infected cells, but their distinct role as virulence factors still needs to be elucidated. Those proteins are CPAF, cHtrA, CT621, CT622, CT311, CT795, *C. trachomatis* glycogen synthase (GlgA), the *C. trachomatis* outer membrane complex protein B, and Pgp3 [12]. Identification of these proteins can elucidate further the mechanism of pathogenic activity of the bacterium [12]. Bacterial antigens present in host cell cytosol are more immunogenic [4].

2.3.1 CPAF

CPAF factor responsible for chlamydial protease/proteasome-like activity is highly conserved [1]. It acts as a zymogen, which means it can self-activate and auto-process via vicinity-dependent homodimerization [1]. It is a secreted serine protease known to cleave a large amount of host proteins. Its role has been described in attacking certain host mechanisms to evade the immune system and to survive and replicate intracellularly. Their targets are the host transcriptional factors USF-1 23, RFX5 24, NF-κB, and HIF-1, the proapoptotic BH3-only proteins, the DNA repairing Poly-ADP-ribose polymerase, cyclin B1, cytoskeleton proteins involved in cell structure like keratin 8, keratin 18 and vimentin, and proteins involved in repairment of Golgi apparatus, proteins involved in cell adhesion like nectin-1 [1, 13]. The secreted CPAF into the cytoplasm of the infected cell degrades the transcription factors RFX5 and USF-1 that are responsible for MHC gene activation. In this way, the microorganism reduces immune recognition by affecting antigen presentation and suppressing IFNγ-inducible MHC class I expression [1, 13]. BH3-only proteins like Puma and Bim that act as intracellular stress sensor molecules via migration to the mitochondria induce apoptosis. The mechanism involves the activation of the multi-domain proapoptotic Bax and Bak to suppress the antiapoptotic function of BcL-2. CPAF degrades the BH3-only domain proteins and acts in favor of antiapoptotic activity. This mechanism still needs elucidation [1, 13]. Another distinct role of CPAF is cleavage of cytoskeletal proteins that lead to depolymerization of the cytoskeleton surrounding the inclusions. In this way the microbe uses the lack of ability of the infected host cells to maintain their cytoskeletal structure, to expand the chlamydial inclusions in favor of their rapid replication [1, 13]. The microbe uses Golgi-derived lipids like sphingomyelin and cholesterol via the chlamydial proteases. Cleavage of golgin-84 leads to recruitment of Golgi fragmentation to acquire nutrients [1, 13].

2.3.2 Chlamydial HtrA

Chlamydial HtrA (cHtrA) is a hexamer with proteolytic activities. It is a periplasmic protein. It acts as a protease that acts on the endoplasmic reticulum of host cells and cleaves the transcription factors ATF6 and SREBP that are involved in cholesterol biosynthesis [14]. It also releases the sE-factor to activate stress response genes and is essential for the survival of the microorganism under high temperature [14]. HtrA is present in the chlamydial inclusion and is secreted in host cell cytosol, a unique property of chlamydial cells.

2.3.3 CT621 and CT622

Chlamydial cells use the type III secretion system to secrete CT621 and CT622 into the host cell cytoplasm [12, 15]. The presence of CT622 and CT621 in host cell cytoplasm should be involved in the pathogenetic mechanism of chlamydial infection, although their role needs to be further studied and elucidated. They seem to follow the same path but different kinetics in expression and secretion, meaning they play different roles in the survival and replication of the bacterium intracellularly [12].

2.3.4 CT311

Protein CT311 of *C. trachomatis* is secreted out of chlamydial inclusion into the cytosol of the infected cell and it enters host cell nucleus, thus it is a sufficient component for nuclear targeting [16]. The presence of this chlamydial component in the nucleus during the late stage of intracellular infection means that it can interact and modulate signal transduction pathways. This is an important tool to induce infection [16]. The most possible role of CT311 is alteration of host cell mechanisms to facilitate exiting of host cell and spreading [16].

2.3.5 CT795

The Chlamydia-specific protein CT795 is detected in the cytoplasm of infected host cells via a sec-dependent mechanism and not by a type III secretion pathway [4].

2.3.6 C. trachomatis glycogen synthase (GlgA)

In recent studies, chlamydial GlgA seems to appear in host cell cytosol and chlamydial inclusion lumen among all *C. trachomatis* serovars and is immunogenic in women urogenital infections. Its specific role in the pathogenicity of chlamydial infections still needs to be elucidated but seems to interfere with the accumulation of glycogen, within the inclusion lumen [17]. Glycogen is a nutritional source but also a TLR2 ligand. In *Chlamydia muridarum* infection plasmid dependent TLR2 activation is related to the promotion of infection and the chronic pathology of oviduct inflammation [18].

2.3.7 The C. trachomatis outer membrane complex protein B

The *C. trachomatis* outer membrane complex protein B (OmcB) is a well-described antigen as far as chlamydial infections are concerned. It is an abundant outer membrane protein, highly conserved among *Chlamydia* species that acts as an adhesin for chlamydial invasion into epithelial cells. It seems to provoke robust antigenic response via the release of the C-terminal region of the molecule (OmcBc) to host cell cytosol [4]. The fragment OmcBc is present in host cell cytosol. The fragment OmcBn stays in the chlamydial inclusions. OmcBc proved to be highly immunogenic in women infected by the microbe. OmcB is therefore a target for the development of diagnostic tools and vaccines [19].

2.4 *Chlamydiae*-induced antiapoptotic activity of infected host cells

Infected cells seem to express antiapoptotic mechanisms like inhibition of caspase 3 activation, blockade of mitochondrial cytochrome c release, inhibition of Bax/Bak NFκB activation. In this way the microbe detours apoptosis, a well-described mechanism of infected cells by intracellular pathogens. CPAF has been described to have an important role in this direction [13].

2.5 Chlamydial cryptic plasmid

The removal of the chlamydial cryptic plasmid in the murine equivalent model of *C. trachomatis, C. muridarum*, has led to reduced bacterial load and upper genital tract and ocular pathologies [1]. The possible mechanisms include the action of two plasmid genes involved in the formation of the antigen Pgp3, a secreted protein component of the outer plasmid membrane, and Pgp4 which is a regulator of both plasmid and chromosomal genes [1]. The products of these genes are related to glycogen production and accumulation, a contributor to virulence [9, 18]. Pgp4 acts also as a transcriptional regulator of both plasmid and chromosomal virulence-associated genes [18]. Both *pgp3* and *pgp*4 genes are essential for in vitro growth of the bacterium, which enforces the aspect that their products are virulence factors [18]. This aspect is enforced by the fact that *pgp*4 is expressed only three hours post-infection [10, 18]. In mice, pGP3 promotes ascending infection and tubal inflammation. The mechanism seems to be via neutralizing the host antimicrobial peptides, like human alpha-defensins, human neutrophil peptide 2, human beta-defensin 3, and cathelicidin LL-37. Host antimicrobial peptides are trapped by pGP3 to form stable complexes. In this way the progeny Elementary Bodies released can safely evade the next host cell [20]. The plasmid-encoded protein CPSIT_P7 of *C. psittaci* via Toll-like receptor 4 and TLR4/Mal/MyD88/NF-κB signaling axis, triggers the expression of interleukin-6, interleukin-8, and monocyte chemoattractant protein-1 [21].

2.6 Protein CT135

Protein CT135 is responsible for persistent urogenital infection in mice and prolonged time to clearance in vivo [1].

2.7 Silencing the NF-κB inflammatory pathway

Chlamydiae seem to suppress NF-κB activation in infected cells. This is in contrast with the production of proinflammatory cytokines that are induced during infection. It appears that the microbe activates MAP kinases in its favor to acquire the needed nutrients for survival. The mechanism seems to be cleavage of NF-κB p65 into the fragments p40 and p20 by a chlamydial protein called tail-specific protease. The over-expression of p40 leads to interaction of the fragment with the cytoplasmic inhibitor of NF-κB I-κBα and blockage of NF-κB pathways [13]. SINC protein of *C. psittaci* targets the inner nuclear membrane of infected host cells. As a result, it is involved in controlling of nuclear structure and gene silencing [7, 22].

2.8 Translocated actin recruiting protein (TarP)

Upon attachment of the elementary body to the host cell, TarP is injected into the host cell. This translocation is made via a chlamydial type 3 secretory system. TarP has three binding sites for vinculin [23]. Additionally, TarP is reported to interact with focal adhesion kinase (FAK) and thus be able to alter cell adhesion signaling [23]. In this way, *Chlamydiae* use extracellular matrix and cell-to-cell junction for their benefit to promote entry to the host cells [23].

2.9 Chlamydial polymorphic outer membrane proteins (Pmps)

Chlamydial polymorphic outer membrane proteins are surface proteins that serve as adhesins, but also have antigenic role. They are present in all chlamydial species. They act as autotransporters that is they can translocate. These proteins are considered virulence factors. *Chlamydia*e in contrast to other Gram-negative bacteria possess more autotransporter proteins. PmpB, C, D, and I of *C. trachomatis* are known to induce strong humoral immune responses in infected patients. Women patients suffering from pelvic inflammatory disease and proved positive for anti-PmpA specific antibodies had a significantly high infertility rate in comparison to women negative for anti-PmpA antibodies. *C. pneumonia* Pmp20 and Pmp21 induce IL-6 and monocyte chemoattractant protein-1 production in human umbilical vein endothelial cells (HUVECs) by activation of NF-kB. The production is dose-dependent and the two Pmps do not act synergistically. *C. trachomatis* PmpD induces strong and dose-dependent IL-8 production from the human monocyte cell line THP-1 [10, 24].

3. Conclusion

Chlamydia spp. are the culprit of many human infections with severe complications, especially involving human eye, reproductive system, and lungs. Many virulence factors of the bacterium have been described in literature. Those virulence factors facilitate invasion in human tissues and provide the microorganism with the ability to hide from immune system and use the host cell mechanisms in its favor. The cell wall structure, Type III secretion systems, chlamydial proteins present in the cytosol of infected cells, induction of antiapoptotic activity of infected host cells, chlamydial cryptic plasmid, protein CT135, silencing of the NF-κB inflammatory pathway, Translocated actin recruiting protein (TarP), chlamydial polymorphic outer membrane proteins (Pmps), are some of them. Elucidation of the mechanisms of pathogenicity may lead to the development of new ways to face this major pathogen.

Funding

None.

Conflicts of interest

We declare no conflict of interest.

Author details

Panagiota Xaplanteri[1*], Nikiforos Rodis[2] and Charalampos Potsios[3]

1 Department of Microbiology, General Hospital of Eastern Achaia, Kalavrita, Greece

2 Department of Surgery, General Hospital of Patras, Patras, Greece

3 University General Hospital of Patras, Patras, Greece

*Address all correspondence to: panagiota.xaplanteri@gmail.com

References

[1] Conrad T, Yang Z, Ojcius D, Zhong G. A path forward for the chlamydial virulence factor CPAF. Microbes and Infection. 2013;**15**(14-15): 1026-1032. DOI: 10.1016/j.micinf. 2013.09.008

[2] Krüll M, Suttorp N. Pathogenesis of *Chlamydophila pneumoniae* infections — Epidemiology, immunity, cell biology, virulence factors. In: Community-Acquired Pneumonia. Birkhäuser Advances in Infectious Diseases. Basel: Birkhäuser; 2007. DOI: 10.1007/ 978-3-7643-7563-8_6

[3] Hsia RC, Pannekoek Y, Ingerowski E, Bavoil PM. Type III secretion genes identify a putative virulence locus of *chlamydia*. Molecular Microbiology. 1997;**25**(2):351-359. DOI: 10.1046/j. 1365-2958.1997.4701834.x

[4] Qi M, Lei L, Gong S, Liu Q, DeLisa MP, Zhong G. *Chlamydia trachomatis* secretion of an immunodominant hypothetical protein (CT795) into host cell cytoplasm. Journal of Bacteriology. 2011;**193**(10):2498-2509. DOI: 10.1128/JB.01301-10

[5] Smieja M, Mahony J, Petrich A, et al. Association of circulating *chlamydia pneumoniae* DNA with cardiovascular disease: A systematic review. BMC Infectious Diseases. 2002;**2**:21. DOI: 10.1186/1471-2334-2-21

[6] O'Connell CM, Ferone ME. *Chlamydia trachomatis* genital infections. Microbial Cell. 2016;**3**(9):390-403. DOI: 10.15698/ mic2016.09.525

[7] Heijne M, Jelocnik M, Umanets A, et al. Genetic and phenotypic analysis of the pathogenic potential of two novel *chlamydia gallinacea* strains compared to *chlamydia psittaci*. Scientific Reports. 2021;**11**:16516. DOI: 10.1038/ s41598-021-95966-9

[8] Stephens RS, Kalman S, Lammel C, Fan J, Marathe R, Aravind L, et al. Genome sequence of an obligate intracellular pathogen of humans: *Chlamydia trachomatis*. Science. 1998;**282**(5389):754-759. DOI: 10.1126/ science.282.5389.754

[9] Hudson AP. A major advance in elucidating the biology/pathobiology of *chlamydia trachomatis*. Infection and Immunity. 2013;**81**(3):622-624

[10] Byrne GI. *Chlamydia trachomatis* strains and virulence: Rethinking links to infection prevalence and disease severity. The Journal of Infectious Diseases. 2010;**201**(S2):S126-S133

[11] Beder T, Saluz HP. Virulence-related comparative transcriptomics of infectious and non-infectious chlamydial particles. BMC Genomics. 2018;**19**:575. DOI: 10.1186/s12864-018-4961-x

[12] Gong S, Lei L, Chang X, Belland R, Zhong G. *Chlamydia trachomatis* secretion of hypothetical protein CT622 into host cell cytoplasm via a secretion pathway that can be inhibited by the type III secretion system inhibitor compound 1. Microbiology (Reading). 2011;**157**(Pt 4):1134-1144. DOI: 10.1099/mic.0.047746-0

[13] Zhong G. Killing me softly: Chlamydial use of proteolysis for evading host defenses. Trends in Microbiology. 2009;**17**(10):467-474. DOI: 10.1016/j. tim.2009.07.007

[14] Wu X, Lei L, Gong S, Chen D, Flores R, Zhong G. The chlamydial

periplasmic stress response serine protease cHtrA is secreted into host cell cytosol. BMC Microbiology. 2011;**11**:87. DOI: 10.1186/1471-2180-11-87

[15] Hobolt-Pedersen AS, Christiansen G, Timmerman E, Gevaert K, Birkelund S. Identification of *chlamydia trachomatis* CT621, a protein delivered through the type III secretion system to the host cell cytoplasm and nucleus. FEMS Immunology and Medical Microbiology. 2009;**57**(1):46-58. DOI: 10.1111/j.1574-695X.2009.00581.x

[16] Lei L, Dong X, Li Z, Zhong G. Identification of a novel nuclear localization signal sequence in *chlamydia trachomatis*-secreted hypothetical protein CT311. PLoS One. 2013;**8**(5):e64529. DOI: 10.1371/journal.pone.0064529

[17] Lu C, Lei L, Peng B, Tang L, Ding H, Gong S, et al. *Chlamydia trachomatis* GlgA is secreted into host cell cytoplasm. PLoS One. 2013;**8**(7):e68764. DOI: 10.1371/journal.pone.0068764

[18] Song L, Carlson JH, Whitmire WM, et al. *Chlamydia trachomatis* plasmid-encoded Pgp4 is a transcriptional regulator of virulence-associated genes. Infection and Immunity. 2013;**81**(3):636-644. DOI: 10.1128/iai.01305-12

[19] Qi M, Gong S, Lei L, Liu Q, Zhong G. A *chlamydia trachomatis* OmcB C-terminal fragment is released into the host cell cytoplasm and is immunogenic in humans. Infection and Immunity. 2011;**79**:2193e2203

[20] Hou S, Sun X, Dong X, Lin H, Tang L, Xue M, et al. Chlamydial plasmid-encoded virulence factor Pgp3 interacts with human cathelicidin peptide LL-37 to modulate immune response. Microbes and Infection. 2019;**21**(1):50-55. DOI: 10.1016/j.micinf.2018.06.003

[21] Chen Q, Li Y, Yan X, Sun Z, Wang C, Liu S, et al. *Chlamydia psittaci* plasmid-encoded CPSIT_P7 elicits inflammatory response in human monocytes via TLR4/mal/MyD88/NF-κB signaling pathway. Frontiers in Microbiology. 2020;**11**:578009. DOI: 10.3389/fmicb.2020.578009

[22] Mojica SA, Hovis KM, Frieman MB, Tran B, Hsia RC, Ravel J, et al. SINC, a type III secreted protein of *chlamydia psittaci*, targets the inner nuclear membrane of infected cells and uninfected neighbors. Molecular Biology of the Cell. 2015;**26**(10):1918-1934. DOI: 10.1091/mbc.E14-11-1530

[23] Whitewood AJ, Singh AK, Brown DG, Goult BT. Chlamydial virulence factor TarP mimics Talin to disrupt the Talin-vinculin complex. FEBS Letters. 2018;**592**(10):1751-1760. DOI: 10.1002/1873-3468.13074

[24] Vasilevsky S, Stojanov M, Greub G, Baud D. Chlamydial polymorphic membrane proteins: Regulation, function and potential vaccine candidates. Virulence. 2016;7(1):11-22. DOI: 10.1080/21505594.2015.1111509

Chapter 3

The Laboratory Diagnosis of *Chlamydia* Infections

Özlem Koca

Abstract

Bacteria of the genus *Chlamydia* belong to the order *Chlamydiales*, within the family *Chlamydiaceae*. These intracellular parasites have a different biphasic reproductive cycle than other bacteria. The important *Chlamydiaceae* are *Chlamydia trachomatis*, *Chlamydophila pneumoniae* and *Chlamydophila psittaci*. *Chlamydia trachomatis* and *Clamydophila pneumoniae* are primary human pathogens. *Chlamydia trachomatis* is transmitted by sexual contact. It is the causative agent of LGV (lymphogranuloma venoreum) and ocular trachoma in humans. *Chlamydophila pneumoniae* causes bronchitis, atypical pneumonia, sinusitis, pharyngitis, and inflammatory atherosclerosis. *Chlamydia psittaci* is the causative agent of psittacosis (pneumonia). It primarily causes infection in birds and domestic animals, and sometimes in humans. *Chlamydia trachomatis* laboratory diagnosis is based on cytological examination (Giemsa), antigen detection (with enzyme-linked immunosorbent assay and direct immunofluorescence staining), nucleic acid-based tests (nucleic acid probe tests and nucleic acid amplification tests—NAAT), cell culture (*in vivo* and *in vitro*), and detection of antibodies (especially microimmunofluorescence—MIF and enzyme immunoassay—EIA, for the diagnosis of LGV). The most specific test in diagnosis is cell culture, and the most sensitive is nucleic acid-based test. NAAT and MIF tests are successful in the diagnosis of *C. pneumoniae* infections. The diagnosis of psittacosis is usually made by serological testing, and species-specific MIF testing should be performed to confirm.

Keywords: *C. trachomatis*, *C. psittaci*, *C. pneumoniae*, Labaratory diagnosis, chlamydia infections

1. Introduction

Chlamydiae are nonmotile, gram-negative, cocci [1]. They are obligate intracellular microorganisms with a biphasic life cycle. They can only grow in live cell cultures [2]. Chlamydias belong to the Chlamydiaceae family, from the order Chlamydiales. Species that cause disease in humans are *Chlamydia trachomatis*, *Chlamydophila psittaci,* and *Clamydophila pneumoniae* [3, 4]. Among them, *C. trachomatis* is among the most common sexually transmitted diseases (STIs) in the world today [5]. According to the World Health Organization (WHO) data, around 90 million new cases of chlamydial infections occur worldwide every year [6]. *Chlamydia trachomatis* has been included in the group D notifiable diseases as a sexually transmitted disease agent in our country since 2005 [7].

There are many diagnostic tests used in the diagnosis of sexually transmitted diseases. Laboratory tests are critical because most of the patients are asymptomatic [8]. Developing countries need cost-effective, fast, reliable, sensitive, and specific laboratory services. The high sensitivity of the tests is important in preventing transmission and complications, directing treatment, and controlling infection [9]. Chlamydia testing is indicated for patients with STIs who have urogenital, anorectal, and ocular symptoms, people who have had sexual contact with patients with STIs, and people who are screened for chlamydia [10].

2. Structure, life cycle

Chlamydia cell wall is rich in lipids like gram-negative bacteria. It does not contain typical bacterial peptidoglycan. It contains N-acetylmuramica acid. They exist in two forms in their life cycle. Elementary body (EC) is the form that is metabolically inactive, resistant to environmental conditions and infective. Reticular Body (RC) is the metabolically active, intracellular proliferative and non-infective form. Elementary bodies show a high affinity for host epithelial cells. Bacterial major outer membrane proteins (major outer membran protein-MOMP, OmcB, PmpD), on the surface of *Chlamydia trachomatis* interact with host cell receptors (heparan sulfate, proteoglycans, mannase-6-phosphate receptors, and growth factor such as receptors) and enter the cell rapidly. They are then taken up into the cell by receptor-mediated endocytosis or pinocytosis. Meanwhile, they are protected from the environment by inhibiting lysosome fusion. In the cell, the EC transforms into a reticular body. The reticular bodies are larger in size and multiply by dividing each into two, forming an intracytoplasmic inclusion. They leave the cell to infect new cells. This cycle takes 24–48 h [10].

3. Staining properties

Chlamydia has different staining characteristics. Elementary bodies are stained purple on blue-stained host cell cytoplasm with Giemsa stain. Reticular bodies are stained blue. Chlamydia stains with gram-negative or variable staining. Therefore, the gram stain is useless in identification. Chlamydia particles and inclusions (with group-specific, species-specific, or serovar-specific antibodies) are stained bright yellow-green by the immunofluorescence dye method. In culture, McCoy cells are stained with iodide when growth occurs. *C. trachomatis* appears with brown-stained inclusions on a yellow background [11].

4. History

Trachoma has been described in BC China and Egypt. The role of chlamydia in genital infections was understood at the beginning of the twentieth century. Inclusion bodies were first demonstrated in 1909 in the conjunctival cells of infants with non-gonococcal ophthalmia neonatorum, in the cervical epithelial cells of their mothers, and in the urethral epithelial cells of male patients. In the samples, they showed intracytoplasmic inclusion bodies with the Giemsa method. Thinking they were protozoa, they named them Chlamydiazoae. In Greek, "chlamys" means a curtain that covers the environment and describes the inclusions that surround the cell nucleus [12]. Lymphogranuloma venereum was first described by scientists in 1913. An epidemic

DOI: http://dx.doi.org/10.5772/intechopen.110464

was studied in Switzerland in 1879 and was named pneumotyphus. Later, in a study on parrots in 1892, the term psittacosis was used. The term psittacosis comes from the Greek "parrot." The psittacosis agent, *C. psittaci*, was first produced in fertilized chicken eggs in 1935 and in cell culture in 1941 [4, 12].

Chlamydia pneumoniae was first isolated from a conjunctival swab of a child participating in the trachoma vaccine trial in Taiwan. It was named TW-183. The agent AR-39, isolated from the throat swab of a student with pharyngitis at Seattle University in 1983, was named. The name TWAR (TW + AR) was formed from the first conjunctival strain and the respiratory strain. *C. pneumoniae* strain was defined by morphological examinations and DNA sequence analysis performed in 1989 [4, 12].

5. Classification

The genus Chlamydia has been described in the Chlamydiaceae family of the order Chlamydiales. Chlamydiae are classified according to their antigenic structures, sulfonamide resistance, host differences, and the diseases they cause. Characteristics of three species infecting humans have been identified:

Chlamydia trachomatis has intracytoplasmic inclusion bodies containing glycogen. They are inhibited by sulfonamides. They cause eye and genital infections in adults and conjunctivitis and pneumonia in infants.

Chlamidiae (Chlamydophila) pneumoniae have intracytoplasmic inclusion bodies that lack glycogen. It is generally resistant to sulfonamides. It causes respiratory tract infections in humans.

Chlamidiae (Chlamydophila) psittaki, contain dense intracytoplasmic inclusions devoid of glycogen. It is generally resistant to sulfonamides. It causes psittacosis in humans and ornithosis in birds [11].

6. *Chlamydia trachomatis*

Clinic: *Chlamydia trachomatis* causes trachoma, adult inclusion conjunctivitis, neonatal conjunctivitis, infant pneumonia, LGV, and urogenital infections. Infections in newborns are directly related to sexually transmitted infections [4].

It is the most common cause of nongonococcal urethritis (NGU) in the sexually active and young population [13]. Although its distribution varies according to region, its prevalence is 20–50% [14]. *Chlamydia trachomatis* is an exclusively sexually transmitted pathogen and has been more isolated in developing countries. Clinically, it usually causes cervicitis in women, and epididymitis and infertility in men. It should be noted that it can be asymptomatic in both men and women. Azithromycin should be considered in the treatment [15].

7. Diseases by serotype

Chlamydia trachomatis, has 15 serotypes due to antigenic variations in MOMP encoded by ompA [16].

1. **A, B, Ba, C serotypes:** It is the cause of endemic trachoma. Hand-eye contact is transmitted by flies.

2. **D, E, F, G, H, I, J, K serotypes:** Causing inclusion conjunctivitis, nongonococcal urethritis, cervicitis, salpingitis, proctitis, epididymitis, neonatal pneumonia, and conjunctivitis. Hand-eye contact, sexually and perinatally transmitted.

3. **L1, L2, L3 serotypes:** Sexually transmitted L1, L2, L3 serotypes cause LGV [7].

8. Trachoma

Clinic: The incubation period of trachoma is 3–10 days. It is a chronic disease that starts in early childhood and progresses insidiously. *Chlamydia trachomatis* serovars A, B, Ba, and C are associated with trachoma. It often accompanies a bacterial conjunctivitis and composes the clinical picture together. Trachoma is chronic keratoconjunctivitis involving the conjunctiva and cornea. At the onset of the disease, lacrimation, mucopurulent discharge, and conjunctival redness are the first findings [11]. It is characterized by advanced ocular signs of trachoma, lymphocyte infiltration in the corneal epithelium, granulations in the conjunctiva, eyelid deformities, and complications that progress to blindness [2].

9. Laboratory diagnosis

Culture: Conjunctival scrapings are taken from the upper tarsal conjunctiva, where inclusion bodies are most common. Conjunctival scrapings taken are inoculated into McCoy cell cultures. Usually, McCoy cell cultures were treated with cycloheximide. The adequate number of viable infectious particles and the application of the centrifugation method increase reproduction. Diagnosis can be made by detecting inclusion bodies by one of the staining methods with fluorescently labeled antibodies against Giemsa, iodine, or chlamydia antigens (LPS or MOMP) after 48–72 hours of incubation of the first passage. Detection by staining with MOMP-specific antibodies is highly specific. The disadvantages of the culture method are the need for a long time, the high workload, and the difficulties in standardization. However, some reference laboratories require a culture method to monitor antibiotic susceptibility or when a highly specific test, such as suspected sexual assault, is required [10, 11]. If cultures are to be cultivated from the samples within 24 hours, they can be kept at +4°C. If it is to be kept for a longer period of time, it should be stored frozen at −70°C. The specificity of the culture is 100% and the sensitivity is below 100% under appropriate conditions. In legal cases, the infectious agent should be determined by culture [17].

Morphological detection of inclusions: In the presence of a large number of chlamydial inclusion bodies, a preliminary diagnosis can be made if the preparations are stained with the Giemsa or Gimenez methods. Inclusions are found in the cytoplasm of epithelial cells, usually in the perinuclear space. The incidence of inclusions in preparations prepared from specimens is the highest in neonatal conjunctivitis, lower in inclusion conjunctivitis and trachoma in adults, and rare in urethritis and cervicitis. Detection of inclusions is a rarely used method in diagnosis. Difficulty in the application, low sensitivity, and specificity are the reasons for not using it [18].

Serology: Among the diagnostic methods other than culture, immunofluorescence and enzyme-based immunological methods (enzyme immunoassay, EIA) are the main ones [18]. Both group antibodies and serovar-specific antibodies are frequently found in the serum and eye secretions of infected patients. Antibodies formed against the cell wall structure of the organism are detected. The microimmunofluorescence method is a sensitive method for measuring antichlamydial antibodies [11].

Molecular methods: Polymerase chain reaction (PCR) and other molecular diagnostic methods are not widely used in the diagnosis of trachoma. In developing countries where trachoma is endemic, there are insufficient resources to perform PCR or other molecular tests. In developed countries, which have the opportunity to apply the tests, trachoma is rare and tests are not needed. These methods are generally used in research studies on trachoma [11].

Treatment and prevention: The primary source in endemic areas is children with ocular infections. Transmission occurs between infected children and their caregivers by hand-eye contact and by the feet of black flies. Hygiene rules such as facial cleaning and reducing flying insects are important in protection [11].

Azithromycin is used in the mass treatment of endemic trachoma. After 6–12 months of treatment, clinical manifestations are greatly reduced. It has replaced erythromycin and doxycycline. Topical therapy is of little value [19].

The World Health Organization initiated the S-A-F-E program to eliminate or reduce trachoma (Surgery-Azithromycin-Face-Environmental). It is a program that covers the treatment of trachoma with surgery and azithromycin, facial cleaning, and environmental cleaning by reducing black flies [11].

10. *Chlamydia trachomatis* genital infections and inclusion conjunctivitis

Clinic: *Chlamydia trachomatis* D-K serovars cause sexually transmitted diseases and eye infections (conjunctivitis with inclusion). Inclusion conjunctivitis in adults is follicular conjunctivitis involving the lower eyelid. In the first two weeks, there are purulent-mucoid discharge and signs of hyperemia in the eye. It is accompanied by keratitis, indistinguishable from ocular trachoma. It usually heals spontaneously. However, if left untreated, it may become chronic and deformities may develop [20].

In newborns, 20–60% are infected as they pass through the birth canal. Conjunctivitis with inclusions (15–20%) and respiratory system infections (10–40%) may develop in infected infants. Neonatal inclusion conjunctivitis begins 7–12 days after birth as mucopurulent conjunctivitis. It tends to improve within weeks to months, either spontaneously or with erythromycin or tetracycline therapy, rarely can become chronic [11].

Most chlamydial endocervical infections are asymptomatic or have mild symptoms such as dysuria, mild abdominal pain, bleeding, and vaginal discharge. Mucopurulent discharge is seen in cervicitis. In women, it causes urethritis, cervicitis, endometritis, pelvic inflammatory disease, and its complications. Ectopic pregnancy, spontaneous abortion, tubal infertility, and chronic pelvic pain are the main complications. Pelvic inflammatory disease can progress to a widespread disease that progresses to perihepatitis and ascites [21].

In men, it causes nongonococcal urethritis and epididymitis. It is the most common cause of nongonococcal urethritis, up to 50% in men and women [22]. The incubation period is 7–14 days. It has clinical signs such as dysuria, non-purulent discharge, and frequent urination [23]. Infected adults infect their conjunctiva by autoinoculation and inclusion conjunctivitis resembling acute trachoma may develop. The most common cause of epididymitis in men over 35 years of age is *Escherichiae coli*, and those under 35 years of age are *C. tachomatis* and *Neisseria gonorrhoeae*. Azoospermia can be seen in the acute phase in the chlamydial epididymitis. It is not known whether it causes infertility or not. It is the most common cause of proctitis and proctocolitis in both men and women, more often in gay men [24]. Patients with proctocolitis have fever, tenesmus, and rectal pain. Asymptomatic rectal carriage can occur in neonates and adults [11, 12]. However, since infections are often asymptomatic, diagnosis cannot be made in most cases [6]. Chlamydial infections trigger reactive arthritis and some of them develop Reiter's Syndrome. Reiter's Syndrome is a disease with urethritis, conjunctivitis, arthritis, mucocutaneous lesions [5, 6]. In addition, chlamydial infections can cause cancerous lesions such as cervical dysplasia [4, 25].

11. Laboratory diagnosis

Taking samples: When taking samples, dacron, rayon (artificial silk), cotton, or calcium alginate swabs with plastic handles should be used. Wooden-handled swabs are toxic to chlamydiae. Because chlamydiae are obligate intracellular bacteria, samples should contain both extracellular material and infected human cells. While collecting samples of the vagina, urethra, endocervix, and conjunctiva, firstly the discharge and secretions are cleaned and then the epithelial cells are scraped with the help of a swab. Samples taken for culture should be placed in chlamydia transport media. It should be kept in the refrigerator until it goes to the laboratory. Urine can be tested to detect the presence of chlamydia. The first 20 ml urine sample can be used for the detection of chlamydia nucleic acid. It may not be detected as it may be diluted in subsequent urine.

12. Molecular methods

Probe tests: There are commercially available hybridization-based tests to detect *Chlamydia trachomatis* directly from clinical specimens. In these tests, a single-stranded DNA probe labeled with a chemiluminescent substance that is complementary to the ribosomal 16sRNA of the target organism can be used. The sensitivity and specificity of this test are good [11].

Nucleic acid amplification test: These tests use molecular methods such as polymerase chain reaction (PCR), chain removal, and transcription-based amplification. NAATs have very high specificity like culture, but differently, it is not dependent on the viability of the causative microorganism and so sample transfer is easier. Today, the results have been accelerated by the use of fluorescent labeled probes and automatic nucleic acid extraction. The use of two target gene regions in NAATs enabled the detection of new variants. Bead-based extraction systems further increased the specificity and sensitivity of the test. Therefore, NAATs have become the gold standard in the diagnosis of *C. trachomatis* infections [10]. For these tests, first urine, vagina, cervix, and urethra swab samples are suitable. Approval studies are ongoing for non-genital (conjunctiva, oropharynx, and rectum) specimens [11]. There are also multiplex real-time PCR tests where other sexually transmitted infectious agents (*Mycoplasma genitalium*, *Tricomonas vaginalis*, *Neisseria Gonorrhoeae* vb.) can be detected [24].

Drekt fluorescent antibody (DFA) tests: These tests are used in newborns, conjunctival samples. They are stained with labeled monoclonal antibodies developed against species-specific antigens on chlamydia major outer membrane protein (MOMP). Stained preparations are examined by fluorescence microscopy and samples containing fluorescent smooth-sided round or oval elementary bodies are considered positive [26].

Enzyme immunoassay (EIA): The enzyme immunoassay detects genus-specific antigens in elementary bodies and is less sensitive than NAAT and is not widely used [26].

Culture: Compared to NAATs, culture is a difficult, costly, delayed, and less sensitive method. Swabs from the endocervix, anal canal, urethra, and conjunctiva are suitable specimens for culture. Swab samples are inoculated into McCoy, HeLa229, and Buffalo Green Monkey Kidney cell lines [10]. Samples are incubated at 35–37°C and 48–72 hours. A second inoculation is performed to increase sensitivity. Intracytoplasmic inclusions are examined by direct immunofluorescence [11].

Serology: An increase in serum antibody titers is observed in acute genital chlamydia infections. Antibodies are raised against the infecting immunotype. Serum antibodies are higher titer than trachoma. In societies with a high prevalence of genital chlamydia infection, there is a high background of antichlamydial antibodies. Therefore, serology is not useful and common in diagnosis [26].

Treatment: In chlamydia infections, simultaneous treatment of sexual partners to prevent reinfection is the basic principle. Tetracyclines (such as doxycycline) are widely used in nongonococcal urethritis and in non-pregnant infected women. Azithromycin is effective and can be used in infected pregnant women. Topical treatment is not helpful in eye infections due to chlamydia so systemic treatment is preferred. Treatment with doxycycline and erythromycin for 2–3 weeks is recommended [16].

13. *Chlamydia trachomatis* and newborn pneumonia

Chlamidia trachomatis can be passed from an infected mother to her baby during birth. In pregnant women, the incidence of chlamydial infection is between 2 and 24% [7]. Infants born to infected mothers may develop inclusion conjunctivitis and pneumonia in the first few weeks after birth. Infants with inclusion conjunctivitis have mucopurulent discharge and conjunctival edema. It can also be asymptomatic [5, 20]. Neonatal pneumonia begins at 3–11 weeks with nasal congestion, tachypnea, and cough. Interstitial infiltrates may be seen in the lungs. If left untreated, respiratory failure may develop. Obstructive lung diseases may be more common in these infants later in life [20].

The first choice in diagnostic methods is the isolation of *C. trachomatis* in respiratory secretion cultures with McCoy or other cell lines. Detection of anti-chlamydia IgM antibodies at higher levels or at titers higher than 1:32 is diagnostic.

Treatment is the same for neonatal inclusion conjunctivitis and pneumonia. Oral erythromycin is effective for 14 days. It also eliminates the carrier [7].

14. Lymphogranuloma venereum

Clinic: Lymphogranuloma venereum is a sexually transmitted disease with suppurative inguinal lymphadenitis and is common in tropical climates.

The first sign of LGV, which is a systemic disease, is a painless papule that can ulcerate at the inoculation site. Later, painful and unilateral regional lymphadenopathy develops and may fistulize. In men, lymph nodes above and below the Poupart ligament are frequently involved. Involved lymph nodes become suppurative, purple, and painful over time. Adhesions may occur in the genital area. Perirectal lymph nodes are mainly involved in homosexual men and women. The disease leads to proctitis and bloody mucopurulent anal discharge. Systemic symptoms such as fever, nausea, vomiting, conjunctivitis, skin rashes, arthralgia, and muscle pains are also accompanied [6].

15. Laboratory diagnosis

Culture: Infected lymph node samples are inoculated into McCoy cell cultures. It can be treated with aminoglycoside to prevent bacterial contamination. The agent is then identified by morphology or serological tests [11].

Serology: Sex-specific antibodies are demonstrated by the complement coupling (CF) test. The test becomes positive 2–4 weeks after the onset of the disease. An increased antibody titer or a single titer greater than 1:64 in a patient with clinical findings is a strong indication of active infection. A decrease in CF titer is observed in patients receiving treatment [11].

Treatment: Treatment with tetracyclines and sulfonamides, especially in the early period, yielded successful results. A significant reduction in complement-binding antibodies was observed in most drug-treated patients. This may indicate that the infectious agent has been eradicated from the body. Surgical treatments may be needed in the late stages [27].

16. *Chlamydia pneumoniae* and respiratory infections

Clinic: *Chlamydia pneumoniae* is known as the TWAR agent. A serotype has been identified. It is pathogenic in humans. It is transmitted by respiratory secretions. They are causative agents of upper and lower respiratory tract diseases, most of which are asymptomatic. They cause atypical pneumonia and inflammatory atherosclerosis and cardiovascular diseases [28]. The seropositivity rate is quite low under the age of five. The incidence begins to increase in school-age children. The incidence in adults and the elderly is around 50–75% [29]. The sex-related seropositivity rate in children is equal. However, it is significantly more common in males than adults. Today, studies are still ongoing to explain this difference [30].

Laboratory diagnosis: Many laboratory tests have been developed for the diagnosis of *Chlamydia pneumoniae*. However, serological tests are frequently used.

Culture: For *Chlamydia pneumoniae*, oropharyngeal swab samples should be transported with a chlamydia transport medium (sucrose phosphate glutamic acid buffer solution). Sputum samples are not suitable. It should be kept in a refrigerator at +4°C before being sent to the laboratory. They die quickly at room temperature. *C. pneumoniae* grows better in HL and Hep-2 cells. They are incubated for three days at 35°C. They are usually detected by fluorescent antibody staining with monoclonal antibodies specific for *C. pneumoniae* [11, 31].

Serology: Microimmunofluorescence (MIF), a serological test method, is the most sensitive method. It is species-specific. IgM increases 2–3 weeks after primary infection and IgG increases 6–8 weeks later. In reinfections, there may be no increase in IgM and after 1–2 weeks there may be an increase in IgG [3].

Nucleic acid amplification methods: The PCR method is used to determine the agents in the pharyngeal swab, bronchoalveolar lavage, and sputum samples. This method is a sensitive and rapid diagnostic test [32].

Treatment: *Chlamydia pneumoniae* are sensitive to macrolides, fluoroquinolones, and tetracyclines. Treatment success is good in patients treated with doxycycline, azithromycin, or clarithromycin. However, after some routine treatments, symptoms of the disease continue or reinfections are observed. Therefore, drugs should be used for 10–14 days [11].

17. *Chlamydia psittaci* and psittacose

Clinic: *Chlamydia psittaci* is the causative agent of psittacosis. It is transmitted by contact with birds and by breathing. Human-to-human transmission is rare. It can survive for months at room temperature. Therefore, environmental cleanliness is important [33]. It can be asymptomatic and pulmonary involvement is seen in humans. It can cause sepsis with severe pneumonia and high mortality. It is accompanied by systemic symptoms such as fever, nausea, vomiting, and muscle aches [34]. In birds, liver, kidney, and pericardium involvement is typical [33].

Laboratory diagnosis: For the isolation of *Chlamydia psittaci* in culture, blood, sputum, and lung tissue samples are suitable. Clinical specimens can be produced by inoculating tissue culture cells, embryonated eggs, and mice. They can be identified by examining them under a microscope. Culture can be dangerous. Molecular and serological tests may be preferred. Antigen detection by DFA or immunoassay (MIF) methods is common and PCR tests are used [11, 34].

Treatment: Since the laboratory diagnosis of *Chlamydia psittaci* infection is difficult, it is usually treated with clinical findings. According to several clinical studies, azithromycin, clarithromycin, and erythromycin (doxycycline in adults) treat most *C. psittaci* infections. Clinical improvement is achieved [11, 33].

Author details

Özlem Koca
Antalya Eğitim ve Araştırma Hastanesi Tıbbi Mikrobiyoloji Laboratuvarı, Antalya, Turkey

*Address all correspondence to: drozlemkoca@gmail.com

References

[1] Sarıer M, Duman İ, Göktaş Ş, Kukul E. Results of multiplex polymerase chain reaction assay to identify urethritis pathogens. Journal of Urological Surgery. 2017;**4**(1):18-22. DOI: 10.4274/jus.1328

[2] Mabey DCW, Solomon AW, Foster A. Trachoma. Lancet (London, England). 2003;**362**(9379):223-229. DOI: 10.1016/S0140-6736(03)13914-1

[3] Özbal Y, Mutlu G, İmir T. Klamidyalar. In: Mete Ö, editor. Temel ve Klinik Mikrobiyoloji. Ankara, Türkiye: Güneş Kitabevi Ltd.; 1999. pp. 705-714

[4] Schachter J, Holmes KK, Sparling PF. Biology of Chlamydia trachomatis, sexually transmitted diseases. In: Lemon MS, editor. Biology of *Chlamydia trachomatis*, Sexually Transmitted Diseases. 3rd ed. New York, USA: McGraw-Hill; 1999. pp. 391-405

[5] Stamm WE, Jones RB, Batteiger BE. Introduction to chlamydial diseases and Chlamydia trachomatis. In: Dolin R, editor. Mandell, Douglas and Benett's Principles and Practice of Infectious Diseases. 6th ed. Philadelphia, USA: Churcill Livingstone; 2005. pp. 2236-2268

[6] Essig A, Murray PR, Baron EJ. Chlamydia and Chlamydophila. In: Pfaller MA, editor. Manual of Clinical Microbiology. 9th ed. Washington, D.C., USA: ASM Press; 2007. pp. 1021-1035

[7] Öztoklu İ, Yücel A. Chlamydia trachomatis Enfeksiyonları. Ankara Medical Journal. 2012;**12**(1):32-36. Available from: https://dergipark.org.tr/en/pub/amj/issue/1741/21437

[8] Sarier M, Demir M, Turgut H, Hizel A, Emek M, Kukul E, et al. New approach to microscopy of gram-stained urethral smear: The kissing slide method. Sexually Transmitted Diseases. 2020;**47**(10):712-715. DOI: 10.1097/OLQ.0000000000001228

[9] Esen B, Gozalan A, Sevindi DF, Demirbas A, Onde U, Erkayıran U, et al. Ureaplasma urealyticum: Presence among sexually transmitted diseases. Japanese Journal of Infectious Diseases. 2017;**70**(1):75-79. DOI: 10.7883/YOKEN.JJID.2015.258

[10] Meyer T. Diagnostic procedures to detect *Chlamydia trachomatis* infections. Microorganisms. 2016;**4**(3):25. DOI: 10.3390/microorganisms4030025

[11] Jawetz MA. Klamidyalar A. In: Yenen OŞ, editor. Jawetz, Melnick & Adelberg's Tıbbi Mikrobiyoloji (Türkçe Çeviri). Ankara, Türkiye: Nobel Tıp Kitabevi; 2015. pp. 359-368

[12] Jones RB, Batteiger B. Chlamydial diseases. In: Dolin R, editor. Principles and Practice of Infectious Diseases. 5th ed. Philadelphia, USA: Churchill Livingstone Elsevier; 2000. p. 1986

[13] Kurahashi T, Miyake H, Nakano Y, Shinozaki M, Oka N, Tanaka K, et al. A comparison of clinical features between chlamydial and non-chlamydial urethritis in men negative for gonococcal infection who attended a urological outpatient clinic in Japan. International Urology and Nephrology. 2007;**39**(3):809-813. DOI: 10.1007/S11255-006-9149-7

[14] Ito S, Yasuda M, Kondo H, Yamada Y, Nakane K, Mizutani K, et al. Clinical courses of herpes simplex virus-induced urethritis in men. Journal of Infection and Chemotherapy : Official Journal

of the Japan Society of Chemotherapy. 2017;**23**(10):717-719. DOI: 10.1016/J.JIAC.2017.03.017

[15] Sarier M, Kukul E. Classification of non-gonococcal urethritis: A review. International Urology and Nephrology. 2019;**51**(6):901-907. DOI: 10.1007/s11255-019-02140-2

[16] O'Connell CM, Ferone ME. Chlamydia trachomatis genital infections. Microbial Cell. 2016;**3**(9):390-403. DOI: 10.15698/mic2016.09.525

[17] Carolyn MB. Current methods of laboratory diagnosis of *Chlamydia trachomatis* infections. Clinical Microbiology Reviews. 1997;**10**(1):160-184. DOI: 10.1128/CMR.10.1.160

[18] Gary PW, Deirdre CL, Geraldine HS. Virüsler, Chlamydia/Chlamydophila, Rickettsia ve İlişkili Organizmalar Tarafından Oluşturulan Enfeksiyonların Tanısı. In: Başustaoğlu A, Us D, editors. Koneman's Color Atlas and Textbook of Diagnostic Microbiology (Türkçe baskısı). 7th ed. Ankara, Türkiye: Hipokrat Kitabevi; 2017. pp. 1571-1575

[19] Bailey RL, Arullendran P, Whittle HC, Mabey DC. Randomised controlled trial of single-dose azithromycin in treatment of trachoma. Lancet (London, England). 1993;**342**(8869):453-456. DOI: 10.1016/0140-6736(93)91591-9

[20] Ward ME, Greenwood D, Slack R. Chlamydia. In: Barer M, editor. Medical Microbiology. 17th ed. Philadelphia, USA: Churchill Livingstone Elsevier; 2007. pp. 375-384

[21] Quan M. Pelvic inflammatory disease: Diagnosis and management. The Journal of the American Board of Family Practice. 1994;**7**(2):110-123. Available from: http://www.ncbi.nlm.nih.gov/pubmed/8184701

[22] Sarıer M. Prevalence of polymicrobial infection in urethritis. Journal of Urological Surgery. 2019;**6**(3):180-183. DOI: 10.4274/jus.galenos.2019.2405

[23] Sarier M, Sepin N, Duman I, Demir M, Hizel A, Göktaş Ş, et al. Microscopy of gram-stained urethral smear in the diagnosis of urethritis: Which threshold value should be selected? Andrologia. 2018;**50**(10):e13143. DOI: 10.1111/and.13143

[24] Sarier M, Sepin N, Emek M, Germen AT, Hoscan MB, Konuk E, et al. Evaluating the utility of the A.F. genital system test for pathogen diagnosis in acute male urethritis. Andrologia. 2022;**54**(4). DOI: 10.1111/and.14377

[25] Ertem E, Topçu AW, Söyletir G. Klamidyaların Genel Özellikleri, Chlamydia trachomatis. In: Doğanay M, editor. Enfeksiyon Hastalıkları ve Mikrobiyolojisi. Ankara, Türkiye: Şti: Nobel Tıp Kitabevleri Ltd.; 2008. pp. 1945-1964

[26] Forbes BA, Sham DF, Weissfeld AS. Obligate intracellular and Nonculturable bacterial agents. In: Forbes AS, Sham BA, Weissfeld DF, editors. Bailey&Scott's 71 Diagnostic Microbiology. 12th ed. Philadelphia, USA: Mosby Elsevier; 2007. pp. 510-518

[27] McLean CA, Stoner BP, Workowski KA. Treatment of lymphogranuloma venereum. Clinical Infectious Diseases. 2007;**44**(Supplement_3):S147-S152. DOI: 10.1086/511427

[28] Ashlesh KM, Weidang L, Kyle HR. Immunopathogenesis of chlamydial

infections. Current Topics in Microbiology and Immunology. 2016;**2016**:183-215. DOI: 10.1007/82_2016_18

[29] Aldous MB, Grayston JT, Wang SP, Foy HM. Seroepidemiology of *Chlamydia pneumoniae* TWAR infection in Seattle families, 1966-1979. The Journal of Infectious Diseases. 1992;**166**(3):646-649. DOI: 10.1093/infdis/166.3.646

[30] Kese D, Hren-Vencelj H, Socan M, Beovic B, Cizman M. Prevalence of antibodies to *Chlamydia pneumoniae* in Slovenia. European Journal of Clinical Microbiology & Infectious Diseases: Official Publication of the European Society of Clinical Microbiology. 1994;**13**(6):523-525. DOI: 10.1007/BF01974652

[31] Kuo CC, Grayston JT. Factors affecting viability and growth in HeLa 229 cells of Chlamydia sp. strain TWAR. Journal of Clinical Microbiology. 1988;**26**(5):812-815. DOI: 10.1128/jcm.26.5.812-815.1988

[32] Dalhoff K, Maass M. Chlamydia pneumoniae pneumonia in hospitalized patients. Clinical characteristics and diagnostic value of polymerase chain reaction detection in BAL. Chest. 1996;**110**(2):351-356. DOI: 10.1378/chest.110.2.351

[33] Schlossberg D. Chlamydia psittaci. In: Bennett JE, Mandell GL, Bennett JE, Dolin R, editors. Mandell Principles and Practice of Infectious Disease. 5th ed. Philadelphia, USA: Churchill Livingstone; 2000

[34] Vanrompay D, Harkinezhad T, van de Walle M, Beeckman D, van Droogenbroeck C, Verminnen K, et al. Chlamydophila psittaci transmission from pet birds to humans. Emerging Infectious Diseases. 2007;**13**(7):1108-1110. DOI: 10.3201/eid1307.070074

Chapter 4

Molecular Approaches to the Diagnosis of *Chlamydia*

Elçin Yenidünya Konuk

Abstract

Chlamydia trachomatis is known as the most common bacterial infection agent to pass with sexual transition. This microorganism is an obligatory intracellular parasite. A variety of infections are caused by *C. trachomatis*, including trachoma, pneumonias in newborns, genital and urinary tract infections, and lymphogranuloma venereum (LGV), which is caused by LGV strains. The diagnosis of *Chlamydia trachomatis* can be made by cultures and isolations, antigens and antibodies (direct fluorescence, enzyme immunoassays), hybridization, or polymerase chain reaction (PCR). Each year, infection and diagnosis rates increase in the developed world. Since *Chlamydia* is mostly asymptomatic, screening, and treatment are a key to detecting cases. Polymerase chain reaction (PCR), ligase chain reaction (LCR), and nucleic acid sequence-based amplification (NASBAa) molecular methods can be used for the detection, low concentration, quantification, and identification of organisms. While the traditional PCR method confirms its existence, it can quantify real-time PCR (RT-PCR). This method (RT-PCR) may have low sensitivity among variants of the same species. Also, PCR scans, which receive urine service, offer great advantages. PCR from initial void urine (FVU) samples is highly sensitive in detecting the organism. Urine Chlamydia screenings are more acceptable in large populations and asymptomatic detections.

Keywords: *Chlamydia*, molecular identification, characterization, chlamydia trachomatis, chlamydia diagnosis

1. Introduction

The Chlamydiaceae family is an obligate intracellular bacterial member. Only the genus *Chlamydia* has 9 species distributed in vertebrates that cause serious effects on human health. The history of *Chlamydia* infection in humankind dates back to 4000 years [1]. *Chlamydia trachomatis* is one of the most common sexually transmitted pathogens worldwide. A *C. trachomatis* infection can cause urethritis, cervicitis, proctitis, and conjunctivitis, depending on the anatomical site of the infection. 50% of men and 70% of women are asymptomatic [2]. When CT infection is not treated, it can cause infertility in men and women, such as epididymitis and pelvic inflammatory disease [3]. If *C. trachomatis* infection increases, it can cause endometriosis of the female upper genital tract, pelvic inflammatory disease and tissue scarring, infertility, ectopic pregnancies, and fibrotic disorder and is also potentially associated with cervical and uterine cancers [4].

Culture methods were first allowed as standards in the 1970s and were developed using McCoy cells. The specificity of this method, originally developed for trachoma and lymphogranuloma venereum (LGV), was 100%, but the overall sensitivity was estimated to be 40–85% lower due to laboratory sensitivity, sampling errors, and variable laboratory standards. In the 1980s, there was a return to the fashion for microscopic identification without culturing using a technique known as direct fluorescence testing, and testing was performed by binding specially produced antibodies to specific sites on the outer membrane of *Chlamydia*. It was used because it was quick and relatively inexpensive, with results being more variable compared to other methods, influenced by many factors, including the recognition of three strains or serotypes of *C. trachomatis*. Because of the revolutionization of the laboratory diagnosis of all diseases using monoclonal antibodies, thanks to many of the advances in molecular biology developed by new biotechnology companies, there are new tests for antibodies (complement fixation and microimmunofluorescence) and new antigen tests (direct fluorescence test and enzyme immunoassay). All were compared to the gold standard of cell culture, but there was growing doubt that this was better than any of the newer tests. In the 1990s, new assays using new DNA technologies, particularly the polymerase chain reaction (PCR) technologies, became available to develop nucleic acid amplification assays (NAATs). In these tests, fragments of *Chlamydia* DNA extracted from clinical samples were amplified in repeated cycles to produce samples large enough for colorimetric evaluations. The first such test was introduced by Roche in 1993. *AMPLICOR C. trachomatis*. An evaluation by doctors in Bordeaux the following year found it to have a sensitivity of 95.3% and a specificity of 100%, concluding that it was superior to culture methods. This was followed by other tests from other companies [1, 5].

Recent taxonomic developments based on 16S and 23S rRNA gene sequences, along with the development of molecular tests, have divided the Chlamydiaceae family into two genera and nine species, including 5 species found to infect humans [6]. Over time, new variants of *C. trachomatis* have emerged, and new test techniques that are inexpensive and easily applicable may emerge to identify them [7]. *Chlamydia* is the most commonly diagnosed bacterium among sexually transmitted diseases [8].

Infection diagnosis rates continue to increase in the developed world. Because *Chlamydia* is largely asymptomatic, screening is the most basic way to detect cases and reduce transmission [9].

2. Target genes used in the identification of *chlamydia*

Recent methods for typing *Chlamydia* have used the Chlamydiaceae 16S and 23S rRNA gene sequences. The gene targets most frequently used in the identification of *Chlamydia* are omp 1 (the gene encoding the major outer membrane protein-MOMP), cryptic plasmid, and 16S and 23S rRNA genes. The omp2 gene has been identified in all Chlamydiaceae except *C. pecorum* strains [6, 10, 11].

3. Molecular techniques used for diagnosing *Chlamydia*

Chlamydia, obligate intracellular bacteria, requires tissue culture techniques to isolate and propagate. Culture in permanent cell lines or embryonated chicken eggs is still widely accepted as the gold standard for chlamydial diagnosis, as it is necessary to demonstrate the viability of a strain of a field and facilitate detailed characterization by molecular and biochemical methods [12].

Culture methods were first allowed as standards in the 1970s and were developed using McCoy cells. This method, originally developed for trachoma and LGV, was approximately 100% specific, but laboratory sensitivity was estimated to be only 70–85%, and overall sensitivity was less than 40–85% due to sampling errors and varying laboratory standards. There are two main approaches to diagnose *Chlamydia* and *Chlamydophila* spp. infections in mammals and birds. The first involves directly detecting its agent in the tissue, and the second includes serological screening of blood samples with anti-chlamydial antibodies [13]. Individual methods of detecting antigen characteristics in sample types sent to the diagnostic laboratory may affect the performance. Tests such as the use of DNA-based PCR offer particular advantages. In the 1980s, there was a return to the fashion of microscopic identification without culturing using a technique known as direct fluorescence testing, where the test was performed by binding specially produced antibodies to specific sites on the outer membrane of *Chlamydia*. Compared to other methods, the results were more variable, and this method was used because it was fast and relatively inexpensive, although it was observed to be influenced by many factors, including the recognition of three strains or serotypes of *C. trachomatis*.

Advances in molecular biology have revolutionized the laboratory diagnosis of all diseases, many of which have been developed by new biotechnology companies and monoclonal antibodies. There are new tests for antibodies (complement fixation and microimmunofluorescence) and new antigen tests (direct fluorescence test and enzyme immunoassay). All were compared to the gold standard of cell culture, but there was a growing suspicion that it was better than any of the newer tests. In the 1990s, new assays using new DNA technologies, particularly the polymerase chain reaction (PCR) technologies, became available to develop nucleic acid amplification assays (NAATs). In these tests, fragments of *Chlamydia* DNA extracted from clinical samples were amplified in repeated cycles to produce samples large enough for colorimetric evaluations. The first test of this type was introduced by Roche in 1993. Abbott Laboratories from Illinois mediated ligase chain reaction and transcription and Gen-Probe, whereas La Jolla from California mediated amplification. A review of the new tests found that although they were based on different molecular strategies, they had equivalent specificity and sensitivity to Roche Amplicor [14].

In recent years, there has been a revolution in diagnostic methodology with the introduction of nucleic acid amplification tests (NAATs). These tests are much more sensitive than the previous non-culture tests [15].

For the first time, diagnostic laboratories have a more sensitive technology in tissue culture than in isolation (TC). While TC, which has long been considered the gold standard for the diagnosis of *C. trachomatis*, is considered to have a specificity approaching 100%, NAAT offers more sensitive tests than culture [14].

In a study published in 1997 where the old enzyme immunoassay methods found a prevalence of 1.6% (0.8–2.7%), 60% sensitivity and 100% specificity and the prevalence of ligase chain reaction was found to be 2.5 (1.5–3.9%) in relation to the improvement offered by new DNA-based techniques; a sensitivity of 90% and specificity of 99.8% were indicated. New technologies not only offer greater specificity, sensitivity, and accuracy but also are cheaper and easier [16].

Therefore, it has become possible to go beyond diagnostic testing to screen for asymptomatic chlamydial infection in both men and women. Paradoxically, NAAT technologies may be responsible for the continued increase in new cases reported, as they enable more testing and greater precision [4].

C. trachomatis infections can be detected using cell culture, immunofluorescence (IF), enzyme immunoassay, direct DNA hybridization, and PCR (identifiable). Laboratory diagnosis of chlamydial infection by culture is limited by the fact that collection of urethral swab specimens is unacceptable for many asymptomatic men. PCR applications using various gene targets, such as various cryptic plasmids, omp 1 (the gene encoding major outer membrane protein-MOMP), and rRNA genes, are more sensitive than culture [3, 4, 6, 9–11, 17–19]. Conventional PCR enables real-time PCR quantification, while it identifies most chlamydial species for the presence and absence of a particular pathogen with the ompB gene, a gene specific to the chlamydia family.

Recent taxonomic advances based on 16S and 23S rRNA gene sequences have divided the Chlamydiaceae family into two genera and nine species, five of which have been found to infect humans. There are several simple methods for detecting and identifying all species precisely and specifically. In this study, the omp2 gene was demonstrated as a target for the molecular identification of suitable Chlamydiaceae. Phylogenetic analysis accepts partial omp2 gene sequences from all nine species based on recently published taxonomic changes. The use of a family-specific PCR primer pair capable of amplifying the 5-end on ribosomal genes is described for the omp2 gene from all *Chlamydiaceae*, except for some strains of *Chlamydophila pecorum*. The identification of all nine species was obtained using restriction fragment length polymorphism analysis with the Alu I enzyme, which was confirmed by DNA sequencing. A PCR enzyme-linked oligonucleotide assay can be developed that can identify mixed human chlamydial infections or a lone chlamydial genome analysis [6].

Another method used for rapid detection of pathogenic bacteria is the DNA microarray method, which is based on DNA hybridization. There are studies examining nine species belonging to the *Chlamydiaceae* family with the help of probes developed to identify species-specific regions such as the ribosomal RNA opreon region. Identification was made both in culture and direct clinical tissue bacteria samples [5].

Isothermal amplification assays such as loop-mediated isothermal amplification (LAMP) are of great utility in the development of rapid diagnostics for infectious diseases, as they have high sensitivity, pathogen specificity, and application potential. However, eliminating nonspecific amplification remains a major challenge for the optimization of LAMP assays [20].

Ocular infections are more difficult to diagnose and confirm than systemic infections or infections of other organs due to their delicate anatomy and fewer sample types and volumes that can be safely collected from the eye. Next-generation sequencing (NGS)-based approaches are revolutionary molecular diagnostics, also called high-throughput. NGS-based approaches can amplify tens to hundreds of samples containing limited genomic content and transcriptomes, allowing characterization of all of them. This technique is of particular interest in clinical diagnosis in ophthalmology, as the sample quantity is limited and difficult to obtain. NGS needs to be developed for clinical applications in ophthalmology by making its use more convenient [14, 17].

The third widely used nucleic acid target amplification method in the United States is isothermal TMA (commercial nucleic acid amplification) based on *C. trachomatis*. Within two hours, the RNA amplification rate increased 10^9-fold. Within four hours, the DNA amplification rate increased 10^6-fold. Nucleic acid amplification assays have been used for verification in previous years because of their high sensitivity, but in recent years, they have been used for screening various samples. Consequently, as nucleic acid-based diagnostic assays continue to evolve, such tests need to be established in both small- and large-scale clinical laboratory settings. Commercial nucleic acid hybridization is nucleic acid hybridization using

DOI: http://dx.doi.org/10.5772/intechopen.109746

oligonucleotide sequences designed to bind to the complementary sequence in the target nucleic acid. It is used in conjunction with cell culture methods to provide optimal conditions due to its low sensitivity. Target and oligonucleotide probe nucleic acid concentrations do not change. It contains target-specific chromosomal and cryptic plasmid sequences for detecting *C. trachomatis* [19].

Due to the lack of a genetic transformation system, studying the molecular biology of Chlamydia, an obligate intracellular bacterium, has been difficult. With genome sequencing, knowledge of the biology of these pathogens has greatly increased. Comparing the seven sequenced genomes of the Chlamydia genome provides an overview of gene content and gene diversity. Genome sequences have allowed general investigations in terms of both transcript and protein content throughout the evolution of the Chlamydial cycle. Chlamydiae form chlamydial inclusions, and the proteins released from this inclusion can interact with host cell proteins and produce changes in the host cell's response to infection. The identification of these proteins is difficult because the cytoplasm of the host cell infected with Chlamydia cannot be purified. This problem has been overcome by comparative proteomics [21].

Ligase chain reactions (LCVs) are among the noninvasive nucleic acid amplification tests and are among the amplification tests that can be used in low-prevalence populations because they are likely to give false positives and need confirmation [22].

4. Use of molecular techniques in chlamydia diagnosis and screening

Since the late 1990s, chlamydia has been the most commonly reported sexually transmitted infection (STI) in Europe and the United States. The infection is caused by the bacterium *C. trachomatis* (*C. trachomatis*), and its common name was given in the late nineteenth century after an infection-causing pathogen. In 2017, there were just over 203,116 new diagnoses in the UK. In contrast, 7137 syphilis and 44,676 gonorrhea and more than 3,126,000 chlamydia diagnoses were made by the National Chlamydia screening program. The disease was equally prevalent in men, and although similar effects on the seminal vesicles are expected, there is as yet no evidence of a strong association between infection and male infertility. The program began in 2004, and the reported incidence of chlamydia has skyrocketed, with journalists warning of "a time bomb for fertility" from these reports. Chlamydia was first recognized as a specific sexually transmitted infection in the 1970s, but in 1988, it became reportable.

There are different types of screening options for chlamydial infections. It has the highest rate of spread on the scale of infectious diseases among youth and late adults. Chlamydia is easily transmitted sexually and can also be transmitted to newborns. A large number of infectious individuals may be overlooked in screening because they do not have symptoms. Although chlamydia can cause serious infections, it can be easily diagnosed with various new tests with high sensitivity. The new urine tests are rapid and noninvasive and give rapid results. It has been shown that scans reduce the rates of pelvic inflammatory disease (PID) and improve birth outcomes when pregnant women are screened and treated. Cost studies, on the other hand, show that screening for women is more cost-effective than no screening. The evidence for screening in men is quite limited. Little is known about how often any of these groups will be screened. Worse health outcomes, such as recurrent infections, PID in women, and ectopic pregnancies, should be followed by conventions, which are currently largely in the domain of public health programs, not clinical practice. As the responsibility for these tasks shifts to public health organizations, clinicians may become more involved in these secondary preventive measures [23]. Increasing evidence suggests that the rate of progression of endocervical chlamydia to pelvic inflammatory disease is lower than previously thought. Population-based studies consistently estimate the incidence rates of pelvic inflammatory disease to be lower than that by clinical-based studies. Therefore, infections detected by screening asymptomatic individuals may have a better prognosis than that of symptomatic infections due to differences in the burden of the organism. However, descriptions of chlamydial infection and its consequences and models of the impact of screening almost always refer to higher estimates [14].

Compared to nucleic acid amplification tests, the sensitivity of conventional methods is very low [19].

Commercial polymerase chain reaction (PCR) uses multiple amplifier product line-based methods to target DNA. This is a cryptic plasmid DNA of 207 nucleotides, which is highly conserved among serotypes for *C. trachomatis.*

Chlamydia species are the leading cause of bacterial STDs, important respiratory pathogens, and the etiologic agent of endemic blinding trachoma, a zoonotic threat. In the last decade, molecular genetic analyses of Chlamydia species have advanced rapidly [24]. *C. trachomatis* (Ct) is the most common sexually transmitted disease worldwide. A Ct infection can cause urethritis, cervicitis, proctitis, and conjunctivitis depending on the anatomical site of the infection. It is asymptomatic in 50% of men and 70% of women. When *C. trachomatis* infection is not treated, it can cause infertility in men and women, such as epididymitis and pelvic inflammatory disease [3].

In the study using DNA enzyme immunoassay (DEAI) and reverse hybridization assay techniques, 19 serovar typing was performed by distinguishing it from other bacteria and chlamydia species or commensal microorganisms in the genital tract with very high sensitivity as a result of the identification of *C. trachomatis*. First, PCR products were hybridized with the probe mixes for the cryptic, plasmid, and omp 1 genes, and *C. trachomatis* was detected [18]. *C. trachomatis* is the most common sexually transmitted bacterial infection in the United States, usually by asymptomatic individuals. FDA-approved molecular methods for diagnosing urogenital *C. trachomatis* include nucleic acid hybridization, signal amplification, polymerase chain reaction, chain displacement amplification, and transcription-mediated amplification [25].

Molecular methods are both rapid and reliable for screening genital species in areas with high disease prevalence. The clinical and analytical sensitivity of some tests is seriously reduced when testing from urine samples. In vitro experiments have shown that transcriptional origin amplification is more sensitive than other molecular-based assays [19].

In the detection of *C. trachomatis*, screening tests without amplification include the direct fluorescent antibody test (DFA), optical immunostaining (OIA), and rapid solid-phase enzyme immunoassay (EIA). The accuracy in the diagnosis of *C. trachomatis* using nonmolecular methods confirms the quality of the reference tests [26].

Commercial nucleic acid hybridization is nucleic acid hybridization using oligonucleotide sequences designed to bind to the complementary sequence in the target nucleic acid. It can be used in conjunction with cell culture methods that do not provide optimal conditions due to low sensitivity. In commercial signal amplification, neither target nor oligonucleotide probe nucleic acid concentrations change. It contains target-specific chromosomal and cryptic plasmid sequences for detecting *C. trachomatis* [19].

C. trachomatis infections can be detected using cell culture, immunofluorescence (IF), enzyme immunoassay, direct DNA hybridization, and PCR (identifiable). Laboratory diagnosis of chlamydial infection by culture is limited by the fact that the collection of urethral swab specimens is unacceptable for many asymptomatic men.

PCR applications using various gene targets, such as cryptic plasmid, omp 1 (the gene encoding major outer membrane protein-MOMP), and rRNA genes, are more sensitive than EIR, IA, and culture [10].

C. trachomatis is the most common sexually transmitted bacterial infection in the United States, usually by asymptomatic individuals. FDA-approved molecular methods for diagnosing urogenital *C. trachomatis* include nucleic acid hybridization, signal amplification, polymerase chain reaction, chain displacement amplification, and transcription-mediated amplification. Molecular methods are both rapid and reliable for screening genital species in areas with high disease prevalence [27]. The clinical and analytical sensitivity of some tests is seriously reduced when testing from urine samples. In vitro experiments have shown that transcriptional origin amplification is more sensitive than other molecular-based assays [19].

Commercial nucleic acid hybridization is nucleic acid hybridization using oligonucleotide sequences designed to bind to the complementary sequence in the target nucleic acid. It can be used in conjunction with cell culture methods that do not provide optimal conditions due to low sensitivity [19]. Samples isolated from 40 patients with *C. trachomatis* infection were transferred to the laboratory, and the methods obtained from the culture method with chlamydial nucleic acids were compared. By PCR, either the characteristic 7.5 kb plasmid DNA or the 16 Cyclic r RNA gene segment was used for identification. All PCR results were validated in Sothern or dot blot format. As a result, 5 *C. trachomatis* were isolated from 6 samples that were PCR positive. More samples (9) were found to be positive, as nucleic acid sequencing showed rRNA-PCR-amplified products in variants. These data showed that *C. trachomatis* infections in patients were either unrecognized or detected variants carrying the *C. trachomatis* plasmid [28].

Epidemiological studies on molecular typing have been conducted since ancient times. Molecular typing and serotyping of 150 *C. trachomatous* specimens isolated from genital sources of 10 different serovars were compared. The most common omp 1 genotypes, E (51.7%), F (17.3%), D (8.8%), and G (8.4%), were determined from the samples collected over 29 months. Molecular biology methods that require molecular biology techniques and equipment allow typing as well as immunology techniques [29].

A different study used rapid antigen identification to identify *C. trachomatis* infections and compared it with direct fluorescent antibody staining and tissue culture. In a study conducted on 507 patients, the sensitivity was found to be 75%, whereas the specificity was 99% [30].

Chlamydia detection and screening methods made from urine samples are commonly used. Sample supply is easier as noninvasive methods are used for sample collection.

However, PCR can also be used because urine specimens are more convenient to collect and more acceptable to patients. Studies have shown that the application of restriction fragment length polymorphism (RFLP), which is another technique in addition to PCR, facilitates the identification of many serovars that are difficult to identify using PCR [31].

PCR is more sensitive and accurate than other methods in chlamydia samples isolated from endocervical swabs. Cell culture PCR results obtained from urine samples as well as the samples collected from the cervix were compared, and the sensitivity was 87% in culture, 92% in cervix PCR, and 95% in urine PCR. Culture from endocervical and urethral swabs is the gold standard for diagnosing chlamydia. However, its sensitivity is affected by many factors, such as conditions during transportation. Recently, PCR amplification methods and ligase chain reactions have been shown to be more sensitive. In recent years, PCR scans from the urine cervix have offered great advantages. Urine

PCR culture is more sensitive than specific culture. Urine chlamydia screenings are more acceptable in large populations and for asymptomatic detection [32].

C. trachomatis (Ct) is an atypical agent for developing acute, subclinical, and chronic conjunctivitis. The chain reaction (PCR) procedure was used for the conjunctivitis test and enzyme-linked fluorescence assay (IFA and ELFA) and molecular analysis of Ct DNA search (Ct DNA) with polymerase among a total of 3520 patients who visited the examination room of the G. d'Annunzio University Eye Clinic between 2006 and 2008 in the study formed with the records of 171 patients with occasional mild, moderate, or severe illness from Chieti, Italy, in a prospective open three-arm study using conventional assays such as immunofluorescence in order to evaluate the presence of *C. trachomatis* against trachoma.

Molecular tests such as the GeneXpert CT/NG test are highly sensitive. However, cost constraints prevent these technologies from being implemented in environments with limited resources. Pooled testing is a strategy to reduce the cost per sample, but the extent of the savings depends on the prevalence of the disease. One study used a pooling strategy based on the identification of sociodemographic and laboratory factors associated with the prevalence of CT/NG in a high-risk area of Zambian female sex workers. Factors associated with positive testing for CT/NG through single mothers' logistic regression modeling conducted from 2016 to 2019 included city, young age, low education, and long-acting reversible contraception. Based on these factors, the study population was divided into high-, medium-, and low-prevalence subgroups. *Trichomonas vaginalis* infection was tested in pools of 3 or 4, respectively, according to bacterial vaginosis and syphilis infection. The fee was reduced from $18 to $9.43 per sample in the low-prevalence subgroup. The described checklist tool and pooling approach can be used in a variety of ways. This is especially valuable in areas where resources are limited. It is also important in treating asymptomatic CT/NG infections missed by traditional syndromic management.

The most attractive DNA amplification methods can be recommended for screening trachomatis infections because of their excellent sensitivity and good performance. This scan has been shown before in the FVU (first-void urine) samples. PCR testing with FVU is cost-effective in a low-prevalence population. A side risk factor for *C. trachomatis* infection is infection exceeding 3.9%. Recent research has shown that neoplasia is a risk factor for pregnancy outcomes other than ectopic pregnancy and possibly for cervical development. The cost-effectiveness of screening the sexually active population with DNA amplification methods can be reassessed.

Pathogens were compared using multiplex real-time polymerase chain reaction (PCR) in men with acute urethritis. Test results were compared in 83 patients using urethral swab samples, multiple real-time PCR, and A.F. Genital System tests in men diagnosed with acute urethritis. The pathogen of urethritis was detected in 69 patients with PCR and in 15 patients with AF. Compared with AF genital tract multiplex PCR, its sensitivity is low in male patients with previous acute urethritis [33]. Urethritis in men is one of the most common sexually transmitted diseases, and although there have been important developments in treatment and diagnosis in recent years, the most common method is the use of polymerase chain reactions [34].

Highly conserved Chlamydial proteins can be used as specific markers in the diagnosis of chlamydial and constitute new targets of drugs specific to these bacteria. In total, 59 Chlamydia proteins, 79 Chlamydiaceae proteins, 20 both Chlamydia and Chlamydophila, and 445 ORFs were found to be specific to Protochlamydia [18].

Studies have been conducted using tandem mass spectrometry and affinity chromatography methods for Chlamydia infections, which do not have an effective vaccine yet and have resulted in significant deaths worldwide [35].

Author details

Elçin Yenidünya Konuk
Faculty of Medicine, Department of Medical Biology, İzmir Bakırçay University, Seyrek, İzmir, Turkey

*Address all correspondence to: elcin.yenidunya@bakircay.edu.tr

References

[1] Nunes A, Gomes J. Evolution, phylogeny, and molecular epidemiology of *chlamydia*. Infection, Genetics and Evolution. 2014;**4**:9-64

[2] Sarier M, Demir M, Turgut H, et al. New approach to microscopy of gram-stained urethral smear: The kissing slide method. Sexually Transmitted Diseases. 2020;**47**(10):712-715. DOI: 10.1097/OLQ.0000000000001228)

[3] Genc M, Mardh PA. A cost-effectiveness analysis of screening and treatment for chlamydia trachomatis infection in asymptomatic women. Molecular and Cellular Probes. 1996;**124**:1-7

[4] Dolat L, Valdivia RH. A renewed tool kit to explore *chlamydia* pathogenesis: From molecular genetics to new infection models [version 1; peer review: 3 approved]. F1000Research. 2019;**8**:935

[5] Sachsea K, Hotzela H, Slickersb P, Ellingerb T. Ehrichtb R: DNA microarray-based detection and identification of chlamydia and Chlamydophila spp. Molecular and Cellular Probes. 2005;**19**:41-50

[6] Hartley JC, Kaye S. Tevenson, Bennett J, RıdgwaY G,: PCR detection and molecular identification of Chlamydiaceae species. Journal Of Clınıcal Mıcrobıology. 2001;**39**:3072-3079. DOI: 10.1128/JCM.39.9.3072-3079.2001

[7] Xiu L, Li Y, Zhang C, Li Y, Zeng Y, Wang F, et al. A molecular screening assay to identify chlamydia trachomatis and distinguish new variants of C. trachomatis from wild-type. Microbial Biotechnology. 2020;**14**(2):668-676. DOI: 10.1111/1751-7915.137242020

[8] Sarier M, Kukul E. Classification of non-gonococcal urethritis: A review. International Urology and Nephrology. 2019;**51**(6):901-907. DOI: 10.1007/s11255-019-02140-2

[9] Hocking JS, Guy R, Walker J, Tabrizi SN. Advances in sampling and screening for Chlamydia. Future Microbiology. 2013;**8**:3

[10] Claas HC, Melchers WJ, Bruijn IH, Graaf M, Van Dijk WC, Lindeman J, et al. Detection of chlamydia trachomatis in clinical specimens by the polymerase chain reaction. European Journal of Clinical Microbiology & Infectious Diseases. 1990;**9**:864-868

[11] Jurstrand M, Falk L, Fredlund H, Lindberg M, Olce'n P, Andersson S, Persson K, Albert J, Ba¨ckman A. Characterization of chlamydia trachomatis omp1 genotypes among sexually transmitted disease patients in Sweden. Journal of Clinical Microbiology. 2001;**39**:3915-3919

[12] Thejls H, Gnarpe J, Gnarpe H, Larsson PG, PlatzChristensen JJ, Ostergaard L, et al. Expanded gold standard in the diagnosis of chlamydia trachomatis in a low prevalence population: Diagnostic efficacy of tissue culture, direct immunofluorescence, enzyme immunoassay, PCR and serology. Genitourinary Medicine. 1994;**70**:300-303

[13] Sachse K, Vretou E, Livingstone M, Borel N, Pospischil A, Longbottom D. Recent developments in the laboratory diagnosis of chlamydial infections. Veterinary Microbiology. 2009;**132**:2-21

[14] Worboys M. Chlamydia the Hidden Affliction: Sexually Transmitted

Infections and Infertility in History NBCI Bookshelf (nih.gov). The Hidden Affliction: Sexually Transmitted. Chapter 5. 2019

[15] Sarier M, Sepin N, Duman I, et al. Microscopy of gram-stained urethral smear in the diagnosis of urethritis: Which threshold value should be selected? Andrologia. 2018;**50**(10):13143. DOI: 10.1111/and.13143

[16] Sarier M, Duman İ, Göktaş Ş, Demir M, Kukul E. Results of multiplex polymerase chain reaction assay to identify urethritis pathogens. Journal of Urological Surgery. 2017;**1**:18-22. DOI: 10.4274/jus.1328

[17] Doan T, Benjamin AP. Current and future molecular diagnostics for ocular infectious diseases. Current Opinion in Ophthalmology. 2016;**27**(6):561-567. DOI: 10.1097/ICU.0000000000000311

[18] Griffiths E, Ventresca MS, Gupta RS. BLAST screening of chlamydial genomes to identify signature proteins that are unique for the *Chlamydiales*, *Chlamydiaceae*, *Chlamydophil* and *chlamydia* groups of species. BMC Genomics. 2006;**7**:14

[19] Harkins AL, Munson E. Molecular diagnosis of sexually transmitted chlamydia trachomatis in the United States. ISRN. Obstetrics and Gynecology. 2011;**2011**:17. DOI: 10.5402/2011/279149

[20] Rolando JC, Jue E, Barlow TJ, IsmagilovR F. Real-time kinetics and high-resolution melt curves in single-molecule digital LAMP to differentiate and study specific and non-specific amplification. Nucleic Acids Research. 2020;**48**(7):42

[21] Vandahl BBS, Birkelund S. Christiansen G 2004. Genome and proteome analysis of chlamydia. Proteomics. 2004;**4**:2831-2842. DOI: 10.1002/pmic.200400940

[22] Zenilman JM, Miller WC, Gaydos C, Rogers SM, Turner CF. LCR testing for gonorrhoea and chlamydia in population surveys and other screenings of low prevalence populations: Coping with decreased positive predictive value. Sexually Transmitted Infections. 2003;**79**:94-97

[23] Nelson HD, Saha S, Helfand M. Rockville Screening for Chlamydial Infection [Internet]. Systematic Evidence Reviews, No. (MD). Agency for Healthcare Research and Quality (US); 2001

[24] Sixt BS, Valdivia RH. Molecular genetic analysis of *chlamydia* species. Annual Review of Microbiology. 2016;**70**:179-198. DOI: 10.1146/annurev-micro-102215-095539

[25] Quint KD, Geraets DT, van den Munckhof HA, de Koning MN, Smelov V, Melchers WJ, et al. Evaluation of a novel chlamydia trachomatis microsphere suspension assay for detection and genotyping of the different Serovars in clinical samples. The Journal of Molecular Diagnostics. 2011;**13**:2

[26] Bandea I, Koumans EH, Sawyer MK, Dover J, O'Connor A, Papp JR, .Unger E R, Braxton J, Black CM, Evaluation of the rapid BioStar optical immunoassay for detection of *chlamydia trachomatis* in adolescent women.Journal of Clinical Microbiology 2009. 47:1

[27] Sarier M. Prevalence of Polymicrobial infection in urethritis. Journal of Urological Surgery. 2019;**6**(3):180-183. DOI: 10.4274/jus.galenos.2019.2405

[28] An Q, Gail R, Vassallo R, Buxton D, O'brıen WJ, Pelletıer DA, et al. Infection

with a plasmid-free variant chlamydia related to chlamydia trachomatis identified by using multiple assays for nucleic acid detection. Journal of Clinical Microbiology. 1992;**30**:2814-2821

[29] Rodriguez P, Barbeyrac BD, Persson K, Dutilh B, Bebear C. Evaluation of molecular typing for epidemiological study of chlamydia trachomatis genital infections. Journal of Clinical Microbiology. 1993;**31**(8):2238-2240. DOI: 10.1128/jcm.31.8.2238-2240.1993

[30] Pol BV, Williams JA, Jones RB. Rapid antigen detection assay for identification f chlamydia trachomatis infection. Journal of Clinical Microbiology. 1995;**3**:1920-1921. DOI: 10.1128/jcm.33.7.1920-1921.1995

[31] Likuan Xiong L, Kong F, Zhou H, Gilbert GL. Use of PCR and reverse line blot hybridization assay for rapid simultaneous detection and Serovar identification of *chlamydia trachomatis*. Journal of Clinical Microbiology. 2006;**44**(4):1413-1418. DOI: 10.1128/JCM.44.4.1413-1418.2006

[32] Livengood CH, Wrenn JW. Evaluation of COBAS AMPLICOR (Roche): Accuracy in detection of chlamydia trachomatis and Neisseria gonorrhoeae by Coamplification of Endocervical specimens. Journal of Clinical Microbiology. 2001;**39**:2928-2932. DOI: 10.1128/JCM.39.8.2928-2932.2001

[33] Sarier M, Sepin N, Emek M, Germen AT, Hoscan MB, Konuk E, et al. Evaluating the utility of the A.F. genital system test for pathogen diagnosis in acute male urethritis. Andrologia Wiley. 2022;**54**(4):14377. DOI: 10.1111/and.1437

[34] Sarier M. Polymerase chain reaction assay in acute urethritis. Andrologia Wiley. 2019. DOI: 10.1111/and.13366

[35] Karunakaran K, Rey-Ladino J, Stoynov N, Berg K, Shen C, Jiang X, et al. Immunoproteomic discovery of novel T cell antigens from the obligate intracellular pathogen *chlamydia*. The Journal of Immunology. 2008;**180**(4):2459-2465. DOI: 10.4049/jimmunol.180.4.2459

Chapter 5

Immune Response to Chlamydia

Gül Aydın Tiğlı

Abstract

Following the chlamydial exposure, a series of events occur in the host belonging to the innate and adaptive immune systems. The first line of defense against chlamydial infections is mucosal secretions contain various antimicrobial peptides. The complement system that can be part of defense is triggered by elementary bodies of Chlamydiae. Chlamydiae that escape from the complement system infect the epithelial cells. Chlamydiae are protected from phagolysosome fusion by generating inclusion formation. However, they are recognized by pattern recognition receptors (PRR), mainly Toll-like receptor 2. Chlamydia-PRR interaction can be resulted by cytokine/chemokine secretion. The first innate immune cells that reach the infection site are natural killer (NK) cells and neutrophils. The most important contribution of NK cells to this pathogen is the production of high levels of IFNγ. Neutrophils are effective in reducing the load of *Chlamydia* and shortening the duration of infection. The relationship of neutrophils with pathology is also discussed. Recognition of MHC class II-restricted Chlamydia peptides presented by dendritic cells *via* CD4 T cells initiates an adaptive immune response. IFNγ-mediated Th1 immune response is essential for *Chlamydia* clearance. CD8 T cells, which are fewer in numbers, have been suggested that they are the main cause of infection-related immunopathology. B cells and antibodies were found to be particularly effective in preventing reinfection.

Keywords: chlamydial infections, innate immunity, adaptive immunity, chlamydial immunology, immune response

1. Introduction

Chlamydia genera belong to the *Chlamydiae* phylum, Chlamydia class, *Chlamydiales* order, and *Chlamydiaceae* family according to phylogenetic classification. *Chlamydiae* are Gram-negative non-motile obligate intracellular bacteria with biphasic developmental cycle. They appear in two different forms called the elementary body (EB) and the reticulate body (RB). EB in the extracellular environment infects susceptible cells. After cell invasion, the disulfide bonds of EB are reduced and the bacteria transform into the RB form. This intracellular form, which is responsible for the persistence of the disease, is metabolically active, replicative, and non-infectious [1–4]. Many species of chlamydia occur as disease agents in humans and animals. The two main species responsible for disease in humans are *Chlamydia trachomatis* and *Chlamydia pneumoniae*. In addition to these two species, which are strictly human pathogens, *Chlamydia psittaci*, whose natural host are birds, also causes infection as a result of transmission to humans [5, 6]. *C. pneumoniae* is primarily associated with bronchitis and pneumonia. Acute infections are usually asymptomatic or mildly clinical. Reinfection is common. In recent years, there has been evidence that *C. pneumoniae* causes some inflammatory diseases. Chronic bronchitis, asthma, atherosclerotic cardiovascular diseases, and cerebrovascular diseases are among the diseases associated with chronic *C. pneumoniae* infection [7]. *C. trachomatis* is grouped into various serovars according to its outer membrane genotype. Serovars A, B, Ba, and C mainly infect the conjunctival epithelium, causing trachoma defects. Recurrent infections can result in corneal damage and blindness [8]. Serovars D, Da, E, F, G, Ga, H, I, Ia, J, and K are causative agents of urogenital chlamydial infection [9]. It causes proctitis and urethritis in men. In women, it causes urethritis, cervicitis, endometritis, and salpingitis. Chronic pelvic pain, ectopic pregnancy, and infertility are common complications, accounting for 20–50% of non-gonococcal urethritis cases [10, 11]. L1, L2, L2a, and L3 serovars spread to the inguinal lymph nodes and cause lymphogranuloma venereum (LGV) [12]. Although sensitive tests such as PCR can be used for the diagnosis of chlamydial infections, their asymptomatic nature delays their diagnosis and increases their spread in the community. Sequelae increase in the long term as a result of not applying timely and appropriate antibiotherapy [13]. Chlamydial infections continue to be an interesting research topic due to their impact on public health. The necessity to understand all aspects of chlamydial infections necessitates the examination of host responses. Various stages of the innate and adaptive immune response have been studied in numerous studies, both in humans and in animals. In this topic, immunological events that occur in the host after chlamydial transmission are summarized based on the literature.

2. Innate immune response

2.1 Physical barriers

Mucosal barriers are physical barriers that form the first line of defense against Chlamydial invasion. They are formed by epithelial cells and the substances they secrete. Mucosal secretions contain various antimicrobial peptides [14].

2.2 Complement system

The complement system, which forms the humoral arm of native immunity, is activated by being stimulated by the EBs. While opsonins such as C3b, which are formed as a result of complement activation, contribute to the removal of EBs, it has been shown that C3a has an immune modulatory effect [15].

Chlamydia that escapes the effect of complement infects epithelial cells. Thanks to the inclusion, they escape phagolysosome fusion, but they cannot avoid being recognized by pattern recognition receptors (PRRs) [16]. The PRRs are an important part of the innate immune response against chlamydia. PRRs are proteins that recognize conserved motifs associated with pathogens called pathogen-associated molecular patterns (PAMPs). More than 20 types of PRRs have been identified in humans, found in epithelial cells as well as innate and adaptive immune cells. PRRs can be located in the cytoplasm or surface of cells [17]. Chlamydial PAMPs are recognized by both intracellular and extracellular PRRs since chlamydia is found in the host cell in the form of reticulate body (RB) and released out of the cell in the form of EB. After PRR activation, soluble antimicrobials, chemokines, and proinflammatory cytokines are secreted from the related cells. The prominent PRRs in chlamydial infections are TLRs, especially Toll-like receptors 2 (TLR2) [18], nucleotide-binding oligomerization domain-like receptors or NOD-like receptors (NLRs) [19], stimulator of interferon genes (STING) [20] and CD14 [21].

TLRs recognize chlamydial components such as lipopolysaccharide (LPS), lipoprotein, Heat Shock Proteins (HSP) [22, 23]. TLR2 is located around inclusion during chlamydial infection. Intracellular signal transmission occurs after recognition of its ligand (LPS, HSP60). In a study demonstrating the role of TLR2 and its adapter myeloid differentiation primary response protein 88 (MYD88), LPS isolated from *C. trachomatis* has been known to activate nuclear factor-kB (NF-kB) *via* TLR2 [24]. Studies in human embryonic kidney 293 (HEK293) cells revealed that TLR2 and its adapter protein MyD88 are required for interleukin-8 (IL-8) production [25]. Darville et al. showed that macrophages from TLR2 knockout mice secrete significantly less IL-6 and TNF-α in response to infection than those from wild-type mice [26].

Where TLR2 is most common in the female genital tract in the uterine tubes and inside the cervix. TLR4 is frequently encountered in the uterine tubes and endometrium [27]. In the study by Bulut et al., it was shown that TLR4-mediated recognition of chlamydial LPS and chlamydial HSP60 during *C. pneumoniae* infection is associated with dendritic cell (DC) maturation and cytokine release [23]. STING, a cytosolic PRR, is activated by recognizing dsDNA, cyclic di-AMP, or di-GMP. STING activation leads to the production of type-I interferon (IFN) [9]. It has been shown that cyclic di-AMP produced by *C. trachomatis* activates STING and causes IFN-β production in infected cells [28]. However, the roles of type-I IFNs in chlamydial infections are not yet clearly understood. In *Chlamydia muridarum* genital infection of genetically deficient mice with type-I IFN receptors, chlamydial shedding and duration of infection were found to be reduced, and there was less chronic oviduct pathology [29]. Type-I IFNs have also been associated with PID and infertility in human studies [30]. These findings suggest that type-I IFNs have a negative effect on chlamydial infection.

CD14, a PRR found in monocytes and macrophages, acts as a receptor for bacterial LPS [21] and mediates the secretion of proinflammatory cytokine during infection with *C. trachomatis*.

NOD-like receptors interact with the LPS and PGN of intracellular bacteria [19]. In a study using HEK293 cells, it was shown that dead *C. pneumoniae* was unable to activate the NOD1 or NOD2 PRRs, indicating that live bacteria are necessary for their stimulation [31].

2.3 Innate immune cells

2.3.1 Neutrophils

Neutrophils are the first immune cells to reach the site of infection [32]. Although they cannot clear the infection on their own, it is predicted that they have effects that reduce the burden of Chlamydia and limit the spread in the initial period of the infection [33]. Studies reporting that neutrophils inactivate *C. trachomatis in vitro* support this view [34]. Some studies do not confirm this assumption. In one study, *C. muridarum* load in the genital tract of neutrophil-depleted mice was 10 times higher than in wild-type mice, while *C. trachomatis* was shown to be eliminated in the same time period in both groups [33]. It has been found to increase chlamydial replication through MYD88-dependent signaling [35].

The relationship of neutrophils with pathology has also been the subject of research. In animal model studies, neutrophils are found to be associated with the development of tissue damage as well as contributing to the development of adaptive immune response [36, 37].

Neutrophils are very short-lived cells compared to other immune cells. They survive for about 5 hours before spontaneous apoptosis. How Chlamydia can persist in such a short-lived cell has been the subject of research. Although uninfected granulocytes become apoptotic within 10 hours, survival of infected granulocytes for up to 90 hours has revealed that Chlamydia can delay neutrophil apoptosis [38]. In a study in which primary human neutrophils were infected with *C. pneumoniae in vitro*, it was reported that the infection activates the ERK1/2 and PI3K/Akt survival signaling pathway, delaying neutrophil apoptosis, and thus prolonging their survival [39]. It has also been shown that granulocyte-macrophage colony-stimulating factor, which supports neutrophil activation and survival, is secreted from epithelial cells infected with *C. trachomatis* [40].

It is thought that the prolongation of neutrophil lifespan may have a negative effect on the outcome of chlamydial infection due to the cytokines they secrete causing tissue damage [41]. In a study performed with human fallopian tube tissue culture, the addition of an IL-1 receptor antagonist prevented tissue damage due to *C. trachomatis*. This study provides evidence that IL-1, a cytokine released mainly by neutrophils and monocytes, causes tissue damage in the genital tract [42].

One of the many mechanisms that Chlamydia spp. uses to break innate immune responses and ensure their persistence is that it causes neutrophil dysfunction. The chlamydial protease-like activity factor (CPAF) affects defense mechanisms such as oxidative burst and formation of extracellular traps by targeting the neutrophil surface receptor formyl peptide receptor 2 [43]. As a result, it is suggested that neutrophils with prolonged lifespans but weakened functions contribute to the pathogenesis of chronic chlamydial infections.

2.3.2 Natural killer cells

Natural killer (NK) cells are a group of innate cells involved in the response against cancer, viral infections, and intracellular bacteria [44]. Their role during chlamydial infection has been studied in various studies [32]. In mice inoculated intravaginally with *C. muridarum*, Tseng and Rank determined that NK cells reached the site of infection within 12–24 hours after inoculation [32, 45].

NK cells produce high levels of interferon-γ (IFN-γ). Hook and colleagues showed that interleukin-18 released from human epithelial and IL-12 produced by dendritic cells after being stimulated by *C. trachomatis* cell (DC) stimulate IFN-γ production in NK cells *in vitro* [46]. IFN-γ is important for the inhibition of Chlamydia growth, as well as one of the main cytokines important for the induction of a Th1 immune response. Animal studies in which NK cells have been experimentally destroyed highlight the importance of these cells. In the study by Tseng and Rank, antibody responses were investigated after intravaginal *C. muridarum* inoculation in mice and wild-type mice treated with anti-NK-cell antibody. In the humoral response to Chlamydia in NK cells depleted mice, Th2-associated antibody IgG1 was found to be significantly higher, while Th1-associated IgG2a antibodies were dominant in mice that did not receive anti-NK-cell antibody treatment. In conclusion, the absence of NK cells was associated with decreased TH1 response and exacerbation of the course of infection [32, 45]. In another study, it was shown *in vitro* that IL-12 secretions were decreased and their CD4 T cell-stimulating capacity decreased in DC obtained after intranasal inoculation of *C. muridarum* in mice with NK cells depleted. In addition, DC cells transferred from NK cell-depleted mice to naive mice failed to induce Th1-mediated immune response against intranasal *C. muridarum* infection [47]. These findings indicate that IFN-γ secreted by the NK cell in the early stages of infection shifts the immune response toward Th1 instead of Th2.

2.3.3 Macrophages

Studies show that macrophages migrate to sites of chlamydial infection [48]. They are attracted to the infection site by chemokines and cytokines secreted from infected epithelial cells [49, 50]. They recognize chlamydial PAMPs through the PRRs they carry, primarily TLR and NOD-like receptors. Chlamydia enters macrophages *via* phagocytosis or receptor-mediated endocytosis [51, 52] and proinflammatory cytokines are secreted [22, 53]. Degradation of ingested bacteria with lysosomes ensures the elimination of bacteria. M66 Host cell autophagy, a process by which cells degrade cytoplasmic proteins and organelles, also makes bacteria the target of lysosomes. There are studies showing that autophagy is important for the clearance of *C. trachomatis* [54, 55]. Far fewer forms of chlamydial RB have been detected in macrophages compared to epithelial cells. Although chlamydia infects macrophages, it does not create a niche for intracellular replication. The reasons for this may be the failure of *C. trachomatis* to inhibit phagosome-lysosome fusion and autophagy [54, 56]. Furthermore, autophagy indirectly enhances cell-mediated and humoral responses against Chlamydia by increasing antigen presentation to T cells as supports [57, 58]. It is also important to note that IFN-γ both enhances autophagy and causes upregulation of MHC class II molecules [59].

2.3.4 Mast cells and eosinophils

After infection of mast cells with Chlamydia, cytokines such as TNF-α and IL-4 are released. As a result of these cytokines opening tight junctions, infiltration of the airways with immune cells occurs. This situation has a negative effect on the spread of Chlamydia [60, 61].

Eosinophils secrete IL-4 in the upper genital tract during genital *C. trachomatis* infection. It has been reported that this cytokine indirectly promotes the proliferation of endometrial stromal cells. In addition, it is thought that IL-4 may regulate the development of Th2 immune response after *C. trachomatis* infection [62].

2.4 Cytokines of the innate immune response

In various animal and human studies, it has been shown that proinflammatory cytokines such as TNF-α IL-8, IL-1, and GM-CSF are associated with the development of tissue damage during the innate immune response to *C. trachomatis* infection [27, 29].

2.5 Dendritic cell

The DCs, which are professional antigen presenting cells (APC), have been shown to activate both CD4 and CD8 T cells through MHC class I/II presentation in Chlamydial infections [63, 64]. In a murine model, DCs appear to harbor infectious *C. muridarum* but can still present antigen to T cells. TLR2, STING, and NLRs in DC lead to the production of proinflammatory cytokines such as IL-6, TNF-a, CCR7, CXCL10, IL-1a, and IL-12 after uptake of Chlamydia. These cytokines ensure DC maturation and optimal antigen presentation [65]. Cytokines produced by DC and process of processing and presenting antigens to T cells determine the Th1/Th2 balance of the adaptive response during chlamydial infection. Upon preferential antigen uptake, preferential production of IL-12 from DC occurs. IL-12 activates naive CD4 T lymphocytes and enables them to differentiate toward the Th1 subgroup [66]. In a study, when DCs stimulated with recombinant chlamydial proteins were adoptively transferred to mice, the predominantly produced antibody became Th2-associated antibody IgG1 [65]. In the study by He et al., Th1 cells were highly activated when Th2-associated cytokine IL-10 knockout DC was stimulated and adoptively transferred [67]. In another related study, Lu and Zhong incubated bone marrow-derived DCs with heat-killed *C. trachomatis* and showed that a Th1 response developed after nasal infection of mice with live *C. trachomatis* [68]. DCs provide a link between innate and adaptive immunity in the control of chlamydial infection. Chlamydiae limit MHC class I/II expression in antigen presenting cells to cope with the immune response at this stage [69]. Chlamydial protease-activating factor (CPAF) released into the cytogel by *C. trachomatis* has been shown to inhibit MHC molecules by degrading the MHC class I transcription factor RFX-5 and the MHC class II transcription factor USF-1 [70, 71].

3. Adaptive immune response

3.1 T cell

Research by Rank et al. in athymic mice demonstrated the importance of T lymphocytes for chlamydial immunity. In this study, after inoculation of *C. muridarum* intravaginally in mice, chronic infection occurred in athymic mice, while wild-type controls were able to eliminate the infection within 20 days [32].

T cells cannot recognize pathogen antigens without MHC molecules. MHC II molecules are only found on professional antigen presenting cells, including DC, macrophage, B cell, while MHC I molecules are expressed on the surface of all nucleated cells. CD4 T cells recognize antigens presented in MHC class II and CD8 T cells are activated by MHC class I antigen complexes [72]. In fact, both T cell subsets have been shown to recognize *C. trachomatis* antigens such as outer membrane protein 2 (Omp2), polymorphic outer membrane protein D (POMP-D), MOMP, heat shock protein 60 (HSP60), chlamydial protease-activating factor (CPAF), PmpG, PmpF, and RplF [58].

4. CD4 t cell

CD4 T cells recognize extracellular antigens from proteins endocytosed by APCs and degraded by endosome proteases. During chlamydial infection, APCs such as DCs and macrophages acquire exogenous chlamydial antigens by phagocytizing EBs in the extracellular space or by capturing infected cells harboring RBs. After phagocytosis, APC cleaves chlamydial components and the peptide-MHC II complex is assembled. This complex is then transferred to the cell surface, where it is recognized by the TCR in CD4 T cells [72].

T cells are detected at the site of infection in mice and humans. The recruitment of CD4 T cells to the infection site occurs by the release of various chemokines as well as the regulation of some surface and adhesion molecules [49, 73–75]. Post-infection APCs also migrate to regions of CD4 T cells. Here, clonal expansion of CD4 T cells recognizing chlamydial antigens is achieved (S. G. [48]).

CD4 T cells play a critical role during chlamydial infection. Evidence from murine non-MHC II models has demonstrated the importance of CD4 T cells in clearing the disease (R. P. [76]). Gondek et al., in their study of murine upper genital *C. trachomatis* infection model studies, suggested that CD4 T cells are necessary and sufficient for clearance of Chlamydia and protection against reinfection [77].

When the cellular immune response against *C. pneumoniae* was examined, proliferation and activation of both CD4 and CD8 T cells were detected during primary infection. However, only the activation of CD4 T cells was detected in the later stage of the infection [78].

CD4 T cells differentiate into subtypes as a result of upregulation of transcription factors that increase the production of specific cytokines after antigen recognition [79]. For example, Th1 cells, which are characterized by the production of large amounts of proinflammatory cytokines, especially IFN-γ, are particularly important for clearance of viral infections and intracellular bacteria [80]. In the context of infection by intracellular bacteria such as Chlamydia, the predominant T cell subset expected to be present is Th1 cells. As stated earlier in the relevant section of this article, Th1 subtype differentiation in CD4+ cells occurs following the production of IFN-γ and IL-12 by innate immune cells early during infection [47, 81].

4.1 T-helper1 responses

Evidence from mouse models indicates that the Th1 subtype is of particular importance in Chlamydia clearance [48]. Observation of increased susceptibility to chlamydial infection in the absence of IL-12 [82, 83] or IFN-γ receptor [84] emphasizes that IFN-γ-producing CD4 T cells are protective against Chlamydia. However, some evidence suggests that a polyfunctional response involving IFN-γ as well as TNF-α can increase immunity [85].

Th1 cells not only activate phagocytic macrophages, but also direct humoral immunity. At the end of the process in which B cells are activated, Th1-related antibodies such as IgG2a and IgG3 are secreted by plasma cells [25, 86, 87]. In addition, the cytotoxic effect of CD4 T cells has also been demonstrated [84].

Th1 responses against *C. pneumonia* predominate, especially during reinfection. Even in mice genetically predisposed to Th2 responsiveness during primary infection, Th1 responses were elicited during reinfection and increased IFN-γ production [88].

4.2 Other T-helper responses

Although the predominant CD4 cells are Th1 in chlamydial infection, other T-helper types such as Th2, Th17, Th22, and Th9 have also been detected. However, the role they play during chlamydial infection cannot be definitively determined [80]. For example, the production of IgG1 antibodies is induced by Th2 cells. However, there is evidence that the Th2 response is not protective and even associated with pathology. The Th2 response during human ocular infection has been associated with disease progression and pathology [89]. Transfer of chlamydia-specific Th2 clones failed to protect mice from genital infection [90]. Another T-helper (Th17) is thought to contribute to the formation of Th1 immunity, but has been associated with both protection and pathogenesis in the mouse model [91, 92].

4.3 Memory CD4 T cells

Memory CD4 T cells are traditionally grouped into two groups: central memory (Tcm) and effector memory (Tem), while CD4 Tcm cells are primarily found in the circulation and lymphatic tissues; peripheral, non-lymphoid tissues host CD4 Tem cells [93]. Therefore, CD4 Tem cells are thought to play a dominant role in clearing genital chlamydial infections. Recently, it has been discovered that a third subset of memory T cells is important in tissue-specific immune responses. Unlike TEM, which recirculates into the lymphatics and blood after pathogen clearance, these cells that remain in non-lymphoid peripheral tissue after pathogen clearance are called tissue resident memory T cells (Trms). Even in the absence of persistent antigen, Trms persist in peripheral tissues for a long time [93]. These cells are found in epithelial tissues in areas that interface with the environment, such as the gut, lungs, skin, reproductive system [94]. They act as the first line of defense when re-exposure to pathogens. They can respond to pathogenic attack faster than other subsets of memory T cells that need tissue traffic.

During secondary *C. trachomatis* infection in mice, memory T cells coming from the circulation to the upper genital tract mucosa together with the CD4 Trm cells present in the tissues provide optimum clearance. Circulating memory T cells contribute to the clearance of secondary infection. However, it has been shown that they cannot clear secondary *C. trachomatis* infection alone without Trm cells [95]. Studies have shown that memory T cells proliferate more rapidly in response to antigen during secondary infection [8, 96].

5. CD8 T cells

CD8 T cells are associated with MHC I. MHC I is expressed in all nucleated cells. Cytosolic proteins, which may originate from intracellular pathogens, are degraded by the proteasome. The degradation product peptides are loaded into the binding groove of MHCI at the end of the process involving TAP and a chaperone protein, tapasin. The MHC I-peptide complex is then exported to the surface of the cell [72]. TCRs on CD8 T cells recognize the endogenous antigen presented on MHC I. The results of this recognition are the expression of various effector cytokines, including IFN-γ, and the release of cytotoxic granzyme and perforin molecules that can lead to target cell death [97]. Because they can kill infected cells, CD8 T cells are thought to play an important role in the immune response to intracellular pathogens.

The role of CD8 T cells in chlamydial infections is controversial. While a broader CD8 T cell response was expected against Chlamydia, an intracellular pathogen, it was determined that the CD8 T cell response against *C. muridarum* in the genital tract was much lower than CD4 cells in mouse experiments. Despite their small number, CD8 T cells are known to migrate to the site of infection, and both human and mouse CD8 T cells have been shown to destroy Chlamydia-infected cells [98]. It has been shown that CD8 T cells recognizing trachomatis proteins class I accessible protein-1 (Cap1) and cysteine-rich protein A (CrpA) can kill target cells in an antigen-dependent manner

[99, 100]. However, there is evidence to suggest that CD8 T cells are not essential for clearance of Chlamydia. It has been observed in past studies that CD8−/− and perforin-deficient mice clear the infection at the same rate as wild-type mice [82, 84]. Murthy and colleagues have also shown in a more recent study that CD8 T knockout mice exhibited similar clearances of C. muridarum as wild-type mice following vaginal exposure. In the same study, less hydrosalpinx formation in CD8 T knockout mice is remarkable in terms of the relationship between pathogenesis and CD8 T [101]. It has been suggested that they are primarily responsible for the immunopathology associated with chlamydial Infection [102]. The association of CD8 T cells with pathogenesis has also been reported in a macaque model [103]. Although CD8 T cells are not critical for *C. trachomatis* elimination and may even cause chlamydial sequelae, antigen-specific CD8 T cell clones can localize to the genital tract and contribute to clearance of infection through IFN-γ production [98].

During *C. pneumoniae* infection, it is observed that the infection progresses rapidly in the absence of CD8 T cells. Unlike *C. trachomatis* infection, CD8 T cells have been suggested to play a very important role in protection against *C. pneumonia* [104].

5.1 Memory CD8 T cells

The memory T cell population formation process of CD8 T cells during *C. trachomatis* infection differs from the responses detected against acute infection agents. Some expansion of CD8 T cells is observed during primary infection in mouse models. However, the fact that *C. trachomatis* CrpA antigen-specific CD8 T cells does not proliferate in the expected number and rate during secondary infection with *C. trachomatis* indicates insufficient formation of memory CD8 T cells [105]. While the elimination of the infected cell will deprive the organism of its intracellular niche, with the deterioration of the adaptive immune response, both the infections cannot be cleared and permanent immunity is not formed.

Differential programming of memory CD8 T cells when stimulated by agents such as *C. trachomatis* that cause persistent infection is attributed to the environment at the onset of infection. Namely, for the activation of Chlamydia-specific naïve T cell clones, both T cell receptors must recognize Chlamydia-derived peptides presented by dendritic cells, and co-stimulatory molecules on the dendritic cell must interact with those on the T cell. Interactions of some of these co-stimulatory molecules cause upregulation of the T cell response, while others cause downregulation of the T cell response [81]. One of the inhibitory interactions is the binding of programmed death ligand 1 (PD-L1) on the dendritic cell with PD-1 on the T cell [106]. A study of murine infection with *C. trachomatis* found PD-L1 upregulation in the uterus and PD-L1 upregulated in *in vitro* infected cells. As a result, CD8 T cell expansion is impaired and the development of CD8 memory responses is inhibited. This upregulation leads CrpA-specific CD8 T cells to the Tcm phenotype, which is found in secondary lymphoid organs and lymphatic vessels but has limited effect in peripheral tissues, instead of the Tem phenotype, which contributes to clearance of pathogens in peripheral tissues. When antibodies that block the interaction of PD-1 with PD-L1 were used during primary infection, or when knockout animals were used in both molecules, there was a marked increase in the number of T cells responding to secondary C. trachomatis infection, with more IFN-γ producing CD8 T cells. The memory CD8 T cell population shifted toward the Tem phenotype, resulting in faster clearance of infection [105].

On the other hand, there are studies suggesting that *C. muridarum* CD8 T cell response contributes to the pathology [101, 107, 108]. For this reason, it has been suggested that PD-L1-mediated inhibition may be a mechanism that prevents cell-mediated uterine pathology by CD8 T cells [101]. In the study by Peng et al., immunoinhibitory molecules TIM3 and PD-L1 were blocked in C. muridarum-infected mice. As a result, it was observed that uterus and oviduct pathology increased [109]. This finding reveals that immunoinhibitory molecules regulate inflammation by preventing T cell activation and cytokine production.

5.2 Interferon-gamma

IFN-γ, which is released from both innate cells such as macrophages and NK cells and CD4 and CD8 T cells in response to chlamydial infection, is a critical cytokine for inhibiting chlamydial growth [104]. Gamma interferon is responsible for the upregulation of some interferon-induced genes that may help control intracellular bacterial replication in infected epithelial cells [110]. As a result, some protective mechanisms emerge in infected cells. Iron metabolism, a critical mineral for Chlamydia, is blocked [111, 112]. Expression of the tryptophan-decyclizing enzyme indoleamine-2,3-dioxygenase (IDO) is induced, which breaks down tryptophan necessary for the survival of most Chlamydia species. Also, IFN-γ enhances the phagocytic abilities of macrophages and also ingestion and destruction of *C. trachomatis* [71, 113].

The effect of IFN-γ on tryptophan metabolism was reviewed by Vasilevsky et al. during *C. trachomatis* infection in humans and the IFN-γ signaling cascade leads to upregulation of the IDO enzyme in genital tract epithelial cells. The enzyme catalyzes the breakdown of tryptophan to N-formylkynurenine and kynurenine, thereby disrupting intracellular tryptophan stores [58]. *C. trachomatis* deprived of this essential amino acid has been shown to die due to tryptophan starvation. There are also chlamydia species that have adapted to tryptophan starvation by transforming into the non-replicating persistent form. After IFN-γ removal and subsequent tryptophan production, these persistent forms rapidly become replicative [76, 114, 115]. Since some genital tract strains also express tryptophan synthase, they can overcome tryptophan depletion by producing their tryptophan using exogenous indole [116]. In addition, kynurenine, a by-product of tryptophan catabolism, inhibits host CD4 T cells, thus reducing IFN-γ production and ultimately limiting its overall production. It has been reported that it can lead to the re-activation of *C. trachomatis* [110].

6. B cells and antibodies

B cells support the immune response in a variety of ways. Effector mechanisms such as antibody-mediated neutralization and opsonization [117], antibody-dependent cellular cytotoxicity (ADCC) [118], induction of phagocytosis, and antigen presentation to CD4 T cells by binding of antigen-antibody complexes to Fc receptors in APC [102] have been identified.

The role of B cells in the immune response against Chlamydia has been the subject of many studies. It is known that many *C. trachomatis* proteins, including the major outer membrane protein, induce the formation of specific antibodies [119]. It has also been shown *in vitro* that anti-chlamydial antibodies are neutralizing [71, 117]. However, there is evidence to suggest that B cells play an important role in the secondary memory response rather than the primary infection. It was determined that primary genital infection with *C. muridarum* in mice lacking B cells did not show a different course than in wild-type mice [120], while mice with B cell deficit were more susceptible to reinfection [121]. Mice that cleared primary genital tract infection were found to be resistant to reinfection even after experimental depletion of CD4 and CD8 T cells. It was observed that B cell-deficient mice were unable to resolve the secondary infection after CD4 T cell depletion [122]. It has been reported that passive immune serum transfer to naïve mice does not provide protection, but CD4 T cells prepared from antigen-experienced mice and immune serum together provide optimum protection [123]. The protective effects of the antibodies are likely due to their ability to activate Th1 cells and enhance cellular immune responses [124]. The detection of high antibody titers associated with infertility rather than infection control in epidemiological studies indicates that the humoral response may also have negative effects [125]. However, data on pathogenic antibodies are limited. One of the antibodies discussed in relation to its contribution to pathology is anti-HSP antibodies. HSPs are a group of chaperones, proteins that ensure the correct folding of intracellular proteins: They are found in both eukaryotic and prokaryotic organisms. Its levels increase when cells are exposed to temperature rises, oxidative stress, and inflammation. HSPs, mainly HSP60, are produced by *C. trachomatis* during infection. HSP60 has high immunogenicity. It is quite similar to human HSP60. Therefore, it is suggested that it may trigger an autoimmune response that leads to pathology. High antibody titers against HSP60 were found to be associated with pelvic inflammatory disease, ectopic pregnancy, and trachoma scar [126].

The effects elicited by the response to HSP60 during *C. trachomatis* infection are thought to be similar in *C. pneumonia* infection. It has been suggested that HSP60 released from infected epithelium and macrophages during recurrent and persistent infection with *C. pneumonia* produces immunopathological results [127].

Antibodies against *C. pneumonia* are also used in seroepidemiological studies investigating the relationship between *C. pneumoniae* infection and inflammatory diseases. It has been suggested that IgA levels are a better marker than IgG, especially in terms of detecting chronic infection [128].

Author details

Gül Aydın Tığlı
Medical Microbiology Department, S.B.U. Antalya Training and Research Hospital, Turkey

*Address all correspondence to: gulaydintigli@gmail.com

References

[1] Bastidas RJ, Elwell CA, Engel JN, Valdivia RH. Chlamydial intracellular survival strategies. Cold Spring Harbor Perspectives in Medicine. 2013;**3**(5):a010256. DOI: 10.1101/cshperspect.a010256

[2] Dautry-Varsat A, Subtil A, Hackstadt T. Recent insights into the mechanisms of chlamydia entry. Cellular Microbiology. 2005;**7**:1714-1722. DOI: 10.1111/j.1462-5822.2005.00627.x

[3] Elwell C, Mirrashidi K, Engel J. Chlamydia cell biology and pathogenesis. Nature Reviews Microbiology. 2016;**14**(6):385-400. DOI: 10.1038/nrmicro.2016.30

[4] Grieshaber S, Grieshaber N, Yang H, Baxter B, Hackstadt T, Omsland A. Impact of active metabolism on chlamydia trachomatis elementary body transcript profile and infectivity. Journal of Bacteriology. 2018;**200**(14): e00065-e00018. DOI: 10.1128/JB.00065-18

[5] Cheong HC, Lee CYQ, Cheok YY, Tan GMY, Looi CY, Wong WF. Chlamydiaceae: Diseases in primary hosts and zoonosis. Microorganisms. 2019;**7**(5):146. DOI: 10.3390/microorganisms7050146

[6] Zhong G. Chlamydial plasmid-dependent pathogenicity. Trends in Microbiology. 2017;**25**(2):141-152. DOI: 10.1016/j.tim.2016.09.006

[7] Porritt RA, Crother TR. Chlamydia pneumoniae infection and inflammatory diseases. Forum on Immunopathological Diseases and Therapeutics. 2016;**7**(3-4):237-254. DOI: 10.1615/ForumImmunDisTher.2017020161

[8] Hu VH, Holland MJ, Burton MJ. Trachoma: Protective and pathogenic ocular immune responses to chlamydia trachomatis. PLoS Neglected Tropical Diseases. 2013;**7**(2):e2020. DOI: 10.1371/journal.pntd.0002020

[9] Bébéar C, de Barbeyrac B. Genital chlamydia trachomatis infections. Clinical Microbiology and Infection. 2009;**15**(1):4-10. DOI: 10.1111/j.1469-0691.2008.02647.x

[10] Sarier M, Kukul E. Classification of non-gonococcal urethritis: A review. International Urology and Nephrology. 2019;**51**(6):901-907. DOI: 10.1007/s11255-019-02140-2

[11] Schust DJ, Ibana JA, Buckner LR, Ficarra M, Sugimoto J, Amedee AM, et al. Potential mechanisms for increased HIV-1 transmission across the Endocervical epithelium during C. trachomatis infection. Current HIV Research. 2012;**10**(3):218-227. DOI: 10.2174/157016212800618093

[12] Stoner BP, Cohen SE. Lymphogranuloma Venereum 2015: Clinical presentation, diagnosis, and treatment. Clinical Infectious Diseases. 2015;**61**(Suppl. 8):S865-S873. DOI: 10.1093/cid/civ756

[13] Sarıer M, Duman İ, Göktaş Ş, Demirorcid.org M, Kukul E. Results of multiplex polymerase chain reaction assay to identify urethritis pathogens. Journal of Urological Surgery. 2017;**4**(1): 18-22. DOI: 10.4274/jus.1328

[14] Madanchi H, Shoushtari M, Kashani HH, Sardari S. Antimicrobial peptides of the vaginal innate immunity and their role in the fight against sexually transmitted diseases. New Microbes and

New Infections. 2020;**34**:100627. DOI: 10.1016/j.nmni.2019.100627

[15] Rattan A, Pawar SD, Nawadkar R, Kulkarni N, Lal G, Mullick J, et al. Synergy between the classical and alternative pathways of complement is essential for conferring effective protection against the pandemic influenza a(H1N1) 2009 virus infection. PLoS Pathogens. 2017;**13**(3):e1006248. DOI: 10.1371/journal.ppat.1006248

[16] Wong WF, Chambers JP, Gupta R, Arulanandam BP. Chlamydia and its many ways of escaping the host immune system. Journal of Pathogens. 2019;**2019**:1-9. DOI: 10.1155/2019/8604958

[17] Li D, Wu M. Pattern recognition receptors in health and diseases. Signal Transduction and Targeted Therapy. 2021;**6**(1):291. DOI: 10.1038/s41392-021-00687-0

[18] Yang X, Joyee A. Role of toll-like receptors in immune responses to chlamydial infections. Current Pharmaceutical Design. 2008;**14**(6):593-600. DOI: 10.2174/138161208783885344

[19] Zou Y, Lei W, He Z, Li Z. The role of NOD1 and NOD2 in host defense against chlamydial infection. FEMS Microbiology Letters. 2016;**363**(17):fnw170. DOI: 10.1093/femsle/fnw170

[20] Wen Y, Li Z. The STING pathway in response to chlamydial infection. Microbial Pathogenesis. 2020;**140**:103950. DOI: 10.1016/j.micpath.2019.103950

[21] Kol A, Lichtman AH, Finberg RW, Libby P, Kurt-Jones EA. Cutting edge: Heat shock protein (HSP) 60 activates the innate immune response: CD14 is an essential receptor for HSP60 activation of mononuclear cells. The Journal of Immunology. 2000;**164**(1):13-17. DOI: 10.4049/jimmunol.164.1.13

[22] Bas S, Neff L, Vuillet M, Spenato U, Seya T, Matsumoto M, et al. The Proinflammatory cytokine response to chlamydia trachomatis elementary bodies in human macrophages is partly mediated by a lipoprotein, the macrophage infectivity Potentiator, through TLR2/TLR1/TLR6 and CD14. The Journal of Immunology. 2008;**180**(2):1158-1168. DOI: 10.4049/jimmunol.180.2.1158

[23] Bulut Y, Faure E, Thomas L, Karahashi H, Michelsen KS, Equils O, et al. Chlamydial heat shock protein 60 activates macrophages and endothelial cells through toll-like receptor 4 and MD2 in a MyD88-dependent pathway. The Journal of Immunology. 2002;**168**(3):1435-1440. DOI: 10.4049/jimmunol.168.3.1435

[24] Erridge C, Pridmore A, Eley A, Stewart J, Poxton IR. Lipopolysaccharides of Bacteroides fragilis, chlamydia trachomatis and Pseudomonas aeruginosa signal via toll-like receptor 2. Journal of Medical Microbiology. 2004;**53**(8):735-740. DOI: 10.1099/jmm.0.45598-0

[25] O'Connell CM, Ingalls RR, Andrews CW, Scurlock AM, Darville T. Plasmid-deficient chlamydia muridarum fail to induce immune pathology and protect against oviduct disease. Journal of Immunology. 2007;**179**(6):4027-4034. DOI: 10.4049/jimmunol.179.6.4027

[26] Darville T, O'Neill JM, Andrews CW, Nagarajan UM, Stahl L, Ojcius DM. Toll-like Receptor-2, but not toll-like Receptor-4, is essential for development of oviduct pathology in chlamydial genital tract infection. The Journal of

Immunology. 2003;**171**(11):6187-6197. DOI: 10.4049/jimmunol.171.11.6187

[27] Hafner LM. Pathogenesis of fallopian tube damage caused by chlamydia trachomatis infections. Contraception. 2015;**92**(2):108-115. DOI: 10.1016/j.contraception.2015.01.004

[28] Barker JR, Koestler BJ, Carpenter VK, Burdette DL, Waters CM, Vance RE, et al. STING-dependent recognition of cyclic di-AMP mediates type I interferon responses during chlamydia trachomatis infection. MBio. 2013;**4**(3):e00018-e00013. DOI: 10.1128/mBio.00018-13

[29] Nagarajan UM, Sikes JD, Yeruva L, Prantner D. Significant role of IL-1 signaling, but limited role of Inflammasome activation, in oviduct pathology during chlamydia muridarum genital infection. The Journal of Immunology. 2012;**188**(6):2866-2875. DOI: 10.4049/jimmunol.1103461

[30] Poston TB, Lee DE, Darville T, Zhong W, Dong L, O'Connell CM, et al. Cervical cytokines associated with chlamydia trachomatis susceptibility and protection. The Journal of Infectious Diseases. 2019;**220**(2):330-339. DOI: 10.1093/infdis/jiz087

[31] Opitz B, Förster S, Hocke AC, Maass M, Schmeck B, Hippenstiel S, et al. Nod1-mediated endothelial cell activation by Chlamydophila pneumoniae. Circulation Research. 2005;**96**(3): 319-326. DOI: 10.1161/01.RES.0000155721.83594.2ci

[32] Rank RG, Lacy HM, Goodwin A, Sikes J, Whittimore J, Wyrick PB, et al. Host chemokine and cytokine response in the Endocervix within the first developmental cycle of chlamydia muridarum. Infection and Immunity. 2010;**78**(1):536-544. DOI: 10.1128/IAI.00772-09

[33] Barteneva N, Theodor I, Peterson EM, de la Maza LM. Role of neutrophils in controlling early stages of a chlamydia trachomatis infection. Infection and Immunity. 1996;**64**(11):4830-4833. DOI: 10.1128/iai.64.11.4830-4833.1996

[34] Register KB, Morgan PA, Wyrick PB. Interaction between chlamydia spp. and human polymorphonuclear leukocytes in vitro. Infection and Immunity. 1986;**52**(3):664-670. DOI: 10.1128/iai.52.3.664-670.1986

[35] Rodriguez N, Fend F, Jennen L, Schiemann M, Wantia N, da Costa CUP, et al. Polymorphonuclear neutrophils improve replication of chlamydia pneumoniae In vivo upon MyD88-dependent attraction. The Journal of Immunology. 2005;**174**(8):4836-4844. DOI: 10.4049/jimmunol.174.8.4836

[36] Lacy HM, Bowlin AK, Hennings L, Scurlock AM, Nagarajan UM, Rank RG. Essential role for neutrophils in pathogenesis and adaptive immunity in chlamydia caviae ocular infections. Infection and Immunity. 2011;**79**(5):1889-1897. DOI: 10.1128/IAI.01257-10

[37] Shah AA, Schripsema JH, Imtiaz MT, Sigar IM, Kasimos J, Matos PG, et al. Histopathologic changes related to fibrotic oviduct occlusion after genital tract infection of mice with chlamydia muridarum. Sexually Transmitted Diseases. 2005;**32**(1):49-56. DOI: 10.1097/01.olq.0000148299.14513.11

[38] van Zandbergen G, Gieffers J, Kothe H, Rupp J, Bollinger A, Aga E, et al. Chlamydia pneumoniae multiply in neutrophil granulocytes and delay their spontaneous apoptosis. The Journal of Immunology. 2004;**172**(3):1768-1776. DOI: 10.4049/jimmunol.172.3.1768

[39] Sarkar A, Möller S, Bhattacharyya A, Behnen M, Rupp J, van Zandbergen G, et al. Mechanisms of apoptosis inhibition in chlamydia pneumoniae-infected neutrophils. International Journal of Medical Microbiology. 2015;**305**(6):493-500. DOI: 10.1016/j.ijmm.2015.04.006

[40] Lehr S, Vier J, Häcker G, Kirschnek S. Activation of neutrophils by chlamydia trachomatis-infected epithelial cells is modulated by the chlamydial plasmid. Microbes and Infection. 2018;**20**(5):284-292. DOI: 10.1016/j.micinf.2018.02.007

[41] Lee HY, Schripsema JH, Sigar IM, Murray CM, Lacy SR, Ramsey KH. A link between neutrophils and chronic disease manifestations of chlamydia muridarum urogenital infection of mice. FEMS Immunology & Medical Microbiology. 2010;**59**(1):108-116. DOI: 10.1111/j.1574-695X.2010.00668.x

[42] Hvid M, Baczynska A, Deleuran B, Fedder J, Knudsen HJ, Christiansen G, et al. Interleukin-1 is the initiator of fallopian tube destruction during chlamydia trachomatis infection. Cellular Microbiology. 2007;**9**(12):2795-2803. DOI: 10.1111/j.1462-5822.2007.00996.x

[43] Rajeeve K, Das S, Prusty BK, Rudel T. Chlamydia trachomatis paralyses neutrophils to evade the host innate immune response. Nature Microbiology. 2018;**3**(7):824-835. DOI: 10.1038/s41564-018-0182-y

[44] Montaldo E, Zotto G, Del Chiesa, Della, Mingari M, Moretta MC, Maria A, et al. Human NK cell receptors/markers: A tool to analyze NK cell development, subsets and function. Cytometry Part A. 2013;**83A**(8):702-713. DOI:

[45] Tseng C-TK, Rank RG. Role of NK cells in early host response to chlamydial genital infection. Infection and Immunity. 1998;**66**(12):5867-5875. DOI: 10.1128/IAI.66.12.5867-5875.1998

[46] Hook CE, Matyszak MK, Gaston JSH. Infection of epithelial and dendritic cells by chlamydia trachomatis results in IL-18 and IL-12 production, leading to interferon-Î³ production by human natural killer cells. FEMS Immunology & Medical Microbiology. 2005;**45**(2):113-120. DOI: 10.1016/j.femsim.2005.02.010

[47] Jiao L, Gao X, Joyee AG, Zhao L, Qiu H, Yang M, et al. NK cells promote type 1 T cell immunity through modulating the function of dendritic cells during intracellular bacterial infection. The Journal of Immunology. 2011;**187**(1):401-411. DOI: 10.4049/jimmunol.1002519

[48] Morrison SG, Morrison RP. In situ analysis of the evolution of the primary immune response in murine chlamydia trachomatis genital tract infection. Infection and Immunity. 2000;**68**(5):2870-2879. DOI: 10.1128/IAI.68.5.2870-2879.2000

[49] Belay T, Eko FO, Ananaba GA, Bowers S, Moore T, Lyn D, et al. Chemokine and chemokine receptor dynamics during genital chlamydial infection. Infection and Immunity. 2002;**70**(2):844-850. DOI: 10.1128/IAI.70.2.844-850.2002

[50] Shi C, Pamer EG. Monocyte recruitment during infection and inflammation. Nature Reviews Immunology. 2011;**11**(11):762-774. DOI: 10.1038/nri3070

[51] Beagley K, Huston WM, Hansbro PM, Timms P. Chlamydial infection of immune cells: Altered function and implications for disease. Critical Reviews™ in Immunology. 2009;**29**(4):275-305. DOI: 10.1615/CritRevImmunol.v29.i4.10

[52] Nans A, Ford C, Hayward RD. Host-pathogen reorganisation during host cell entry by chlamydia trachomatis. Microbes and Infection. 2015;**17**(11-12):727-731. DOI: 10.1016/j.micinf.2015.08.004

[53] Yilma AN, Singh SR, Fairley SJ, Taha MA, Dennis VA. The anti-inflammatory cytokine, Interleukin-10, inhibits inflammatory mediators in human epithelial cells and mouse macrophages exposed to live and UV-inactivated chlamydia trachomatis. Mediators of Inflammation. 2012;**2012**:1-10. DOI: 10.1155/2012/520174

[54] Al-Zeer MA, Al-Younes HM, Lauster D, Abu Lubad M, Meyer TF. Autophagy restricts chlamydia trachomatis growth in human macrophages via IFNG-inducible guanylate binding proteins. Autophagy. 2013;**9**(1):50-62. DOI: 10.4161/auto.22482

[55] Yasir M, Pachikara ND, Bao X, Pan Z, Fan H. Regulation of chlamydial infection by host autophagy and vacuolar ATPase-bearing organelles. Infection and Immunity. 2011;**79**(10):4019-4028. DOI: 10.1128/IAI.05308-11

[56] Sun HS, Eng EWY, Jeganathan S, Sin AT-W, Patel PC, Gracey E, et al. Chlamydia trachomatis vacuole maturation in infected macrophages. Journal of Leukocyte Biology. 2012;**92**(4):815-827. DOI: 10.1189/jlb.0711336

[57] Crotzer VL, Blum JS. Autophagy and its role in MHC-mediated antigen presentation. The Journal of Immunology. 2009;**182**(6):3335-3341. DOI: 10.4049/jimmunol.0803458

[58] Vasilevsky S, Colino J, Puliaev R, Canaday DH, Snapper CM. Macrophages pulsed with Streptococcus pneumoniae elicit a T cell-dependent antibody response upon transfer into naive mice. The Journal of Immunology. 2008;**181**(3):1787-1797. DOI: 10.4049/jimmunol.181.3.1787

[59] Cao H, Wolff RG, Meltzer MS, Crawford RM. Differential regulation of class II MHC determinants on macrophages by IFN-gamma and IL-4. Journal of Immunology. 1989;**143**(11):3524-3531

[60] Chiba N, Shimada K, Chen S, Jones HD, Alsabeh R, Slepenkin AV, et al. Mast cells play an important role in chlamydia pneumoniae lung infection by facilitating immune cell recruitment into the airway. The Journal of Immunology. 2015;**194**(8):3840-3851. DOI: 10.4049/jimmunol.1402685

[61] Oksaharju A, Lappalainen J, Tuomainen AM, Pussinen PJ, Puolakkainen M, Kovanen PT, et al. Pro-atherogenic lung and oral pathogens induce an inflammatory response in human and mouse mast cells. Journal of Cellular and Molecular Medicine. 2008;**13**(1):103-113. DOI: 10.1111/j.1582-4934.2008.00285.x

[62] Vicetti Miguel RD, Quispe Calla NE, Dixon D, Foster RA, Gambotto A, Pavelko SD, et al. IL-4–secreting eosinophils promote endometrial stromal cell proliferation and prevent chlamydia -induced upper genital tract damage. Proceedings of the National Academy of Sciences. 2017;**114**(33):E6892-E6901. DOI: 10.1073/pnas.1621253114

[63] Jiang X, Shen C, Rey-Ladino J, Yu H, Brunham RC. Characterization of murine dendritic cell line JAWS II and primary bone marrow-derived dendritic cells in chlamydia muridarum antigen presentation and induction of protective immunity. Infection and Immunity.

2008;**76**(6):2392-2401. DOI: 10.1128/IAI.01584-07

[64] Matyszak MK, Young JL, Gaston JSH. Uptake and processing of chlamydia trachomatis by human dendritic cells. European Journal of Immunology. 2002;**32**(3):742. DOI: 10.1002/1521-4141(200203)32:3<742::AID-IMMU742>3.0.CO;2-9

[65] Shaw JH, Grund VR, Durling L, Caldwell HD. Expression of genes encoding Th1 cell-activating cytokines and lymphoid homing chemokines by chlamydia-pulsed dendritic cells correlates with protective immunizing efficacy. Infection and Immunity. 2001;**69**(7):4667-4672. DOI: 10.1128/IAI.69.7.4667-4672.2001

[66] Labuda JC, McSorley SJ. Diversity in the T cell response to chlamydia-sum are better than one. Immunology Letters. 2018;**202**:59-64. DOI: 10.1016/j.imlet.2018.08.002

[67] He Q, Moore TT, Eko FO, Lyn D, Ananaba GA, Martin A, et al. Molecular basis for the potency of IL-10-deficient dendritic cells as a highly efficient APC system for activating Th1 response. The Journal of Immunology. 2005;**174**(8):4860-4869. DOI: 10.4049/jimmunol.174.8.4860

[68] Lu H, Zhong G. Interleukin-12 production is required for chlamydial antigen-pulsed dendritic cells to induce protection against live chlamydia trachomatis infection. Infection and Immunity. 1999;**67**(4):1763-1769. DOI: 10.1128/IAI.67.4.1763-1769.1999

[69] Ibana JA, Schust DJ, Sugimoto J, Nagamatsu T, Greene SJ, Quayle AJ. Chlamydia trachomatis immune evasion via downregulation of MHC class I surface expression involves direct and indirect mechanisms. Infectious Diseases in Obstetrics and Gynecology. 2011;**2011**:1-8. DOI: 10.1155/2011/420905

[70] Dong F, Pirbhai M, Zhong Y, Zhong G. Cleavage-dependent activation of a chlamydia-secreted protease. Molecular Microbiology. 2004;**52**(5):1487-1494. DOI: 10.1111/j.1365-2958.2004.04072.x

[71] Zhong G, Fan P, Ji H, Dong F, Huang Y. Identification of a chlamydial protease–like activity factor responsible for the degradation of host transcription factors. Journal of Experimental Medicine. 2001;**193**(8):935-942. DOI: 10.1084/jem.193.8.935

[72] Neefjes J, Jongsma MLM, Paul P, Bakke O. Towards a systems understanding of MHC class I and MHC class II antigen presentation. Nature Reviews. Immunology. 2011;**11**(12):823-836. DOI: 10.1038/nri3084

[73] Davila SJ, Olive AJ, Starnbach MN. Integrin α4β1 is necessary for CD4+ T cell-mediated protection against genital chlamydia trachomatis infection. Journal of immunology. 2014;**192**(9):4284-4293. DOI: 10.4049/jimmunol.1303238

[74] Kelly KA, Wiley D, Wiesmeier E, Briskin M, Butch A, Darville T. ORIGINAL ARTICLE: The combination of the gastrointestinal integrin (α4β7) and selectin ligand enhances T-cell migration to the reproductive tract during infection with chlamydia trachomatis. American Journal of Reproductive Immunology. 2009;**61**(6):446-452. DOI: 10.1111/j.1600-0897.2009.00705.x

[75] Olive AJ, Gondek DC, Starnbach MN. CXCR3 and CCR5 are both required for T cell-mediated protection against C. trachomatis infection in the murine genital mucosa. Mucosal Immunology. 2011;**4**(2):208-216. DOI: 10.1038/mi.2010.58

[76] Morrison RP, Feilzer K, Tumas DB. Gene knockout mice establish a primary protective role for major histocompatibility complex class II-restricted responses in chlamydia trachomatis genital tract infection. Infection and Immunity. 1995;**63**(12):4661-4668. DOI: 10.1128/iai.63.12.4661-4668.1995

[77] Gondek DC, Olive AJ, Stary G, Starnbach MN. CD4+ T cells are necessary and sufficient to confer protection against chlamydia trachomatis infection in the murine upper genital tract. The Journal of Immunology. 2012;**189**(5):2441-2449. DOI: 10.4049/jimmunol.1103032

[78] Halme S, Latvala J, Karttunen R, Palatsi I, Saikku P, Surcel HM. Cell-mediated immune response during primary chlamydia pneumoniae infection. Infection and Immunity. 2000;**68**(12):7156-7158. DOI: 10.1128/IAI.68.12.7156-7158.2000

[79] O'Shea JJ, Paul WE. Mechanisms underlying lineage commitment and plasticity of helper CD4+ T cells. Science (New York, N.Y.). 2010;**327**(5969):1098-1102. DOI: 10.1126/science.1178334

[80] Zhu J. T helper cell differentiation, heterogeneity, and plasticity. Cold Spring Harbor Perspectives in Biology. 2018;**10**(10):a030338. DOI: 10.1101/cshperspect.a030338

[81] Chen L, Lei L, Zhou Z, He J, Xu S, Lu C, et al. Contribution of Interleukin-12 p35 (IL-12p35) and IL-12p40 to protective immunity and pathology in mice infected with chlamydia muridarum. Infection and Immunity. 2013;**81**(8):2962-2971. DOI: 10.1128/IAI.00161-13

[82] Perry LL, Feilzer K, Caldwell HD. Immunity to chlamydia trachomatis is mediated by T helper 1 cells through IFN-gamma-dependent and -independent pathways. Journal of Immunology. 1997;**158**(7):3344-3352

[83] Wang S, Fan Y, Brunham RC, Yang X. IFN-gamma knockout mice show Th2-associated delayed-type hypersensitivity and the inflammatory cells fail to localize and control chlamydial infection. European Journal of Immunology. 1999;**29**(11):3782-3792. DOI: 10.1002/(SICI)1521-4141(199911)29:11<3782::AID-IMMU3782>3.0.CO;2-B

[84] Johnson RM, Kerr MS, Slaven JE. Plac8-dependent and inducible NO synthase-dependent mechanisms clear chlamydia muridarum infections from the genital tract. The Journal of Immunology. 2012;**188**(4):1896-1904. DOI: 10.4049/jimmunol.1102764

[85] Yu H, Karunakaran KP, Kelly I, Shen C, Jiang X, Foster LJ, et al. Immunization with live and dead chlamydia muridarum induces different levels of protective immunity in a murine genital tract model: Correlation with MHC class II peptide presentation and multifunctional Th1 cells. The Journal of Immunology. 2011;**186**(6):3615-3621. DOI: 10.4049/jimmunol.1002952

[86] Bancroft GJ, Schreiber RD, Bosma GC, Bosma MJ, Unanue ER. A T cell-independent mechanism of macrophage activation by interferon-gamma. Journal of Immunology. 1987;**139**(4):1104-1107

[87] Olivares-Zavaleta N, Whitmire W, Gardner D, Caldwell HD. Immunization with the attenuated plasmidless chlamydia trachomatis L2(25667R) strain provides partial protection in a murine model of female genitourinary tract infection. Vaccine. 2010;**28**(6):1454-1462. DOI: 10.1016/j.vaccine.2009.11.073

[88] Penttilä JM, Anttila M, Puolakkainen M, Laurila A, Varkila K, Sarvas M, et al. Local immune responses to chlamydia pneumoniae in the lungs of BALB/c mice during primary infection and reinfection. Infection and Immunity. 1998;**66**(11):5113-5118. DOI: 10.1128/IAI.66.11.5113-5118.1998

[89] Holland MJ, Bailey RL, Conway DJ, Culley F, Miranpuri G, Byrne GI, et al. T helper type-1 (Th1)/Th2 profiles of peripheral blood mononuclear cells (PBMC); responses to antigens of chlamydia trachomatis in subjects with severe trachomatous scarring. Clinical and Experimental Immunology. 2003;**105**(3):429-435. DOI: 10.1046/j.1365-2249.1996.d01-792.x

[90] Hawkins RA, Rank RG, Kelly KA. A chlamydia trachomatis-specific Th2 clone does not provide protection against a genital infection and displays reduced trafficking to the infected genital mucosa. Infection and Immunity. 2002;**70**(9):5132-5139. DOI: 10.1128/IAI.70.9.5132-5139.2002

[91] Frazer LC, Scurlock AM, Zurenski MA, Riley MM, Mintus M, Pociask DA, et al. IL-23 induces IL-22 and IL-17 production in response to chlamydia muridarum genital tract infection, but the absence of these cytokines does not influence disease pathogenesis. American Journal of Reproductive Immunology. 2013;**70**(6):472-484. DOI: 10.1111/aji.12171

[92] Scurlock AM, Frazer LC, Andrews CW, O'Connell CM, Foote IP, Bailey SL, et al. Interleukin-17 contributes to generation of Th1 immunity and neutrophil recruitment during chlamydia muridarum genital tract infection but is not required for macrophage influx or Normal resolution of infection. Infection and Immunity. 2011;**79**(3):1349-1362. DOI: 10.1128/IAI.00984-10

[93] Mueller SN, Gebhardt T, Carbone FR, Heath WR. Memory T cell subsets, migration patterns, and tissue residence. Annual Review of Immunology. 2013;**31**:137-161. DOI: 10.1146/annurev-immunol-032712-095954

[94] Clark RA. Resident memory T cells in human health and disease. Science Translational Medicine. 2015;**7**(269):269rv1. DOI: 10.1126/scitranslmed.3010641

[95] Stary G, Olive A, Radovic-Moreno AF, Gondek D, Alvarez D, Basto PA, et al. A mucosal vaccine against chlamydia trachomatis generates two waves of protective memory T cells. Science. 2015;**348**(6241):aaa8205. DOI: 10.1126/science.aaa8205

[96] Whitmire JK, Eam B, Whitton JL. Tentative T cells: Memory cells are quick to respond, but slow to divide. PLoS Pathogens. 2008;**4**(4):e1000041. DOI: 10.1371/journal.ppat.1000041

[97] Halle S, Halle O, Förster R. Mechanisms and dynamics of T cell-mediated cytotoxicity In vivo. Trends in Immunology. 2017;**38**(6):432-443. DOI: 10.1016/j.it.2017.04.002

[98] Wizel B, Nyström-Asklin J, Cortes C, Tvinnereim A. Role of CD8+T cells in the host response to chlamydia. Microbes and Infection. 2008;**10**(14-15):1420-1430. DOI: 10.1016/j.micinf.2008.08.006

[99] Fling SP, Sutherland RA, Steele LN, Hess B, D'Orazio SE, Maisonneuve J, et al. CD8+ T cells recognize an inclusion membrane-associated protein from the vacuolar pathogen chlamydia trachomatis. Proceedings of the National Academy of Sciences of the United States of America. 2001;**98**(3):1160-1165. DOI: 10.1073/pnas.98.3.1160

[100] Starnbach MN, Loomis WP, Ovendale P, Regan D, Hess B, Alderson MR, et al. An inclusion membrane protein from chlamydia trachomatis enters the MHC class I pathway and stimulates a CD8+ T cell response. Journal of Immunology. 2003;**171**(9):4742-4749. DOI: 10.4049/jimmunol.171.9.4742

[101] Murthy AK, Li W, Chaganty BKR, Kamalakaran S, Guentzel MN, Seshu J, et al. Tumor necrosis factor alpha production from CD8 + T cells mediates oviduct pathological sequelae following primary genital chlamydia muridarum infection. Infection and Immunity. 2011;**79**(7):2928-2935. DOI: 10.1128/IAI.05022-11

[102] Igietseme JU, Eko FO, He Q, Black CM. Antibody regulation of T-cell immunity: Implications for vaccine strategies against intracellular pathogens. Expert Review of Vaccines. 2004;**3**(1):23-34. DOI: 10.1586/14760584.3.1.23

[103] Van Voorhis WC, Barrett LK, Sweeney YT, Kuo CC, Patton DL. Repeated chlamydia trachomatis infection of Macaca nemestrina fallopian tubes produces a Th1-like cytokine response associated with fibrosis and scarring. Infection and Immunity. 1997;**65**(6):2175-2182. DOI: 10.1128/iai.65.6.2175-2182.1997

[104] Rottenberg ME, Gigliotti Rothfuchs AC, Gigliotti D, Svanholm C, Bandholtz L, Wigzell H. Role of innate and adaptive immunity in the outcome of primary infection with chlamydia pneumoniae, as analyzed in genetically modified mice. Journal of Immunology. 1999;**162**(5):2829-2836

[105] Fankhauser SC, Starnbach MN. PD-L1 limits the mucosal CD8+ T cell response to chlamydia trachomatis. The Journal of Immunology. 2014;**192**(3):1079-1090. DOI: 10.4049/jimmunol.1301657

[106] Francisco LM, Sage PT, Sharpe AH. The PD-1 pathway in tolerance and autoimmunity. Immunological Reviews. 2010;**236**(1):219-242. DOI: 10.1111/j.1600-065X.2010.00923.x

[107] Manam S, Nicholson BJ, Murthy AK. OT-1 mice display minimal upper genital tract pathology following primary intravaginal chlamydia muridarum infection. Pathogens and Disease. 2013;**67**(3):221-224. DOI: 10.1111/2049-632X.12032

[108] Vlcek KR, Li W, Manam S, Zanotti B, Nicholson BJ, Ramsey KH, et al. The contribution of chlamydia-specific $CD8^+$ T cells to upper genital tract pathology. Immunology and Cell Biology. 2016;**94**(2):208-212. DOI: 10.1038/icb.2015.74

[109] Peng B, Lu C, Tang L, Yeh I-T, He Z, Wu Y, et al. Enhanced upper genital tract pathologies by blocking Tim-3 and PD-L1 signaling pathways in mice intravaginally infected with chlamydia muridarum. BMC Infectious Diseases. 2011;**11**(1):347. DOI: 10.1186/1471-2334-11-347

[110] Helble DJ, Starnbach MN. T cell responses to chlamydia. Pathogens and Disease. 2021;**79**(4):ftab014. DOI: 10.1093/femspd/ftab014

[111] Al-Younes HM, Rudel T, Brinkmann V, Szczepek AJ, Meyer TF. Low iron availability modulates the course of chlamydia pneumoniae infection. Cellular Microbiology. 2001;**3**(6):427-437. DOI: 10.1046/j.1462-5822.2001.00125.x

[112] Ryu SY, Jeong KS, Kang BN, Park SJ, Yoon WK, Kim SH, et al. Modulation of transferrin synthesis, transferrin

receptor expression, iNOS expression and NO production in mouse macrophages by cytokines, either alone or in combination. Anticancer Research. 2000;**20**(5A):3331-3338

[113] Fernandez-Boyanapalli R, McPhillips KA, Frasch SC, Janssen WJ, Dinauer MC, Riches DWH, et al. Impaired phagocytosis of apoptotic cells by macrophages in chronic granulomatous disease is reversed by IFN-γ in a nitric oxide-dependent manner. The Journal of Immunology. 2010;**185**(7):4030-4041. DOI: 10.4049/jimmunol.1001778

[114] Beatty WL, Belanger TA, Desai AA, Morrison RP, Byrne GI. Tryptophan depletion as a mechanism of gamma interferon-mediated chlamydial persistence. Infection and Immunity. 1994;**62**(9):3705-3711. DOI: 10.1128/iai.62.9.3705-3711.1994

[115] Beatty WL, Byrne GI, Morrison RP. Morphologic and antigenic characterization of interferon gamma-mediated persistent chlamydia trachomatis infection in vitro. Proceedings of the National Academy of Sciences. 1993;**90**(9):3998-4002. DOI: 10.1073/pnas.90.9.3998

[116] Aiyar A, Quayle AJ, Buckner LR, Sherchand SP, Chang TL, Zea AH, et al. Influence of the tryptophan-indole-IFNÎ³ axis on human genital chlamydia trachomatis infection: Role of vaginal co-infections. Frontiers in Cellular and Infection Microbiology. 2014;**4**:72. DOI: 10.3389/fcimb.2014.00072

[117] Bartolini E, Ianni E, Frigimelica E, Petracca R, Galli G, Berlanda Scorza F, et al. Recombinant outer membrane vesicles carrying chlamydia muridarum HtrA induce antibodies that neutralize chlamydial infection in vitro. Journal of Extracellular Vesicles. 2013;**2**(1):20181. DOI: 10.3402/jev.v2i0.20181

[118] Moore T, Ananaba GA, Bolier J, Bowers S, Belay T, Eko FO, et al. Fc receptor regulation of protective immunity against chlamydia trachomatis. Immunology. 2002;**105**(2):213-221. DOI: 10.1046/j.0019-2805.2001.01354.x

[119] Finco O, Frigimelica E, Buricchi F, Petracca R, Galli G, Faenzi E, et al. Approach to discover T- and B-cell antigens of intracellular pathogens applied to the design of chlamydia trachomatis vaccines. Proceedings of the National Academy of Sciences. 2011;**108**(24):9969-9974. DOI: 10.1073/pnas.1101756108

[120] Ramsey KH, Soderberg LS, Rank RG. Resolution of chlamydial genital infection in B-cell-deficient mice and immunity to reinfection. Infection and Immunity. 1988;**56**(5):1320-1325. DOI: 10.1128/iai.56.5.1320-1325.1988

[121] Su H, Feilzer K, Caldwell HD, Morrison RP. Chlamydia trachomatis genital tract infection of antibody-deficient gene knockout mice. Infection and Immunity. 1997;**65**(6):1993-1999. DOI: 10.1128/iai.65.6.1993-1999.1997

[122] Morrison SG, Morrison RP. Resolution of secondary chlamydia trachomatis genital tract infection in immune mice with depletion of both CD4 + and CD8 + T cells. Infection and Immunity. 2001;**69**(4):2643-2649. DOI: 10.1128/IAI.69.4.2643-2649.2001

[123] Morrison SG, Morrison RP. A predominant role for antibody in acquired immunity to chlamydial genital tract reinfection. The Journal of Immunology. 2005;**175**(11):7536-7542. DOI: 10.4049/jimmunol.175.11.7536

[124] Brady LJ. Antibody-mediated immunomodulation: A strategy to improve host responses against microbial antigens. Infection and Immunity.

2005;**73**(2):671-678. DOI: 10.1128/IAI.73.2.671-678.2005

[125] Russell AN, Zheng X, O'Connell CM, Taylor BD, Wiesenfeld HC, Hillier SL, et al. Analysis of factors driving incident and ascending infection and the role of serum antibody in chlamydia trachomatis genital tract infection. Journal of Infectious Diseases. 2016;**213**(4):523-531. DOI: 10.1093/infdis/jiv438

[126] Linhares IM, Witkin SS. Immunopathogenic consequences of chlamydia trachomatis 60 kDa heat shock protein expression in the female reproductive tract. Cell Stress and Chaperones. 2010;**15**(5):467-473. DOI: 10.1007/s12192-010-0171-4

[127] von Hertzen LC. Role of persistent infection in the control and severity of asthma: Focus on chlamydia pneumoniae. European Respiratory Journal. 2002;**19**(3):546-556. DOI: 10.1183/09031936.02.00254402

[128] Dowell SF, Peeling RW, Boman J, Carlone GM, Fields BS, Guarner J, et al. Standardizing chlamydia pneumoniae assays: Recommendations from the Centers for Disease Control and Prevention (USA) and the Laboratory Centre for Disease Control (Canada). Clinical Infectious Diseases. 2001;**33**(4):492-503. DOI: 10.1086/322632

Section 2

Chlamydia as a Zoonosis and the Treatment of Chlamydial Infection

Chapter 6

Chlamydias as a Zooonosis and Antibiotic Resistance in Chlamydiae

Gül Banu Çiçek Bideci

Abstract

Chlamydiosis is a disease that can be seen in different forms in the animals. In the genus *Chlamydia*, two species have been reported in the studies. The first is *C. trachomatis*, which is responsible for infections in humans and *C. psittaci*, which has a wide host distribution, including many animals and humans. *C. psittaci* is usually transmitted from poultry to humans. Along with causing flu-like conditions in humans, it has also caused abortions in pregnant women by contact with sheep and goats that have been infected and have offspring. The likelihood of pregnant women contracting the *Chlamydia* pathogen through contact with sheep and goats increases the zoonotic importance of the disease. There are few reports documenting antibiotic resistance in Chlamydiae. Furthermore, there are no examples of natural or permanent antibiotic resistance in strains that cause disease in humans. In some strains, the detected antibiotic resistance cannot be identified in vitro, which hinders the recognition and interpretation of antibiotic resistance.

Keywords: chlamydias, zoonoz, ovine enzootic abortion, psittacosis, antibiotic resistance

1. Introduction

The most important characteristic that distinguishes *Chlamydia* genus bacteria from other bacteria is their biphasic growth cycle and their status as obligate intracellular pathogens. The *Chlamydia* genus belongs to the Chlamdiaceae family within the Chylamdiades order. In classification, their antigenic structures, intracellular inclusion bodies, sulfonamide sensitivity, and disease presentations are taken into account. Their three-layered outer membrane makes them resemble Gram-negative bacteria because they have a non-peptidoglycan envelope. The proteins they encode are referred to as major outer membrane proteins, which all *Chlamydia* species produce. *Chlamydia*'s reproduction is unique to itself, and in its growth cycle, it has infectious and reproductive forms known as EC: Elementary Body and RC: Reticulate Body. The *Chlamydia* genus includes *C. pneumonia*, *C. Trachomatis*, *C. pisittaci*, and *C. pecorum* [1, 2].

In previous years, the Chlamydiaceae family was divided into several classes, but recently, it has been assessed that it may be separated into two possible genera. Genus

IntechOpen

1 includes *Chlamydia trachomatis*, *Chlamydia suis*, and *Chlamydia muridarum*. Genus 2 includes *Chlamydophila abortus* (*Chlamydia psittaci* serotype 1), *Chlamydophila caviae*, *Chlamydophila felis*, *Chlamydophila pecorum*, *Chlamydophila pneumoniae*, and *Chlamydophila psittaci* [3].

C. pneumoniae is involved in respiratory tract infections such as sinusitis, pharyngitis, bronchitis, asthma, pneumonia, and atherosclerotic diseases in the heart, brain, and peripheral arterial system. It also plays a role in most cases of acute ischemia [4]. The bacteria *C. trachomatis* causes psittacosis/ornithosis in humans, urogenital infections, and lymphogranuloma venereum (LGV) [5].

Serological tests are often used for the diagnosis of the disease because the causative agent can only be produced in vitro environments. This requires living environments such as cell culture and embryonated eggs, which are difficult and time-consuming. This is the main reason why serological tests are used in the diagnosis of the disease [3, 6].

The tests used in the diagnosis of the disease are immunofluorescence assay (IFA), enzyme-linked immunosorbent assay (ELISA), and complement fixation test (CFT). The IFA is used to diagnose and differentiate *Chlamydia* species, as its sensitivity and specificity are high. However, ELISA and CFT have limitations in diagnosis and species identification [3, 6].

2. Potential Danger *Chlamydia* family

The Chlamydiaceae family is made up of bacteria that can only survive inside other cells and are unable to survive outside of them. These Gram-negative bacteria can cause various illnesses in humans, animals, and birds infections in animals can lead to a variety of negative effects on reproductive health, such as causing abortions or infertility. It can also cause issues with the digestive system, such as enteritis, and can affect the brain and nervous system, resulting in encephalomyelitis. Additionally, it can cause eye inflammation, known as conjunctivitis, inflammation in the joints, arthritis, and respiratory diseases [7–9].

Chlamydiae are a type of bacteria that can cause a variety of health problems in humans, including preventable blindness, sexually transmitted diseases, respiratory infections, and potentially cardiovascular disease. They are a common cause of preventable blindness and sexually transmitted diseases. They also can cause respiratory infections and have been linked to cardiovascular disease [9, 10].

3. Discovery of chlamydial organisms from past to present

Chlamydial organisms, first described by Halberstaedter and von Prowazek in 1907, were isolated from human trachoma. During isolation, conjunctival cells were injected into orangutan cells, and intracellular inclusion bodies were identified in this way [11, 12]. These organisms were classified as protozoa, not bacteria, and given the name Chlamydozoa. The Greek word “chlamys” means a cloak, referring to the red elementary bodies (EBs) embedded in a blue matrix in bacteria [13].

Psittacosis, a zoonotic disease, was first described by Ritter in 1879. In 1985, Harris and Williams identified respiratory disease in people who had contact with tropical pet birds, which was found to be psittacosis [13]. The disease was named Psittokos after an outbreak in parrots in 1892. The etiologic agent was isolated in 1930, and research was carried out on lovebirds. In the same year, *Chlamydia*, the etiologic agent of lymphogranuloma venereum (LGV) in humans, was isolated, and the two agents, which had similar characteristics, were known as psittacosis-LGV group viruses [5, 13].

Until the 1930s, *Chlamydia psittaci* was known to cause disease only in exotic and psittacine birds. With the reporting of new cases, it was discovered that the agent could also cause disease in other birds, including fulmar petrels, domestic pigeons, and ducks. The term ornithosis was used to describe the disease that developed in non-psittacine birds. By the 1950s, the zoonotic importance of *Chlamydia* was further understood, as outbreaks of human psittacosis-related ornithosis were seen in people in contact with ducks and turkeys [14].

The first notable case in farm animals occurred in 1936 when researcher Greig observed reproductive disorders and abortions in a flock of sheep, which he called enzootic abortion of ewes. He argued that the disease was caused by nutritional disorders, as he could not identify the etiologic agent. However, in the 1950s, it was proven by Stamp et al. that the etiologic agent of this disease was the psittacosis-LGV group organism. In addition, a respiratory disease seen in cats was also associated with this group of organisms in later years [13].

After all these developments, it was proven that *Chlamydia* was not a virus. They had a cell wall containing RNA and DNA, their cell wall structure was similar to Gram-negative bacteria, their reproductive cycle was different from viruses, and they had ribosomes sensitive to antibiotics. These characteristics classify them as part of the prokaryotic family [13].

4. Taxonomy of Clamydiae

The taxonomy used for classifying living organisms was discovered by Carl von Linne (Linnaeus) in 1735. This system, which is used by all biologists, still remains the basis for classifying living organisms today. In this classification, Chlamydiae, which have a prokaryotic cell structure, were initially considered as bacteria-like organisms. In the taxonomic classification, Chlamydiae belong to the domain bacteria and the order Chlamydiales [2].

Classification	**Old**	**Last**	
Order	Chlamydiales	Chlamydiales	
Family	Chlamydiaceae	Chlamydiaceae-Simkaniaceae	Parachlamydiaceae; Waddliaceae
Genus	Chlamydia	Chlamydia	Chlamydophila
Species	*C. trachomatis*	*C. trachomatis*	*C. pneumoniae*
	C. pneumoniae	*C. muridanum*	*C. psittaci*
	C. psittaci	*C. suis*	*C. abortus*
			C. felis
	C. pecorum		*C. caviae*
			C. pecorum

Table 1.
Chlamydial taxonomy [2, 13].

Until the molecular studies conducted by Everet, Bush, and Anderson, Chlamydiae, considered a single family, was divided into four different families and included in the classification (**Table 1**). These families are Chlamydiaceae, Simkaniaceae, Parachlamydiaceae, and Waddliaceae within the Chlamydiales order. Within the Chlamydiaceae family, based on the sequence analysis of the 16S and 23S rRNA genes, two genera (*Chlamydia* and *Chlamydophila*) and nine species were reclassified [15].

The truth is that the changes in the taxonomic classification of *Chlamydia* proposed by Everett and Everett et al. (1999) are not accepted by many. The fact that this new classification is not used in studies conducted in the field of human medicine is an indication of this. The use of more molecular markers in classification can eliminate these uncertainties. However, there is no confusion in the classification of *Chlamydia* agents in animals [13].

5. Animal diseases

Chlamydia, as a host, selectively infects humans, other mammals and birds by colonizing certain systems and causing various health issues. Some of these species are zoonotic and can cause human and animal diseases. In this regard, *C. abortus* and *C. psittaci* are essential. *C. abortus* causes abortion, while *C. psittaci* causes a respiratory disease known as psittacosis [13].

The *Chlamydia* diseases in animals that have been confirmed to be transmitted to humans to date are Ovine Enzootic Abortion, and Avian Chlamyiosis. All disease factors are listed below.

1. *C. abortus*: Causes abortion in animals and pregnancy-related diseases such as endometritis and placentitis in humans.

2. *C. psittaci*: Causes psittacosis, a respiratory infection.

3. *C. trachomatis*: Causes a sexually transmitted infection in humans and can cause conjunctivitis in animals.

4. *C. pneumoniae*: Can cause respiratory infection in humans and animals.

5. *C. suis*: Causes swine enzootic pneumonia, a respiratory infection in pigs.

6. *C. caviae*: Causes guinea pig enzootic abortion, triggers abortions in cavy.

7. *C. muridarum*: Causes murine pneumonitis, a respiratory infection in mice.

5.1 Clamidya abortus at Ovine

C. abortus is responsible for causing Ovine enzootic abortion, a disease that is encountered in almost every region of the world. It is a major factor in lamb losses in sheep herds. Countries that engage in sheep breeding, particularly in Europe, have recognized *C. abortus* as one of the responsible factors for these losses [7, 8].

After 1 or 2 weeks of sheep contracting the disease, discharge related to birth disappears. Pregnant animals that have had a miscarriage due to this disease will not be affected by the disease again. They will not encounter another abortion due to *Chlamydia*. Animals that are infected but have not had an abortion do not fully develop immunity to this agent, so they spread the agent to their surroundings during other breeding seasons and lambing periods. Sheep flocks can always be infected with *Chlamydia*, but the most vulnerable period for them to the disease is during lambing [16]. *Clamydia* can survive for weeks or months at low temperatures but has a shorter lifespan at higher temperatures and in harsher environments. There is no evidence that sheep can get infected through sexual transmission [9, 13]. However, if a sheep encounters infection during mating season, the resulting low-weight live offspring or abortion during lambing season suggests sexual transmission. Experimental studies have shown that infection with *C. abortus* did not result in abortion when sheep were artificially inseminated with infected semen or mated with infected rams. However, the infection was still detected in the flock even though it did not result in abortion [15].

Male animals are thought to contribute more to the spread of the disease, as they are not always housed with female animals. Experiments have shown that an infected ram can infect a healthy ewe and her offspring [16]. The presence of *C. abortus* has been detected in the semen of infected 12-month-old rams. When *C. abortus* enters a flock, the first symptoms are not necessarily abortions; general discomfort and discharge from the genital organs within 48 hours are more common. Later on, abortions 2–3 weeks before normal birth indicate that the flock is infected [17]. The waste material is either normal in appearance or has swelling in the umbilical area. The placental membranes have thickened and become reddened. Seven to 10 days after the waste is produced, the infected ewe may have a dirty pink vaginal fluid, which spreads the disease. If the agent remains in the birth canal, it can lead to general discomfort and metritis. Secondary infections result in death. In goats and cattle, vaginitis, endometritis, and placental retention are most commonly seen [15].

The fleece of a lamb that has been aborted may be discolored with a pink-brown substance from placental secretions. In addition to abortion, premature or full-term delivery of stillborn, sickly, or weak lambs can also occur, and most weak lambs do not survive more than 48 hours, even with nursing. Some infected ewes may give birth to healthy lambs, and it is not uncommon for an infected ewe to deliver both a dead and a weak or healthy lamb [16]. The normal pattern of infection in a previously unaffected flock is that a small number of abortions occur in the first year, usually due to the addition of infected replacement female sheep, followed by a sudden increase in abortions in the second year, affecting 30% or more of the female sheep population [7, 8].

The pattern of infection in a previously unaffected flock usually begins with a small number of abortions in the first year, caused by the addition of infected replacement female sheep. In the second year, there is a sudden increase in abortions affecting 30% or more of the female sheep population. Then, in the third year, there is a final enzootic phase in which younger ewes are mainly affected and are generally in their second year of lambing after becoming infected in their first [16]. If adequate control measures are not introduced, the annual incidence of abortion is likely to be around 5–10% [7]. In flocks with an extended lambing season, this pattern may be different, as infected ewes can infect other pregnant ewes later in the same season. In general, the current pregnancy is not at risk unless more than 3–4 weeks remain until lambing [15].

It is believed that the primary infection in sheep is initially established in the tonsils and then spreads to other organs via blood or lymph. In non-pregnant animals, a latent infection is formed, likely in lymphoid tissue, through a process that is influenced by cytokines, especially the pro-inflammatory cytokine interferon-gamma (IFN-g). IFN-g produced in response to infection with *C. abortus* restricts the organism's growth in living organisms and in the laboratory by inducing the enzyme indolamine 2,3-dioxygenase, which breaks down tryptophan. The *Chlamydia* static effect can be reversed by adding exogenous L-tryptophan [16].

Latently infected sheep do not show any signs of having chlamydial organisms [16]. During pregnancy, the immune system may become weakened, allowing the organisms to multiply and cause a low-grade chlamydaemia, leading to placental infection. In sheep, the placenta is structured with cotyledons, is non-deciduous, and has a syndesmo-epitheliochorial design [16]. Around day 60 of gestation, the mother develops haematomas at the interface between the mother and fetus in the hilus of each placentome these haematomas are believed to allow the Chlamydiae to come into contact with the chorionic epithelium and infect the fetus. No significant changes occur until after day 90 of gestation [13]. The Chlamydiae invade the fetal trophoblastic cells in the hilus of the cotyledon and replicate, causing visible cytoplasmic chlamydial inclusions [8, 13]. Once the infection has taken hold in the trophoblastic cells in the hilus of several placentomes, it spreads to the peri-placentome and intercotyledonary regions of the chorion, causing inflammation, edema, and damage to the epithelial cells and resulting in red, thickened placental membranes. Not all placentomes will become infected, and the degree of inflammation and necrotic damage to the cotyledons and intercotyledonary membrane can vary. In the fetus, the primary pathological changes occur in the liver and can also occur in the lung, spleen, brain, and lymph nodes, although less frequently [16].

The mechanisms behind abortions in sheep infected with *Chlamydia abortus* are not well understood. However, it is believed that the destruction of the chorionic epithelium and related damage may be the cause. A partial impairment of the placentomes can affect the transfer of oxygen and nutrients between the mother and fetus, leading to fetal death [13]. Examination of the infected placental tissues shows a mixture of inflammatory cells, with inflammation and blood clots in the intercotyledonary membranes. The infected tissues also have high levels of TNF-alpha, which is not present in normal ovine placentas. This TNF-alpha is believed to cause damage to the placenta and contribute to abortion or premature birth. In vitro studies have shown that the infected trophoblast cells produce PGE2, which may be induced by chlamydial lipopolysaccharide (LPS) through TNF-alpha. The levels of hormones like progesterone, 17b-estradiol, and PGE2 change during chlamydial infection of the placenta and may also play a role in triggering premature labor [13].

5.1.1 Effects on people

Compared to the human infections caused by *C. psittaci*, which is more commonly found in birds, infection with *C. abortus* is relatively uncommon. A study of 1157 cases of human chlamydiosis in Scotland from 1967 to 1987 showed that only 11 cases were linked to sheep and cattle, while 94 cases were linked to birds [1]. However, a survey of antibody levels in an area in northwest England found no significant difference between the frequency of chlamydial infections in adults working in sheep farming and those in other types of farming or non-farming [8]. Nevertheless, there have been reports of respiratory illness in laboratory staff and workers in vaccine plants and abattoirs, indicating a potential risk for those working in such environments [7, 13].

Pregnancy poses the greatest risk of human infection due to the ability of *C. abortus* to settle in the human placenta. Cases of transmission have been reported in various countries, including the United Kingdom, France, the Netherlands and the United States. Although the number of cases each year is low, the potential danger to the pregnant woman and her unborn baby is significant. In the first trimester of pregnancy, human infection will likely lead to spontaneous abortion, while later infections can result in stillbirths or premature labor. These conditions usually follow several days of flu-like symptoms. Pregnant women with the infection may also experience kidney failure, liver problems, and a spreading blood clotting disorder, which can be fatal. Diagnosing *C. abortus* infection can be done through tests such as cell culture or PCR of swabs and fetal samples [7, 8].

Humans can experience abortion caused by *C. abortus* due to exposure to infected sheep or goats, usually transmitted through oral contact, such as handling infected animals or contaminated clothing. Other causes include contaminated food, smoking with unwashed hands, or mouth-to-mouth resuscitation of weak lambs, as well as inhaling contaminated air, for instance from infected lambs placed in front of fan heaters [13].

5.1.2 Diagnosis

The early and correct identification of the reason for an abortion during pregnancy is essential to implement appropriate measures to limit or stop the spread of the infection. If an abortion occurs in the final two to three weeks of pregnancy and is accompanied by inflamed and necrotic placental membranes, it suggests a potential chlamydial infection, although other microorganisms such as *Coxiella burnetii*, *Campylobacter fetus* ssp. *fetus*, and *Toxoplasma gondii* may also lead to placental damage [7, 8].

Placentae and dead lambs should be immediately sent to a national veterinary laboratory for examination [13]. The process involves placing the samples into strong plastic bags with the use of disposable gloves. The placentae are examined for necrotic placentitis, and stained smears of infected cotyledons are analyzed under a microscope for chlamydial organisms. In case of a possible delay, a piece of affected placental tissue containing an infected cotyledon should be removed and placed in a *Chlamydia* transport medium called SPG. This medium contains 10% fetal calf serum and antibiotics such as streptomycin and gentamicin, but not penicillin. If the placenta is not available, swabs should be taken from the vagina and the moist coats of the lambs to detect any organisms. Suitable staining procedures include Macchiavello, Giemsa, or MZN, with MZN being the preferred choice for routine use. Positive MZN staining, under high-power microscopy, should reveal many small, round, coccoid EBs, either individually or in clusters, stained red against a blue background of cellular debris. Under dark field illumination, the organisms will appear as bright, pale green, round objects [7, 8].

C. abortus can be grown from samples of infected tissues, such as eggs from infected hens, endocervical swabs, intercervical membranes, fetal liver, vaginal tampon samples, embryonic eggs of laying hens, and cell cultures. It is important to avoid gut contamination, as there is evidence of enteric *C. abortus* non-pathogenic or commensal strains in ovine infections, and another chlamydial species, *C. pecorum*, is frequently found in feces. Tissue samples or tampons should not be preserved or dried in SPG. *C. abortus* can be isolated from many cell types, but the most commonly used are McCoy, L929, and baby hamster kidney cells [6, 7]. The growth of *C. abortus* in cell culture can be improved by the presence of cycloheximide in the infection inoculum, pre-treatment of cells with emetine, or exposure of cells to 5-iodo-2-deoxyuridine. After growth, Chlamydiae can be detected by staining smears made from infected yolk sac membranes with Giemsa or staining growing cells in culture with MZN or Giemsa [8, 10].

5.1.3 Control and prevention

It is necessary to isolate sheep immediately after abortion. As the lambing process continues, attention should be paid to promptly identify and isolate all affected sheep, particularly those giving birth to live lambs instead of stillborns. All dead lambs, placentas, and bedding must be properly disposed of, and lambing pens must be cleaned and disinfected in order to reduce the risk of contamination. It is crucial to thoroughly clean one's hands after handling infectious material before caring for other animals [7, 8].

Long-acting oxytetracycline can be given to reduce the severity of OEA infection in pregnant ewes, but it should only be used in exceptional circumstances. The treatment should start as soon as possible after day 95 of gestation, and multiple doses should be given every 2 weeks until lambing. However, it is important to note that this treatment will not eliminate the infection and cannot undo any damage that has already been done to the placenta. Controlling OEA through proper flock management and vaccination is more effective than relying solely on antibiotics [13].

Pregnant women are recommended to avoid working with sheep, particularly during the lambing period, and to keep away from any potential sources of infection, such as contaminated work clothing. People with compromised immune systems should also exercise caution to avoid contact with sources of infection during the lambing season [7, 8]. Basic hygiene practices like washing hands before eating, drinking, or smoking, and using disinfectants are general steps to be taken but should be strictly followed if an infection is suspected. Disposable gloves should always be used when handling placentas, and under no circumstances should mouth-to-mouth resuscitation be performed on a lamb. Early diagnosis is crucial in treating the infection, which is responsive to antibiotics like tetracyclines and erythromycin when given early [13].

5.2 Avian Chlamydiosis (Psittacosis, Ornithosis)

Chlamydophila psittaci infections can be found all over the world and the bacteria has been found in a wide range of birds, both wild and domesticated, including psittacine birds such as parrots and macaws, game birds, seabirds, garden birds, pigeons, and poultry [14]. These infections are most commonly found in psittacine birds, and the disease is referred to as psittacosis. In other bird species, the same disease is referred to as ornithosis. However, since the disease is similar in all bird species, the term avian chlamydiosis can be used to describe all bird infections caused by *Chlamydophila psittaci* [8, 9].

Studies by Schwartz and Fraser (1982), Bracewell and Bevan (1986), Grimes and Clark (1986), Dorrestein and Wiegman (1989), and Vanrompay et al. (1992) show that the highest incidence of *C. psittaci* infection occurs in psittacine birds. Meanwhile, according to research by Panigrahy et al. (1982), Chiba (1984), Bracewell and Bevan (1986), and Alexander et al. (1989), pigeons have the highest rates of *C. psittaci* infection [13]. Additionally, several economically significant outbreaks of chlamydiosis have been reported in turkeys, and wild birds. Human infections have also been linked to some of these outbreaks [9, 14].

The spread of *C. psittaci*, a type of microorganism, occurs mostly among birds through breathing in dried-up excrement and secretions, including both eye and nose, from infected birds or by ingesting contaminated feces [13, 14]. The parent birds that are shedding the organism can also pass the infection to their young in the nest, and there is evidence that it can also be transmitted through eggs [14]. *C. psittaci* can also be spread from bird to bird through blood-sucking ectoparasites like lice, mites, and flies, or less frequently through bites or wounds. To avoid the spread of infection, contact between wild birds and poultry should be prevented, as wild birds can act as a potential source of infection [7–8].

Exposure to *C. psittaci* can lead to a variety of infections with varying symptoms, depending on factors like the bird species, virulence, and bird health and stress. The onset of symptoms can range from 3 days to several weeks. In turkeys, the organism can be detected within 48 hours, but symptoms may not appear until 5–10 days later. While subclinical infections may not display symptoms, infected birds can act as carriers and intermittently shed the organism. Acute avian chlamydiosis is a serious infection that affects all major organs, causing symptoms like respiratory distress, lethargy, reduced appetite, ruffled feathers, diarrhea, and discharges from the eyes and nose. The mortality rate from this infection can vary greatly [13].

In summary, birds belonging to the psittacine species can display several clinical signs when infected with *Chlamydia*, such as anorexia, diarrhea, respiratory issues, sinusitis, conjunctivitis, yellow droppings, and central nervous system disturbances [7, 9]. Pigeons can exhibit anorexia, diarrhea, conjunctivitis, swollen eyelids, and rhinitis in acute cases and lameness, torticollis, opisthotonus, tremor, and convulsions in chronic cases [13, 14]. Turkeys infected with highly virulent serovar D strains can experience severe symptoms such as anorexia, cachexia, yellow-green diarrhea, low egg production, conjunctivitis, sinusitis, and sneezing, with mortality rates ranging from 10 to 30% [15]. If turkeys are infected with a virulent B serovar instead of a serovar D, the infection will run a milder course. Symptoms such as mild anorexia and diarrhea may be noticeable [7, 15]. Ducks can show symptoms such as trembling, unsteady gait, conjunctivitis, nasal discharge, and depression. Chickens tend to be relatively resistant to *Chlamydia*, but in some cases, they may develop blindness, weight loss, and an increase in mortality rate [13].

5.2.1 Effects on people

Psittacosis or ornithosis is a disease that can be transmitted from birds to humans. The largest group affected by this disease are bird fanciers and pet bird owners, as well as people whose jobs put them at risk of exposure such as pet shop employees, aviary workers, veterinarians, laboratory workers, poultry processing plant employees, farmers, and zoo workers [13]. From 1996 to 2001, there were reports of 1620 cases of human psittacosis in the United Kingdom, 661 in Germany, and 165 in the United States. These figures are believed to underestimate the actual number of cases, as psittacosis can be difficult to diagnose. The disease is considered to be an occupational hazard and is recognized as a prescribed disease for Industrial Injuries Disablement Benefit in the United Kingdom [15]. The OIE Central Bureau maintains a world database of animal diseases and zoonoses, which can be accessed through the Handistatus web interface [13].

Infection with *C. psittaci* can occur through inhaling dried feces or respiratory secretions from infected birds, or by having direct contact with their feathers, tissues, or secretions, including through mouth-to-beak contact or open skin wounds. Some virus strains are very contagious to humans, and even a short exposure could lead to infection. Although there have been suggestions for person-to-person transmission, it is not considered a common occurrence [7, 8].

The human disease known as psittacosis has an incubation period that is generally estimated to be between 5 to 14 days, but in some instances, it may last up to a month. Symptoms of psittacosis can be either mild, with flu-like symptoms such as fever, headache, joint and muscle pain, photophobia and sore throat, or severe, with symptoms of atypical pneumonia including a non-productive cough and difficulty breathing [14]. During the acute phase of the illness, the white blood cell count is often normal, although a decrease in white blood cells, known as leucopenia, can occur in approximately 25% of cases. The pulse rate is typically slow relative to the elevated body temperature, and a rash may also be present. Chest X-rays often reveal signs of pneumonia [14, 15].

In addition to affecting the respiratory system, psittacosis can also result in complications in other organs, such as myocarditis, endocarditis, hepatitis, encephalitis, meningitis, and kidney and neurological issues [7, 8]. Those most at risk of developing these complications are the very young, the elderly, and individuals with weakened immune systems [13].

In order to diagnose chlamydiosis in birds, it is important to detect the presence of the *Chlamydia* organism or antibodies to the infection. Symptoms such as an increased white blood cell count, changes in liver enzyme activity, radiographic signs of liver and spleen enlargement, and air sac inflammation may indicate the presence of chlamydiosis. However, a definitive diagnosis requires the detection of the organism or the presence of antibodies. The tests used to diagnose avian chlamydiosis are similar to those used to diagnose other chlamydiosis [15].

The most effective methods for detecting antigens involve the use of PCR technology. There are several PCR tests mentioned in the scientific literature that target different genes such as ompA (MOMP), pmp (or pomp) genes, and 16S and 23S rRNA [15]. These tests have been successfully used on bird samples, but more research is needed to fully validate their use for diagnosing psittacosis. These PCR tests and the MIF test can be used to differentiate infections caused by the bacterium *C. psittaci* [13, 15].

The methods for diagnosing human psittacosis are similar to those for birds. The organism may be cultured from bodily fluids such as sputum, blood, pleural fluid, or biopsy material, but this is not typically done. Instead, infection is usually diagnosed based on a serological analysis of paired sera taken at least 2 weeks apart. Chest X-rays can also help with the diagnosis and may show signs of lobar, patchy, or interstitial infiltrates. MIF assays and several PCR tests can be used to differentiate *C. psittaci* infections from other chlamydial infections like *C. pneumoniae* and *C. trachomatis* in human patients [15].

5.2.2 Control and prevention

In short, controlling human psittacosis requires controlling the disease in birds. This can be done by maintaining high standards of aviary husbandry, including daily cleaning and disinfection of cages with effective disinfectants such as 70% isopropyl alcohol, 1% lysol, or a 1 in 100 dilutions of household bleach. All waste feed and litter must be disposed of as they can remain infectious for several months. Minimizing aerosols can be done by using litter that does not produce dust, spraying floors with disinfectant or water, and providing sufficient exhaust ventilation [13].

These measures are aimed at reducing the risk of infection with avian influenza or bird flu, which is a highly contagious virus that can cause severe disease in birds and in some cases, can be transmitted to humans [7, 8]. The use of protective clothing and respirators helps to prevent airborne transmission of the virus, while the use of biological safety cabinets and local exhaust ventilation helps to minimize the risk of exposure to the virus through contaminated surfaces and respiratory droplets. The use of detergent and water when performing necropsies helps to reduce the spread of the virus through aerosols, while heat-treating birds and providing respiratory protection in poultry processing plants helps to reduce the risk of exposure to the virus for workers handling infected birds [8, 14].

Treatment for avian chlamydiosis typically involves the use of tetracycline drugs, as recommended by Vanrompay et al. and the Centers for Disease Control [13]. This treatment involves the administration of CTC through medicated feed, which is commercially available as pellets for larger birds and millet for smaller ones. However, it is important to monitor the bird's food consumption, as acceptance of the medicated feed may be variable. The diet should not have a calcium content higher than 0.07% as it interferes with the uptake of CTC. Most companion birds should receive the medicated diet for a minimum of 45 days, while poultry should receive it for a minimum of two weeks, but it should be discontinued two days before slaughter. In cases where the bird is severely ill, oral or parenteral treatment may be necessary, with doxycycline being the preferred drug for oral treatment with a recommended dosage of 25 to 50 mg/kg once a day on an empty crop to aid absorption [14]. Injectable formulations of doxycycline or oxytetracycline may be given intramuscularly, but the latter should only be given to stabilize severely ill birds as it can cause tissue necrosis. Enrofloxacin, a quinolone approved for use in domestic animals, is also being evaluated for the treatment of avian chlamydiosis. During treatment, supportive care such as intravenous fluid therapy and a heated, uncrowded environment may be necessary. It is important to eliminate the possibility of reinfection by thoroughly cleaning and disinfecting the environment after recovery [13].

Currently, there are no commercially available vaccines for avian chlamydiosis. However, research has been done in the past, and some promising results have been seen. In the 1970s, a vaccine was created using an inactivated form of the bacteria that causes chlamydiosis, *Chlamydia psittaci*, which successfully induced a cell-mediated immune response and protected 90% of turkeys against the disease after being challenged [15]. More recently, another vaccine was developed using DNA from *Chlamydia psittaci*, which has resulted in a significant level of protection in turkeys, generating both humoral and cell-mediated responses [13].

5.3 Other Animal Chlamydioses

In simpler terms, *Chlamydia psittaci* and *Chlamydia abortus* are both known to cause human illnesses, but *Chlamydia felis* is the only other type of *Chlamydia* that has been linked to human infections. This type of *Chlamydia* is commonly found in cats and can cause eye infections, especially in young kittens [7, 8].

In simpler terms, there have been several reports of people getting sick from being in close contact with cats, including eye infections, abnormal liver function, heart and kidney problems, and atypical pneumonia [4]. A recent study showed that a patient with a chronic eye infection and one of the patient's cats had the same type of *Chlamydia* (*C. felis*), which suggests that the infection was transmitted from the cat to the person. However, such infections are not commonly reported, which could be because they are rare or because they are not properly diagnosed [13].

Although we have some knowledge about the potential of *C. abortus*, *C. psittaci*, and *C. felis* to cause disease in humans, we do not know much about the disease-causing potential of other chlamydial agents in humans [13]. *C. pecorum*, which causes significant diseases in animals, affects many domestic farm animals such as sheep, goats, cows, horses, and pigs, causing pneumonia, conjunctivitis, polyarthritis ("stiff lamb disease"), inapparent intestinal infections, mastitis, metritis, and encephalomyelitis [8]. However, no zoonotic cases have been reported so far. *C. suis* in pigs causes conjunctivitis, enteritis, and pneumonia. *C. pneumoniae*, which causes disease in humans' respiratory tract, has also been isolated from frogs, koalas, and horses [7, 8]. It has been associated with chronic heart disease, Alzheimer's disease, reactive arthritis (Reiter's syndrome), and asthma [7]. Waddlia chondrophila, recently isolated from aborted bovine fetuses, belongs to the Chlamydiales order, and more data is needed to determine its zoonotic potential [13].

6. Antibiotic resistance in Chlamydiae

There are few reports documenting antibiotic resistance in Chlamydiae. Furthermore, there are no examples of natural or permanent antibiotic resistance in strains that cause disease in humans. In some strains, the detected antibiotic resistance cannot be identified in vitro, which hinders the recognition and interpretation of antibiotic resistance. This is due to differences in laboratory procedures for chlamydial culture, low recovery rates of clinical isolates, and the unknown significance of heterotypic resistance observed in culture [4]. Although antibiotic resistance in Chlamydiae has not been reported throughout history, a few reports indicate that they have the ability to develop resistant phenotypes to a significant extent. In vitro antibiotic resistance in Chlamydiae is demonstrated by contemporary examples of mutagenesis, recombination, and genetic transformation. In addition, tetra-cyclone-resistant *Chlamydia* strains can be isolated from pigs, producing tetra-cycline-resistant genes under extreme pressure [17].

In *Chlamydia* infections without any complex infections present, tetracyclines (TETs) and azithromycin (AZM) are commonly used as they are highly effective in treating these diseases [8]. However, data obtained so far indicate that *Chlamydia* may develop long-term infections that are resistant to antibiotic treatment and involve persistence in the reproductive cycle of the microorganism, leading to a deterioration of the infection. Further data is required to confirm these descriptions [10].

Antibiotic treatment may fail due to the development of chlamydial persistence in laboratory studies, where the infection can become unresponsive to antibiotics. The use of penicillin, in particular, can trigger this persistence, which hinders the differentiation of reticulate bodies into elementary bodies and interrupts cell division [15]. Distinguishing between persistence or phenotypic resistance and antibiotic resistance is a difficult task. However, in vivo evidence suggests that persistence is a common occurrence, with the presence of chlamydial RNA, DNA, and abnormal reticulate bodies often found in culture-negative cases [1].

In *Chlamydia*, there is no one-size-fits-all method to test for antibiotic resistance. The accuracy of antibiotic susceptibility analysis can be affected by several factors, including the type of cell lines utilized, the passage number of both the host cells and *Chlamydia*, the size of the inoculum, and the time at which antibiotics are added. In addition, due to the bacteria's fastidious nature, the success rate of isolating clinical samples for culture-based diagnostic methods can vary, making them less favorable when compared to nucleic acid amplification tests with high sensitivity [17].

Stable strains of *C. suis* that are resistant to tetracycline have been discovered in the United States and Italy. Researchers have identified seven isolates that contain genomic islands of varying lengths and compositions. These genomic islands encode a tetracycline efflux pump called tet(C) and a novel insertion sequence element that likely helps integrate the genomic islands into the chlamydial genome at specific sites [17].

Growing *Chlamydia* bacteria in conditions with sub-inhibitory or excessively high concentrations of six different types of antibiotics can encourage the development of mutations and genetic resistance in various *Chlamydia* strains. Some spontaneously occurring mutations that cause resistance have minimal impact on the chlamydial growth characteristics, while others may cause competitive disadvantages in resistant strains [6].

A technique was developed to facilitate the transfer of genes in the laboratory by using chlamydial strains with mutations that make them resistant to antibiotics and infecting them simultaneously with tetracycline-resistant *C. suis* strains. This process, which involves introducing dissimilar antibiotic-resistant markers into co-infecting strains, can cause genetic exchange between different species of *Chlamydia* and result in genomic rearrangement and mosaicism. Researchers demonstrated the first successful transformation of *Chlamydia*, both naturally and using electroporation, by introducing spontaneous mutations that conferred aminoglycoside resistance. However, significant limitations are still associated with the techniques used for *Chlamydia* recombination and transformation [17].

7. Conclusion

The Chlamydiales order is a diverse group of organisms that are important for human and animal health and have a significant economic impact worldwide. The zoonotic potential of these organisms requires further investigation by studying animal chlamydiosis and evaluating the risks to human health from contact with domestic, wild, and synanthropic animals. There is still much to learn about these organisms in terms of biology, immunology, and disease pathogenesis in order to improve diagnosis and vaccines to control and prevent infections in humans and animals. Antibiotics are also important in treating these infections, as overuse can lead to antibiotic resistance.

Conflict of interest

"The author declare no conflict of interest."

Author details

Gül Banu Çiçek Bideci
Republic of Turkey Ministry of Agriculture and Forestry, Kastamonu, Turkey

*Address all correspondence to: gulbanu.cicekbideci@tarimgov.tr

References

[1] Kaplan SL, Steinbach WJ, Hotez P, editors. Feigin and Cherry's Textbook of Pediatric Infectious Diseases. 7th ed. Philadelphia: Elsevier Saunders; 2014. pp. 2631-2645

[2] Everett KD, Bush RM, Andersen AA. Emended description of the order Chlamydiales, proposal of Parachlamydiaceae fam. nov. and Simkaniaceae fam. nov., each containing one monotypic genus, revised taxonomy of the family Chlamydiaceae, including a new genus and five new species, and standards for the identification of organisms. International Journal of Systematic Bacteriology. 1999;**49**:415-440. DOI: 10.1099/00207713-49-2-415

[3] Verkooyen RP, Willemse D, Hiep-van Casteren SC, et al. Evaluation of PCR, culture, and serology for diagnosis of Chlamydia pneumoniae respiratory infections. Journal of Clinical Microbiology. 1998;**36**:2301-2307

[4] Ashkenazi H, Rudensky B, Paz E, et al. Incidence of immunoglobulin G antibodies to Chlamydia pneumoniae in acute myocardial infarction patients. The Israel Medical Association Journal. 2001;**3**:818-821

[5] Ward ME, Treharne JD, Murray A. Antigenic specificity of human antibody to chlamydia in trachoma and lymphogranuloma venereum. Journal of General Microbiology. 1986;**132**:1599-1610. DOI: 10.1099/00221287-132-6-1599

[6] Tuuminen T, Palomaki P, Paavonen J. The use of serologic tests for the diagnosis of chlamydial infections. Journal of Microbiological Methods. 2000;**42**:265-279

[7] Schachter J. Overview of human diseases. In: Barron AL, editor. Microbiology of Chlamydia. Boca Raton, Florida: CRC Press; 1988. pp. 153-165

[8] Storz J. Overview of animal diseases induced by chlamydial infections. In: Barron AL, editor. Microbiology of Chlamydia. Boca Raton, Florida: CRC Press; 1988. pp. 167-192

[9] Schachter J. Infection and disease epidemiology. In: Stephens RS, editor. Chlamydia: Intracellular Biology, Pathogenesis, and Immunity. Washington, D.C: ASM Press; 1999. pp. 139-169

[10] Saikku P, Leinonen M, Mattila K, Ekman M-R, Nieminen MS, MaÈkelaÈ PH, et al. Serological evidence of an association of a novel Chlamydia, TWAR, with chronic coronary heart disease and acute myocardial infarction. Lancet. 1988;**ii**:983-986

[11] Halberstaedter L, von Prowazek S. U È ber ZelleinschluÈ sse parasitaÈrer Natur beim Trachom. Arbeiten aus dem Kaiserlichen Gesundheitsamte. 1907a;**26**:44-47

[12] Halberstaedter L, von Prowazek S. Zur Aetiologie des Trachoms. Deutsche Medizinische Wochenschrift. 1907b;**33**:1285-1287

[13] Longbottom D, Coulter LJ. Animal chlamydiosis and zoonotic implications. Journal of Comparative Pathology. 2003;**128**:217-244

[14] Meyer KF, Eddie B. Human carrier of the psittacosis virus. Journal of Infectious Diseases. 1951;**88**:109-125

[15] Everett KDE, Andersen AA. Identification of nine species of the Chlamydiaceae using PCR-RFLP.

International Journal of Systematic Bacteriology. 1999;**49**:808-813

[16] Papp JR, Shewen PE. Localization of chronic Chlamydia psittaci infection in the reproductive tract of sheep. Journal of Infectious Diseases. 1996a;**174**:1296-1302

[17] Sandoz K, Rockey DD. Antibiotic resistance İn Chlamydiae. Future Microbiology, 2010;**5**(9): 1427-1442 doi:10.221/fmb.10.96

Chapter 7

Treatment of Chlamydial Infections

Hande Berk Cam

Abstract

Sexually transmitted infections (STIs) are a major health problem with an estimated burden of disease transmission as high as one million new cases per day globally. *Chlamydia trachomatis,* a member of the genus *Chlamydia*, is one of the most common and curable causative agents of STIs. *C. trochomatis* infections usually affect sexually active young adults and adolescents; and are composed of a broad spectrum of diseases varying from asymptomatic infection to severe genito-urinary infection leading to infertility and acute or chronic ocular infection (trachoma), which may result in blindness and pneumonia. Among the members of the genus *Chlamydia,* there are also two pathogenic species, *Chlamydia pneumoniae* and *Chlamydia psittaci* which are responsible for acute respiratory tract infections and febrile illness in humans. The incidence, pathophysiology, and diagnostic methods are discussed in detail in the previous chapters. The purpose of this chapter is to elucidate the management of infections due to *C. trachomatis, C. pneumoniae,* and *C. psittaci* including antibiotic susceptibility and resistance mechanisms, treatment recommendations for ocular infections, genito-urinary and respiratory tract infections, and management of sex partners, pregnant women, neonates, and children according to the latest data.

Keywords: *Chlamydia trachomatis*, *C. pneumoniae*, *C. psittaci*, chlamydial infection, antibiotic treatment

1. Introduction

Chlamydia spp. (order *Chlamydiales*; family *Chlamydiaceae*; genus *Chlamydia*) are obligatory intracellular gram-negative bacteria that cause acute and chronic infections in humans and animals. Genus *Chlamydia* is the sole member of the family *Chlamydiaceae* and includes nine different species. Among them, *C. trachomatis* and *C. pneumoniae* are primarily human pathogens, whereas *C. psitacii*, *Chlamydia abortus,* and *Chlamydia felis* mainly infect animals but occasionally cause zoonotic diseases [1, 2].

Sexually transmitted infections (STIs) are a major health problem with an estimated burden of disease transmission as high as one million new cases per day globally. *C. trachomatis* is one of the most common curable causative agents of STIs and usually affects sexually active young adults and adolescents. The pathogen is the causative agent of a disease called chlamydia, which constitutes a broad spectrum of illnesses varying from asymptomatic infection to severe genital infection leading to infertility, especially in women. Apart from the spread by sexual activity, direct personal contact with shared contaminated items may also cause a chronic ocular infection called trachoma and result in blindness if left untreated. Finally, perinatal transmission of the agent is another undesired entity with adverse clinical outcomes. *C. pneumoniae* and *C. psittaci* are two other pathogens in the genus *Chlamydia* and are responsible for acute respiratory tract infections and febrile illness in humans. However, *C. trachomatis* draws much attention as chlamydial infections account for significant morbidity worldwide. The global control of chlamydia faces some difficulties such as diagnostic challenges, social stigma, and the necessity of routine screening programs due to the asymptomatic course of the disease also concerns about treatment adherence and antibiotic efficacy in extra-genital involvements. The incidence, pathophysiology, and diagnostic methods of chlamydial infections are discussed in detail in the previous chapters. The purpose of this chapter is to elucidate the management of human chlamydial infections in every aspect including antibiotic susceptibility and resistance mechanisms, treatment recommendations for ocular infections, genito-urinary and respiratory tract infections, and also the management of sex partners, pregnant women, neonates, and children according to the latest data.

2. Antibiotic susceptibility and resistance mechanisms in human chlamydial infections

Chlamydiae are obligate intracellular bacteria that have a distinctive bi-phasic life cycle that typically lasts 40–72 hours [3]. The extracellular infectious form is called the elementary body (EB); however, EB does not have metabolic activity and is resistant to antibiotics. On the other hand, the intracellular form, the reticulate body (RB), is the replicative element that synchronously duplicates every 2 to 3 hours and is the target for antibacterial agents [2, 3]. To achieve optimal bacterial clearance, antibiotics with good intracellular penetration and preservation of antibiotic concentration throughout the life-cycle of the organism are needed.

Chlamydiae are sensitive to a wide range of antibiotics such as tetracyclines, macrolides, fluoroquinolones, rifamycins, and clindamycin, which prevent deoxyribonucleic acid (DNA) and protein synthesis and have good activity against intracellular bacteria. Beta-lactam antibiotics and especially penicillins may exhibit *in vitro* efficacy but are linked to the persistence of chlamydial infection and therefore are not recommended for treatment. However, studies revealed that amoxicillin may exhibit higher efficacy than erythromycin in pregnant women with chlamydia disease and due to the paucity of antibiotic options in this period amoxicillin might be offered as an alternative therapy during pregnancy [4–6]. Among other antibacterial classes, aminoglycosides and glycopeptides are ineffective against chlamydial infections since *Chlamydiae* are constitutively resistant. Also, trimethoprim is not effective against *Chlamydia* spp. but *C. trachomatis* is susceptible to sulfonamides [7].

Despite having a severely condensed genome of only about 1 megabase, *Chlamydia* spp. have a highly reserved genomic structure and evidence of horizontally acquired foreign DNA is scarce. Antibiotic resistance is not common in human chlamydial infections but significant resistance phenotypes such as heterotypic resistance, which is characterized by few organisms (less than 1%) that are resistant to antibiotics at concentrations higher than their minimal inhibitory concentrations (MIC), might be expressed [8]. Currently, *in vitro* susceptibility testing of *Chlamydia* spp. is not methodized because resistant clinical isolates are rare; without host cells, the organism cannot be recovered; the identification and interpretation of antibiotic resistance are not standard; and the impact of heterotypic resistance is uncertain [3].

In vitro studies have shown that antibiotic exposure can lead to the accumulation of point mutations, which result in antibiotic resistance in *Chlamydiae.* Stable genetic resistance and transmission of resistance genes across strains have not been reported for human chlamydial infections; however, genetically stable tetracycline resistance has been detected in *Chlamydia suis* (which causes disease in pigs) isolates and acquired tetracycline resistance (Tet^R) has been shown *via* horizontal gene transfer and homologous recombination mechanisms [3, 6, 9, 10].

As mentioned above, the mechanisms that might be related to antibiotic resistance in human chlamydial infections are the persistence of the microorganism, heterotypic resistance, and antibiotic point mutations, which will be detailed as follows:

2.1 Chlamydial persistence

When exposed to stressful circumstances such as beta-lactam antibiotics, interferon-gamma (IFN-γ), a lack of iron supplements, or amino acids, *Chlamydia* spp. exhibit characteristics of chlamydial persistence [3, 11]. Among them, beta-lactam antibiotics constitute a major problem since they are among the groups of antibiotics that are most frequently used for the treatment of various infections [12]. Similar to gram-negative bacteria, *Chlamydia* spp. have an outer membrane but they lack peptidoglycan while having genes that code for proteins necessary for its formation [13]. Studies have shown that *C. pneumoniae* and *C. trachomatis* can synthesize an unusual truncated type of peptidoglycan, which may serve as a target for beta-lactam antibiotics. However, following antibiotic exposure, the pathogen enters a stage known as persistence in which the stressed *Chlamydiae* remain viable but non-culturable. Moreover, it was shown that the persistence of *Chlamydiae* may remain in culture for months and result in clinical treatment failure because of phenotypic resistance to antibiotics, which are often quite efficient [3, 14]. As an example azithromycin, phenotypic resistance emerged in *C. trachomatis* isolates after pre-exposure to penicillin in experimentally infected endometrial epithelial cells *in vitro*, rendering the pathogen refractory to the given medication [15]. Azithromycin and ofloxacin resistance in *C. pneumoniae* and doxycycline resistance in *C. trachomatis* have both been demonstrated to increase in response to environmental changes [16, 17]. More importantly other than phenotypic resistance, recent data indicate that chlamydial persistence may potentially be associated with chronic diseases such as reactive arthritis, chronic prostatitis, asthma, and atherosclerosis [3, 7].

2.2 Heterotypic resistance

Although many antibiotics are effective against chlamydial infections, antibiotic failure rates that vary between 5 and 23% of cases have been reported in chlamydia disease. However, chlamydial resistance is not frequent in humans. Much of these failures have been connected to re-infection and antibiotic compliance issues [6]. In the literature, antibiotic-resistant, *C. trachomatis* clinical isolates are scarce and displayed characteristics of heterotypic resistance as previously explained [3]. It was hypothesized that heterotypic resistance may be due to the slow growth of the organism in certain environments or the exhibition of an adaptive response that makes the pathogen resistant to antibiotics [9]. On the other hand, resistant isolates exhibited reduced fitness, which impaired long-term survival or led to the loss of resistance pattern upon serial passaging. It is considered that this phenotypic alteration seems to impair the transmission and therefore prevents the emergence of non-susceptible clones [3, 18, 19].

2.3 Genes and mutations associated with human chlamydial infections

For the treatment of chlamydial infections, tetracyclines and macrolides are quite effective. It is commonly acknowledged that antibiotic misuse or overuse increases the chance of microorganisms' developing antibiotic resistance, which poses a critical and dangerous public health issue globally [20, 21]. However, human chlamydial infections have not been associated with persistent and heritable genetic resistance. *In vivo* studies have shown that *Chlamydiae* may acquire resistance through several mutations to antimicrobials [3]. Additionally, it has been demonstrated that the serial passage of *Chlamydia* spp. leads to the selection of resistant isolates if exposed to sub-inhibitory antibiotic doses [21].

Tetracyclines are bacteriostatic antibiotics that prevent aminoacyl tRNAs from binding with ribosomal 30S subunit, hence inhibiting bacterial protein production [3]. Doxycycline is a semisynthetic tetracycline and is recommended as the primary therapeutic option against *C. trachomatis* infections. Apart from human infections tetracyclines are widely used in veterinary medicine. The emergence of genetically stable TetR resistance is first described in the 1990s and observed in *C. suis* isolates recovered from pigs both healthy and sick. Since then, the threat of transmission of TetR resistance to other members of *Chlamydiae* is of great concern [10]. Although *in vitro* tests have shown that TetR may be horizontally transmitted from *C. suis* to clinical isolates of *C. trachomatis* during co-culture; to date, antibiotic failure due to stable TetR has not been reported in human chlamydial infections. In a study by O'Neill et al., a porB gene mutation was discovered in two clinically resistant isolates but the isolates were reported to be phenotypically sensitive to tetracyclines *in vitro* and stable genetic resistance was not evident [22].

Macrolides are a group of antimicrobials that bind to bacterial 50S ribosomal subunit and impair bacterial growth due to the inhibition of protein synthesis. They are also effective front-line classes of antibiotics used for the treatment of chlamydia infections. The size of the macrocyclic lactone ring determines whether the group is classified as having a 12-, 14-, 15-, or 16-membered ring. Among macrolides, erythromycin (14-membered first generation), clarithromycin (14-membered second generation), and azithromycin (15-membered) are widely used for chlamydial infections [23]. The 23S rRNA gene alterations that make antibiotics less able to bind to the 50S ribosomal subunit, which is necessary for bacteriostatic action, usually cause macrolide resistance. It has been demonstrated that mutations to the 23S rRNA gene can cause *C. trachomatis* and *C. psittaci* to become resistant to macrolides. In addition by means of alterations in the rplD and rplV genes, *C. trachomatis* may also exhibit macrolide resistance [21].

Fluoroquinolones are broad-spectrum widely used bactericidal antibiotics that function by blocking the DNA gyrase and DNA topoisomerase IV enzymes needed for bacterial DNA synthesis [24]. The first-generation fluorinated quinolones include norfloxacin, ciprofloxacin, and ofloxacin. The usage of norfloxacin is restricted to the treatment of STIs and urinary tract infections because of its relatively low serum levels and inadequate tissue penetration. On the other hand, ciprofloxacin is an effective antibiotic that is still being widely used for the treatment of a number of gram-negative systemic infections. The more recent fluoroquinolones, such as levofloxacin (an isomer of ofloxacin) and moxifloxacin, have improved efficacy against gram-positive respiratory tract infections [25]. Fluoroquinolones generally have good activity against chlamydial infections; however, *in vitro* experiments have shown that sub-inhibitory antibiotic concentrations may lead to resistance in various *Chlamydia* spp. including *C. trachomatis*. It was discovered that mutations in the gyrA, parC, and ygeD genes may cause *C. trachomatis* to become resistant to fluoroquinolones, while changes in the gyrA gene may cause *C. pneumoniae* to become resistant [21].

Bactericidal drugs known as rifamycins selectively bind to the β-subunit of RNA polymerase, which result in the inhibition of the transcription process. Although they have strong *in vitro* activity, these medicines are not the first-line treatments for chlamydial infections. *In vitro* studies have demonstrated that *Chlamydia* spp., such as *C. pneumonia*, *C. trachomatis*, and *C. psittaci*, rapidly establish a resistance to rifamycins following exposure to sub-inhibitory antibiotic concentrations [3, 26]. In most research, rifampin (RIF) serves as a representative of rifamycins and rifampin resistance mostly results from rpoB gene nucleotide mutation [21].

Resistance to lincomycin, a bacteriostatic protein synthesis inhibitor, is noted in *in vitro*-generated *C. trachomatis* strains exposed to sub-inhibitory antibiotic concentrations. It was revealed that resistant strains exhibit mutations in 23S rRNA genes [3, 27].

3. Management of human chlamydial infections

Management of human Chlamydial infections will be discussed as separate sections and will include the most common etiological agents: *C. trochomatis, C. pneumoniae*, and *C. psittaci*, respectively.

3.1 Management of *C. trochomatis* infections

Infections due to *C. trochomatis* are caused by 19 serovars, which affect the ocular, genito-urinary tract, and pulmonary systems. Ocular infections mainly result from serovars A-C, which led to trachoma and to a lesser extent serovars D-K which led to inclusion conjunctivitis and sometimes infant pneumonia [28]. On the other hand, genito-urinary tract infections include chlamydia and lymphogranuloma venereum (LGV), which are caused by serovars D-K and serovars L1-L3, respectively [2, 18, 29].

In most men and women, chlamydia maintains an asymptomatic course and becomes a silent reservoir for infection [5, 30]. Spontaneous clearance of the pathogen may occur gradually over years but if chlamydia is not treated effectively, major medical conditions with both immediate and long-term complications could arise [3, 31, 32]. These health problems include clinical or subclinical pelvic inflammatory disease (PID) leading to chronic pelvic pain, infertility, ectopic pregnancy and Fitzhugh-Curtis syndrome in women; pre-term delivery, inclusion conjunctivitis, and pneumonia in the newborn; and reactive arthritis in both sexes [5, 33, 34]. It was also shown that untreated chlamydia may promote the spread of other STIs, such as human immunodeficiency virus (HIV) [35]. Therefore to prevent chlamydia-associated diseases and to decrease the degree of transmission to susceptible populations, presumptive or guided therapy should be started in all suspected or confirmed chlamydia infections including asymptomatic diseases.

3.1.1 Treatment of ocular infections due to C. trachomatis

The most prevalent infectious etiology of blindness all over the world is *C. trachomatis*, which leads to ocular illnesses known as trachoma and adult/neonatal inclusion conjunctivitis. Trachoma is transmitted through direct or indirect contact with objects such as hands, fomites, bed sheets, eye-seeking insects, and polluted towels in unsanitary settings [28]. On the other hand, inclusion conjunctivitis is spread by perinatal transmission in neonates or by hand-to-eye inoculation of infected genital secretions in adults.

3.1.1.1 Treatment of trachoma

Trachoma specifically targets the world's poorest regions. According to data from June 2022 provided by the World Health Organization (WHO), 125 million people reside in areas where trachoma is an endemic disease [36]. Trachoma is initiated in early childhood and recurrent ocular infection leads to conjunctival scarring and eventually blindness. Trachoma incidents decreased as a result of general improvements in living conditions, but recent predictions show that 1.9 million individuals worldwide are blind or have significant vision problems as a result of trachoma. The WHO is implementing the SAFE strategy as part of a global initiative to eradicate blinding trachoma. The SAFE strategy includes early surgical intervention for trichiasis (contact between the eyelids and the eye that results in blindness), widespread use of antibiotics like azithromycin to manage infections, regular facial hygiene, and advancements in living conditions to minimize bacterial spread.

The World Health Organization divides trachoma into five stages, with Stages 1 and 2 characterized by trachomatous inflammation that is follicular (TF) or intense (TI), respectively; Stage 3 by trachomatous scarring (TS); Stage 4 by trachomatous trichiasis (TT); and Stage 5 by corneal opacity (CO), which results in visual impairment and blindness.

Antibacterial treatment is advised in the first two stages of trachoma's inflammatory phase (stages 1 and 2) and before scarring sets in, which is Stage 3 [37, 38]. The antibacterial drug of choice is oral azithromycin because it can be taken as a single dose, has a relatively long half-life, and is more concentrated in tissue than in plasma [39]. Adults and children are given a single oral dose of azithromycin at doses of 1 g and 20 mg/kg, respectively. In case of antibiotic failure, topical 1% tetracycline eye ointment, twice a day, for 6 weeks or erythromycin, 20 mg/kg (maximum 1 gr), orally, twice a day, for 14 days can be given. In stages 3 and 5, no treatment option exists but in Stage 4 surgical treatment is advocated for the protection of the cornea from abrasion.

Because trachoma is a major public health issue, the WHO recommends widespread administration of antibiotics in places with populations of 100,000–250,000 people and when the prevalence of the active trachoma, Stage 1 (TF), is greater than 5% in children aged 1–9 years. According to the most recent estimate of TF prevalence and until the percentage falls below 5%, it is advised that all inhabitants receive antibiotic therapy on an annual basis. It is also recommended that all inhabitants receive antibiotic medication annually up until the most current estimate of the prevalence of TF drops below 5% [40].

3.1.1.2 Treatment of neonatal inclusion conjunctivitis

Neonatal inclusion conjunctivitis is a preventable yet an undesired complication of active maternal chlamydial infection that affects newborns. Perinatal transmission of

C. trachomatis to neonates during vaginal delivery occurs as high as 60% of the cases [41]. Though neonatal infection may retain an asymptomatic course, the infection is usually progressive and mostly affects the conjunctiva, nasopharynx, and lungs. Among infants presenting with conjunctivitis, the likelihood of neonatal-acquired inclusion conjunctivitis varies between 20 and 64% [41, 42]. Conjunctivitis that is left untreated can last for months and cause corneal and conjunctival scarring. Also, the disease may spread to the lungs and cause infantile pneumonia [41]. To prevent the systemic spread of the agent, all infants infected with *C. trachomatis* should receive treatment even if they are asymptomatic.

The neonatal inclusion conjunctivitis incubation period is generally 5–12 days after birth. Conjunctivitis in newborns younger than 30 days should be investigated for chlamydial infection, particularly if the mother has a past history of illness. Infection with ophthalmia neonatorum should also be considered and ocular samples should be examined for *Neisseria gonorrhoeae* [43].

Neonatal inclusion conjunctivitis is treated with oral erythromycin base or ethyl succinate, 50 mg/kg/day in four divided doses for 14 days. The alternative treatment is oral azithromycin 20 mg/kg/day for 3 days [44]. Both antimicrobials have been associated with infantile hypertrophic pyloric stenosis (IHPS) in infants less than 6 weeks of age; consequently, newborns medicated with any of these antimicrobials should be monitored for IHPS [45]. Compared to oral therapy, topical medication has been demonstrated to be ineffective in eliminating nasopharyngeal colonization and linked to persistent infection [46].

There is currently no effective prophylaxis for the prevention of newborn inclusion conjunctivitis, and neonatal gonococcal ophthalmia neonatorum prophylaxis does not offer protection against chlamydial conjunctivitis. Implementing health policies for routine antenatal testing and treatment of pregnant women at risk for chlamydia is advocated as a substitute, however, due to the financial burden of the strategy the screening programs cannot be utilized globally [47].

3.1.1.3 Treatment of adult inclusion conjunctivitis

Adult inclusion conjunctivitis, a self-limiting condition, is brought on by the inoculation of the eye with infected vaginal fluids. Without treatment, the infection might resolve spontaneously in 6–18 months but more frequently the disease progresses to complicated/uncomplicated chlamydia or impair reproductive health. Also, ocular complications such as conjunctival scarring, punctate keratitis, and iritis may take place. To prevent morbidity and related complications, treatment should be given to all patients. Topical antibiotics alone are not sufficient due to the possible concomitant urogenital infection; therefore, combined therapy with systemic antibiotics is necessary. Systemic oral antibiotic therapy options include azithromycin 1 g, single-dose; doxycycline 100 mg, twice a day for 7 days; tetracycline 100 mg, four times a day for 7–10 days; or erythromycin 500 mg, four times a day for 7 days. Of note, the usage of tetracycline and doxycycline during pregnancy is contraindicated and should be avoided. Adjunctive topical treatment of adult inclusion conjunctivitis includes antibacterial drugs such as erythromycin, gentamicin, tetracycline, and fluoroquinolones [48].

3.1.2 Treatment of urogenital and extra-genital infections due to C. trachomatis

In this section, the management of chlamydia and LGV will be discussed in detail.

3.1.2.1 General approach to chlamydia disease and treatment options

The key to the management of chlamydia starts with clinical suspicion. Patients who have chlamydia disease may present with urinary symptoms and might be misdiagnosed as urinary tract infections. Also, patients who experienced sexual assault or sexually active adolescents may be reluctant to give the right information or may be unaware of the situation. Therefore in case of doubt about chlamydia, clinicians should immediately initiate diagnostic methods and send appropriate clinical specimens to the laboratory for testing. Moreover, co-infection with other STIs including gonorrhea, HIV, and syphilis must be investigated [49]. Early appropriate antibiotic therapy is important and the patient's age, pregnancy status, access to medication, and treatment compliance should all be taken into account. In case of severe PID, consultation with obstetrics/gynecology and in case of ocular involvement consultation with ophthalmology should be performed. In order to prevent reinfection, patients should be informed about safe sex practices and the necessity of partner management. Finally, a patient-based follow-up test strategy should be determined after the completion of treatment [45].

For treatment purposes, chlamydia is mainly categorized into two forms according to the anatomical site involved. Oropharyngeal and lower genital tract involvement (cervicitis/urethritis/epididymitis/anorectal infection) are defined as uncomplicated disease, whereas upper genital tract involvement [salpingitis/endometritis/pelvic inflammatory disease (PID), Fitzhugh-Curtis syndrome] is defined as a complicated disease.

The laboratory diagnosis of chlamydia has significantly improved as a result of the switch from culture-based to molecular-based testing procedures [50]. Because of its high sensitivity, high specificity, and convenience to be utilized on a variety of clinical specimen types, nucleic acid amplification testing (NAAT) is the most efficient method [45, 51, 52]. Unfortunately, NAAT may not always be available in every facility and patients who are at risk for STIs may sometimes be unlikely to return for test results; therefore, WHO recommends consideration of a syndromic approach (to detect and treat patients with STIs based on particular symptoms and signs, which are indicators of infection) in these situations [43, 53]. Also when administering single-dose or multidose regimens to patients, medicine should be given with the first dosage being closely monitored on-site and in the clinic [43].

Doxycycline 100 mg, orally, twice a day for 7 days (or delayed release 200 mg tablet, once a day for 7 days) is the recommended regimen for non-pregnant adults and adolescents with uncomplicated chlamydia involving cervical, urethral, rectal, and oropharyngeal sites. Oral azithromycin 1 g single-dose is the alternative treatment regimen for uncomplicated chlamydia. Previously, single-dose azithromycin had been another preferred option due to its high efficacy against *C. trachomatis,* better adherence due to once-daily usage, and similar adverse effect profiles. However, mounting evidence suggests that azithromycin has a lesser rate of microbiologic cure than doxycycline especially in treating rectal and oropharyngeal infections, and currently, it is accepted as the alternative treatment option [45].

According to a meta-analysis and a Cochrane systematic review that included men with urogenital chlamydia, a 7-day course of doxycycline achieved higher success rates than single-dose azithromycin regimens [54, 55]. Furthermore, as shown by two randomized, double-blind clinical trials and several nonrandomized studies doxycycline regimen may be 20% more effective than azithromycin in managing rectal *C. trachomatis* infection in both women and men who have sex with men (MSM) [54, 56–59].

Similar findings have been published from prospective, open-label research involving individuals with oropharyngeal chlamydia and a 7-day doxycycline regimen showed less treatment failure when compared with azithromycin single-dose treatment [60]. Urogenital *C. trachomatis* infections may be accompanied by concomitant anorectal and oropharyngeal chlamydia, which might remain asymptomatic for that reason doxycycline regimen should be chosen as the primary treatment regimen in adults and adolescents with chlamydia except in patients who are unlikely to be able to complete the 7-day doxycycline course and pregnant women. In such cases, azithromycin regimen should be considered [45, 61, 62].

Among other therapeutic options erythromycin base 500 mg, orally, four times a day for 7 days, is also an effective alternative regimen but gastrointestinal side effects are frequent and nonadherence might be observed. Fluoroquinolones are highly active against *C. trachomatis* infections and levofloxacin 500 mg, orally, once a day for 7 days or ofloxacin 200–400 mg, orally, twice a day for 7 days are other alternative medications yet the regimens are more expensive and cannot be offered during pregnancy and breastfeeding periods [43].

3.1.2.2 Treatment of cervicitis due to C. trachomatis

Chlamydia majorly presents as cervicitis in women. The majority of patients who have chlamydia cervicitis are asymptomatic or present with mild nonspecific symptoms such as irregular vaginal discharge, intermenstrual or post-coital bleeding, and dyspareunia. Patients should be evaluated for PID since cervicitis may be a marker of upper genital tract involvement [43]. In order to prevent the complications that impair reproductive health and to avoid sexual and perinatal transmission to susceptible people, all women with chlamydia cervicitis should receive treatment for chlamydia. However, under the following circumstances, presumptive antibiotic treatment for *C. trachomatis* should be administered:

- The patient is prone to contracting *C. trachomatis* infection (e.g., women under 25 years old, women who have a new sex partner, a sex partner with multiple partners, or a sex partner with an STI) and testing with NAAT/quality-assured rapid test with a minimum sensitivity of 80% and specificity of 90% are not possible.

- The patient is prone to contracting *C. trachomatis* infection as above and NAAT/ quality-assured rapid tests are accessible in the facility but the results are not obtainable at the same appointment, and patient follow-up cannot be assured [43, 53].

- The suggested treatment for chlamydia cervicitis in non-pregnant adults and adolescents is a 7-day course of doxycycline. Alternative treatment plans include a single dosage of azithromycin or a 7-day course of either erythromycin or ofloxacin [53]. Patients should also be assessed for concomitant gonococcal infection and other STIs.

3.1.2.3 Treatment of urethritis due to C. trachomatis

It was shown that nearly all women who have chlamydia cervicitis also have concomitant urethritis [63]. In men, chlamydia disease generally involves the male urethra. *C. trachomatis* is a frequent cause of acute urethritis in young, sexually active individuals and is responsible for more than half of all instances of non-gonococcal urethritis [43, 64, 65]. Most cases of chlamydia urethritis in both men and women go unnoticed. In women, urinary symptoms such as frequent urination and dysuria are common, whereas in male patients additional complaints of urethral discharge and discomfort are prevalent [66]. Ideally, treatment should be given after pathogen detection but quick access to diagnostic data might not always be possible; therefore, presumptive treatment should begin for non-gonococcal urethritis (NGU) for those who have symptoms of urethral discharge from the penis, and patient follow-up cannot be assured or test results are not accessible on the same day. Evaluation and treatment of NGU should also include gonococci. For gonococci, a single intramuscular dose of ceftriaxone (500 mg [or 1 gr for individuals ≥150 kg]) might be considered but the choice of appropriate treatment regimen should be guided according to the local antibiotic resistance patterns [43, 53]. The recommended and alternative treatment options for urethritis due to *C. trachomatis* are the same as other uncomplicated chlamydia infections mentioned above.

3.1.2.4 Treatment of rectal infections due to C. trachomatis

Acute proctitis and proctocolitis are two distinct manifestations of chlamydia in individuals who have anal exposure to *C. trachomatis* by oral, genital, or digital interaction. Proctitis is the inflammation of the distal part of the rectum and presents with anorectal discomfort, tenesmus, or rectal discharge, whereas proctocolitis is the extension of proctitis to the colonic mucosa above the anus and additional symptoms such as diarrhea or abdominal cramps may be seen [43]. Rectal *C. trachomatis* infection rates in MSM and women are similar and range from 1 to 18%. It was shown that in women, the rectal disease may accompany urogenital infection in up to 83% of cases and can occur regardless of receptive anal sexual behavior [61]. In MSM, the incidence of asymptomatic rectal infection is high and reaches above 80% [62].

Either asymptomatic or not, microbial eradication at the rectal site is crucial for treating urogenital chlamydia. Due to its higher microbiologic cure rates and asymptomatic nature of rectal chlamydia disease, doxycycline is the recommended antibiotic choice for anal infections caused by *C. trachomatis* [54, 59].

A 7-day course of doxycycline 100 mg orally, twice a day is the suggested regimen for proctitis and proctocolitis due to chlamydia. Doxycycline treatment should be extended to 21 days if symptoms indicating lymphogranuloma venereum such as anal bloody discharge, tenesmus, perianal or mucosal ulcers are present. Erythromycin 500 mg, orally, 4 times a day for 14 days is the alternative regimen. Treatment of patients with sexually acquired proctitis should also include treatment for gonococci. For gonococci, a single intramuscular dose of ceftriaxone (500 mg [or 1 gr for individuals ≥150 kg]) should be added. WHO advises a syndromic approach in cases with anorectal discharge and a reported history of receptive anal sex to allow treatment on the day of the visit in regions that have little to no molecular testing or laboratory capacity [53].

3.1.2.5 Treatment of oropharyngeal infections due to C. trachomatis

C. trachomatis can lead to oropharyngeal infection in those having receptive oral intercourse, same as gonorrhea [43]. The prevalence of oropharyngeal chlamydia infection approximately ranges from 1 to 3% in MSM and women [61]. Without therapy, oropharyngeal chlamydia can spread to other genital locations *via* sexual contact [67, 68]. The optimal antibiotic regimen for oropharyngeal chlamydia has not been thoroughly investigated. It was revealed that doxycycline is more efficient in treating oropharyngeal chlamydia than azithromycin similar to rectal chlamydia infections. The recommended treatment is a 7-day course of oral, twice a daily 100 mg doxycycline [45].

3.1.2.6 Treatment of epididymitis due to C. trachomatis

An uncomfortable, swollen, and inflamed epididymis is symptom of the clinical illness known as epididymitis. Unilateral testicular pain and palpable swelling are common in patients with acute epididymitis. The disease sometimes involves the testicles and is called epididymo-orchitis. Testicular torsion is a complication of epididymitis that requires emergency surgery. Acute epididymitis caused by STIs is a typical complication of young, sexually active men, and the condition frequently coexists with urethritis. Gonococci and *C. trachomatis* testing should be performed on all suspected instances of acute epididymitis. If patients are unable to follow the prescribed antibiotic regimen or if significant pain or fever points to complications such as testicular torsion, abscess, or necrotizing fasciitis, patient evaluation for hospitalization should be considered. All sexually active men who have acute epididymitis should get presumptive therapy Doxycycline 100 mg orally, twice a day for 10 days, is the recommended treatment for acute epididymitis caused by *C. trachomatis*. The therapy should include treatment for gonococci and a single intramuscular dose of ceftriaxone (500 mg [or 1 g for individuals ≥150 kg]) should be added [43]. In patients who report insertive anal sex, enteric organisms might be involved in epididymitis. In such cases, fluoroquinolones are effective against both gram-negative enteric bacteria and chlamydia therefore ofloxacin 300 mg orally, twice a day for 10 days or levofloxacin 500 mg orally, once a day for 10 days (plus ceftriaxone for gonococci) can be offered [43, 69].

3.1.2.7 Treatment of PID due to C. trachomatis

PID is an inflammatory disease affecting female upper genital tract organs including endometritis, salpingitis, tubo-ovarian abscess, and pelvic peritonitis. PID is often caused by STIs, with *N. gonorrhoeae* or *C. trachomatis* as the etiological agent in up to half of the cases [43]. Women with PID frequently exhibit mild and vague symptoms such as abnormal vaginal discharge, spotting, and dyspareunia but may also be asymptomatic. Untreated PID might impair reproductive health and lead to complications such as tubal infertility and ectopic pregnancy [53]. Moreover, PID can also extend to abdominal organs and cause Fitzhugh-Curtis syndrome, which requires in-patient treatment and is characterized by peritonitis and inflammation of the liver capsule [32]. Since PID is related to severe morbidity, presumptive therapy should begin for sexually active women at risk for STIs who complain of pelvic or lower abdominal discomfort and there is tenderness on pelvic examination [43].

The women who present with PID should also be evaluated for the need for hospitalization when there is suspicion of surgical emergency, presence of tubo-ovarian abscess, pregnancy status, severe illness [nausea, vomiting, and fever >38.5°C (101°F)], or no clinical benefit from oral antibiotic treatment. Broad-spectrum antibiotics against probable agents should be initiated as soon as possible. Antibiotics should cover *C. trachomatis* and *N. gonorrhoeae* even if endocervical testing is negative as upper genital tract infection cannot be fully ruled out [43]. The recommended regimen for *C. trachomatis*-related PID is doxycycline 100 mg, orally, twice a day for 14 days combined with antibiotics active against gonococci. Facultative anaerobic bacteria and enteric gram-negative rods are among other etiologic agents that should be considered for the treatment of PID [43].

3.1.2.8 Treatment of LGV

C. trachomatis serovars L1, L2, or L3 are the culprits behind LGV and are responsible for a more invasive form of the chlamydial disease called LGV characterized by genital ulcer disease, lymphadenopathy, and proctocolitis. Among them, proctocolitis is a frequent finding in LGV and is especially seen in MSM. Inflammatory bowel disease-like symptoms, such as mucoid or hemorrhagic rectal discharge, anal pain, constipation, fever, or tenesmus, might be clinical indicators of proctocolitis. Until recently, LGV was exclusively a problem in tropical and subtropical regions of the globe with little resources. Since 2003, endemic LGV cases have been observed in MSM across Europe [70, 71]. If untreated, rectal LGV may be invasive and cause chronic colorectal fistulas and strictures. LGV can also cause inguinal or femoral lymphadenopathy with suppurated bubo formation and the condition may lead to genital elephantiasis. Consequently, presumptive treatment should be started if a patient with proctocolitis exhibits symptoms or signs such as bloody discharge, tenesmus, or ulceration at the rectal site; if a patient with a recent history of genital ulcer displays severe inguinal lymphadenopathy with bubo formation; or if the patient has genital ulcer disease and other causes have been ruled out [43, 72].

The most effective antibiotic for the treatment of LGV is doxycycline but unlike uncomplicated chlamydia caused by serovars D-K, treatment of LGV needs a prolonged course of therapy. Doxycycline 100 mg twice a day for 21 days is the standard course of treatment for LGV. Azithromycin 1 g orally once a week for 3 weeks and erythromycin base 500 mg orally four times a day for 21 days are two alternate regimens. Unfortunately, the LGV-specific azithromycin regimen has not been confirmed, and a follow-up test with *C. trachomatis* NAAT is advised about 4 weeks after the end of therapy [43]. Patients who have LGV should be observed until all symptoms and signs have disappeared [43].

3.1.2.9 Treatment of chlamydia and LGV during pregnancy and breastfeeding

The tetracycline group of antibiotics including doxycycline which is the primary antibiotic option for chlamydia and LGV is contraindicated during pregnancy and breastfeeding due to the possibility of tooth discoloration [43]. In pregnant and breastfeeding women suffering from chlamydia disease, azithromycin, erythromycin, and amoxicillin are the safer antibiotic options [73]. The recommended antibiotic regimen for pregnant and breastfeeding adults and adolescents with cervical, urethral, rectal, and oropharyngeal chlamydia is azithromycin 1 g orally given as a single-dose. As a secondary option amoxicillin 500 mg orally, three times a day for 7 days can be used. Beta-lactam antibiotics are associated with the persistence of chlamydia; therefore, caution must be given for re-emergence of viable pathogen after discontinuation of amoxicillin therapy [43]. Erythromycins 500 mg orally, four times a day for 7 days, or erythromycin 500 mg orally, twice a day for 14 days, are two alternative possibilities for pregnant and nursing women with uncomplicated chlamydia. Of note, estolate formulation of erythromycin is contraindicated in pregnancy due to the risk for drug-related hepatotoxicity, and erythromycin base or erythromycin ethyl succinate should be prescribed instead [53, 74, 75].

For many years, macrolides including azithromycin and erythromycin have been frequently utilized as safe antibiotic options during pregnancy; however, in a recent population-based cohort study it was found that first-trimester usage of macrolides (mainly erythromycin given over several days) was associated with a higher incidence of congenital abnormalities than penicillins [76]. It was also shown that erythromycin medication during 7 weeks of delivery or while breastfeeding has been linked to a higher incidence of IHPS [7]. The impact of azithromycin single-dose regimen on a fetus is unknown but it is considered that the advantages of azithromycin therapy outweigh any potential risks. Finally, although fluoroquinolones can be used in non-pregnant patients, its usage is restricted during pregnancy and breastfeeding due to fetal and neonatal adverse effects [43].

For pregnant women with LGV, the optimum dose and duration of antibiotic therapy are not known. Azithromycin 1 g orally, once a week for 3 weeks, can be used. Erythromycin 500 mg orally, four times a day for 21 days is another option for use in pregnancy and nursing women but gastrointestinal adverse effects are frequent [43, 74].

All pregnant women should get a NAAT retest around 4 weeks following the end of their therapy since the infection can remain and cause serious side effects in both mothers and neonates [45]. Also to detect re-infection, retesting should be repeated in pregnant women 3 months after completing therapy [45].

To prevent maternal complications and infant chlamydial infections, it is advised that pregnant women under 25 years old, pregnant women who have a new sex partner, a sex partner with multiple partners, or a sex partner with an STI, should be checked at the first antenatal control and retested in the third trimester. However, routine antenatal screening of pregnant women at risk for chlamydia disease cannot be utilized in all countries [31, 77].

3.1.2.10 Treatment of chlamydia disease among infants and children

C. trachomatis acquired in the perinatal period can persist for up to 3 years. Any prepubertal youngster with chlamydia disease should be evaluated for the possibility of sexual abuse. In case of a suspect of sexual abuse, local authorities should be notified. The recommended regimens for chlamydia disease among infants and children are as follows:

- For infants and children weighing less than 45 kg: erythromycin base or ethyl succinate 50 mg/kg/day orally divided into four doses daily for 14 days;

- For children weighing more than 45 kg but aged under 8 years old: azithromycin 1 g orally, in a single dose; and

- For children aged above 8 years: azithromycin 1 g orally in a single dose or doxycycline 100 mg orally, two times a day for 7 days.

3.1.2.11 Follow-up recommendations for chlamydia and LGV

Sexual activity should be avoided by people with *C. trachomatis* (LVG or non-LGV serotypes) and their partners until treatment is complete (7 days after single-dose therapy or after completion of a multiple-dose regimen) and all current partners have recovered [43, 74].

A test of cure to detect therapeutic failure (repeated testing 4 weeks after finishing therapy) is not advocated for non-pregnant patients with uncomplicated chlamydia disease. But if therapeutic adherence is not assured, the patient has persistent symptoms, regimens with low efficacy (such as erythromycin or amoxicillin) have been implemented, or re-infection is suspected, clinician can offer a follow-up visit and retest the patient. Nonviable organisms may persist up to 4 weeks after completion of therapy and may cause false positive test results therefore testing with chlamydial NAATs at less than 4 weeks following the conclusion of medication is not advised [45].

In order to detect re-infection, all patients should be retested for chlamydia in 3 months (or retesting at 3 months is not feasible, within 12-months) after completion of therapy. It is suggested to schedule the follow-up appointment at the time of treatment [43].

If the patient has complaints of chronic or recurring symptoms, non-adherence to the given medication, re-infection, completion of sex partner treatment, and coinfection with other STIs should be questioned and evaluated. Assuming that *C. trachomatis* is found on repeat testing, treating with the same regimen (preferably doxycycline regimen) is advised since drug resistance to doxycycline (or azithromycin) has not yet been proven in *C. trachomatis* as explained previously in the Subsection 2.

3.1.2.12 Management of sex partners of patients who have chlamydia and LGV

If a patient with chlamydia or LGV had intercourse with a partner within 60 days of the onset of their symptoms or chlamydia diagnosis, the partner should be referred for screening for *C. trachomatis*. A 7-day doxycycline regimen should be presumptively given to asymptomatic partners. In addition, co-infection with other STIs such as gonorrhea, HIV, and syphilis should be investigated in individuals and their sex partners who had a diagnosis of chlamydia or LGV [43]. However, if the clinician is worried that sex partners are unable to access evaluation and treatment services, a strategy termed "expedited partner therapy" (EPT) can be applied as permitted by law. In this strategy, treatment is delivered to the sex partner without examination by either giving an antibiotic/prescription to the index patient (so they can give it to their partners) or by calling in a prescription directly for the partner. Partners who will receive EPT should be informed about the significance of treatment, potential side effects of the medications, and complications of the disease [43].

3.1.3 Treatment of infantile chlamydial pneumonia

Chlamydial pneumoniae is subacute pneumonia that mainly affects newborns between the ages of 1–3 months. *C. trachomatis* testing should be performed in all newborns aged 1–3 months who are suspected of having pneumonia especially if there is a risk for chlamydia infection in the mother such as pregnant women under 25 years old and pregnant women who have a new sex partner, more than one sex partner, a sex partner with multiple partners, or a sex partner with an STI [43].

Erythromycin base or ethyl succinate 50 mg/kg/day orally divided into four doses every day for 14 days is the recommended regimen for infantile chlamydial pneumonia. Azithromycin suspension 20 mg/kg/day orally, once a day for 3 days is the alternative regimen that can be given presumptively when there is a strong suspicion of chlamydia infection and there are limited laboratory resources or infant follow-up is not possible [43]. It is advised to monitor infants for resolution of pneumonia symptoms as the efficacy of erythromycin against *C. trachomatis* pneumonia is approximately 80% [43, 78]. Additionally, mothers of babies with infantile chlamydial pneumonia should be assessed, screened, and treated for chlamydia disease [43].

3.1.4 Reactive arthritis due to C. trachomatis *infection*

Reactive arthritis is a type of arthritides known as the spondyloarthritides that usually develops following an enteric or venereal infection. Both men and women can develop reactive arthritis after infection due to *C. trachomatis* whether they are symptomatic or not. Moreover, reactive arthritis can occasionally be one of the three symptoms that used to be known as Reiter's syndrome, which also includes urethritis and conjunctivitis [34]. Although randomized studies for long-term anti-chlamydial antibiotic treatment for reactive arthritis showed varied results, the majority of studies showed no benefit. Therefore, antibacterial medication is not recommended in reactive arthritis related to *C. trachomatis* [79, 80].

3.2 Treatment of infections due to *C. pneumoniae*

C. pneumoniae is another important human pathogen in the family *Chlamydiaceae* that mainly infects the respiratory tract. The agent causes upper or lower respiratory tract infections including pharyngitis, laryngitis, and community-acquired pneumoniae (CAP). Most *C. pneumoniae*-related respiratory infections are asymptomatic or mild; however, severe complications such as exacerbation of asthma, encephalitis, and myocarditis can occur, which may require hospitalization [81]. *C. pneumoniae* prevalence rates in individuals with CAP range from 1 to 20% of cases [82, 83]. Therefore, empiric treatment of CAP frequently includes the usage of antibiotics effective against *C. pneumoniae* [84].

Among antibacterial medications, beta-lactam antibiotics, aminoglycosides, glycopeptides (such as vancomycin), and sulfonamides are not effective against *C. pneumoniae*, whereas macrolides, doxycycline, and fluoroquinolones are effective options [72, 85]. Acquired and heritable antibacterial resistance have not been revealed in *C. pneumoniae* and laboratory tests for the detection of *C. pneumoniae* are not routinely recommended in CAP management. Decisions for testing can be individualized on a case-by-case basis and the availability of microbiological tests [3, 84]. In the literature, clinical trials that show the efficacy of antibacterial medications on outcomes of pneumonia due to *C. pneumoniae* are limited [86]. However, the performance of antibacterial agents in eradicating nasopharyngeal *C. pneumonia* has been evaluated in several studies. The efficiency of eradicating microorganisms was shown as around 80% in those trials using a 5-day course of azithromycin and between 70% and 100% when using 7 to 10-day courses of clarithromycin, erythromycin, moxifloxacin, or levofloxacin. The authors revealed that the majority of patients improved despite the organism's persistence in the nasopharynx; therefore, the significance of bacterial eradication for treatment success is still controversial [86–90]. Studies have shown that in patients who remained culture positive after treatment, antibiotic failure is the result of the persistent state of the organism and not due to drug resistance [72, 91].

Numerous researchers have questioned the ideal length of antibiotic treatment in CAP. Historically at least 7 days of treatment was recommended for CAP; however, in the last decades there is a tendency toward shorter courses of therapy in both adults and children due to the abundant evidence showing non-inferior efficacy compared to longer courses [84, 92–95]. In recent years, guidelines have changed their recommendations to the usage of shorter duration of antibiotic regimens for CAP. But not all patients respond to a standard duration of therapy; therefore, it is advised that clinicians should use clinical stability indicators such as the return of normal vital sign patterns, the capacity to eat, and mental function to determine the length of antibiotic therapy. The recommendation is that the treatment is administered for a minimum of 5 days overall and until the patient reaches stability [84, 95, 96].

In adult patients where *C. pneumonia* is the confirmed etiological agent for pneumonia the following therapy regimens can be given as a 5-day course of antibiotic therapy and according to the patients' clinical stability [84, 95]. The necessity of eradication of *C. pneumoniae* from clinical isolates for treatment success is not known but treatment might be extended up to 10 days in selected cases due to the previously mentioned studies about post-treatment bacterial eradication rates.

- Azithromycin 500 mg orally once a day on the first day then 250 mg daily on the following days for up to 5 days,
- Clarithromycin 500 mg orally two times a day (or clarithromycin extended-release tablet 1 g once a day),
- Erythromycin 500 mg four times a day (for pregnant women),
- Doxycycline 100 mg orally two times a day,
- Levofloxacin 500 or 750 mg orally once a day,
- Moxifloxacin 400 mg orally once a day and
- Gemifloxacin 320 mg orally once a day.

Intravenous (IV) formulations of levofloxacin and moxifloxacin can be given in the same oral dosages to severe patients who are hospitalized and unable to take oral medication [84, 95]. All patients should be reassessed within 3 days for improvement of symptoms and the possibility of transition to oral medication [95].

For children, the recommendations for assessing the duration of antibiotics for pneumonia are the same as the adult patients [95, 97]. The treatment options for confirmed *C. pneumonia* in pediatric patients are:

- Azithromycin 10 mg/kg orally or IV once a day on the first day then 5 mg/kg once daily for up to 5 days,
- Erythromycin 40 mg/kg/day orally divided into four doses or erythromycin lactobionate 20 mg/kg/day IV four times a day,
- Clarithromycin 15 mg/kg/day orally divided into two doses,
- Levofloxacin 16–20 mg/kg/day IV divided into two doses for children 6 months to 5 years old and 8–10 mg/kg/day once a day for children 5 to 16 years old and levofloxacin 500 mg/day orally once a day for adolescents with skeletal maturity (the pediatric dosage of levofloxacin should not exceed 750 mg/day),

- Moxifloxacin 400 mg/day once a day for adolescents with skeletal maturity, and
- Doxycycline 2–4 mg/kg/day orally divided into two doses for children>7 years old (the pediatric dosage of doxycycline should not exceed 200 mg/day).

Similar to adult patients response to therapy and decision to transition to oral therapy should be assessed within 3 days of treatment [97]. Due to the paucity of clinical trials directly evaluating the efficacy of antibiotics on clinical outcomes in children with *C. pneumoniae* pneumonia, the medications might be lengthened to 10 days according to the physician's decision [97].

3.2.1 C. Pneumonia*-related chronic diseases*

The connection between chronic persistent *C. pneumoniae* infection and chronic inflammatory disorders is still up for debate. In addition to contributing to respiratory tract infections, a growing body of research suggests that *C. pneumoniae* may also be involved in the pathogenesis of several inflammatory diseases, including atherosclerosis, arthritis, asthma, chronic obstructive pulmonary disease (COPD), lung cancer, and some neurological conditions such as Alzheimer's disease, multiple sclerosis, and schizophrenia [98]. Among them, patients who have asthma/COPD and present with symptoms of confirmed *C. pneumonia* airway infection should be treated according to the treatment recommendations for acute respiratory infections mentioned above. Due to a paucity of data, there are presently no recommendations for treating any other chronic diseases associated with *C. pneumoniae* infection, other than asthma and COPD [3, 72, 98].

3.3 Treatment of infections due to *C. psittaci*

C. psittaci causes a zoonotic disease called psittacosis, also known as ornithosis. Psittacosis is frequently transmitted to humans predominantly from birds *via* inhalation of dried droppings, feather dust, or respiratory secretions [99, 100]. The disease can manifest clinically in a variety of ways, ranging from asymptomatic disease or non-specific flu-like illness to severe systemic illness with pneumonia [100, 101]. Other complications that may require hospitalization are cardiac infections (such as endocarditis and myocarditis), hepatitis, arthritis, encephalitis, and sepsis [102]. The most typical illness manifestation is an upper respiratory infection. It is assumed that about 1–8% of CAP is caused by psittacosis [101, 103]. The laboratory diagnosis of psittacosis is usually difficult. Clinical application of traditional pathogen culture is uncommon since it takes a long time and requires high-standard laboratory conditions to culture *C. psittaci* in cells. Serological testing is primarily utilized in retrospective research and is not very useful for the earlier detection of severe patients. *C. psittaci* is easily identified by NAAT and metagenomic next-generation sequencing; however, these procedures are not routinely utilized in most hospitals [104]. Therefore, a patient with a history of bird contact who exhibits atypical pneumonia symptoms or unexplained fever without localizing signs, clinicians should consider a diagnosis of psittacosis, and treatment should not await a definitive diagnosis.

Beta-lactam antibiotics are not effective in psittacosis, whereas tetracyclines and macrolides are both effective against *C. psittaci*. Tetracyclines and especially doxycycline is the preferred medication for the treatment of *C. psittaci* pneumoniae [104, 105].

As an alternative or in situations where tetracyclines are prohibited, such as in pregnant women or young children under the age of eight, macrolides such as erythromycin and azithromycin may be utilized [106]. Doxycycline 100 mg orally two times a day for 7 to 10 days is the suggested regimen for psittacosis. Also, a 5 to 7-day regimen of azithromycin (if a clinical response is observed) can be used alternatively. The third-line antibiotics for *C. psittaci* are fluoroquinolones, which have less potency than tetracyclines and macrolides [95, 104, 107]. With proper and early treatment overall prognosis is good and death occurs in less than 1% of patients [102, 104].

4. Conclusions

Chlamydial infections are one of the most prevalent infectious diseases reported worldwide. The spectrum of diseases varies from asymptomatic silent infection to severe disease affecting ocular, genito-urinary, and pulmonary systems. Without proper management, the infections might progress and result in blindness, infertility, sepsis, or death. Antibacterial medications such as tetracyclines, macrolides, and quinolones, which have been used for many years to treat a variety of infections that are also effective for human infections caused by *C. pneumoniae*, *C. trachomatis*, and *C. psittaci*. Although persistent and heritable antibacterial resistance is common in some *Chlamydia* spp. such as *C. suis*, genotypic stable resistance has not been reported in human chlamydial infections. Phenotypic antibacterial resistance might result from the persistence of microorganisms or heterotypic resistance, whereas antibiotic failure might result from non-adherence to medication, re-infection, or choice of regimens with lower success. The laboratory diagnosis of chlamydial infections might be challenging in many centers and patient follow-up cannot be assured on some occasions; therefore, in case of doubt of chlamydial infection early presumptive treatment with recommended regimens, proper follow-up of the patients, prevention of re-infection via patient and partner counseling and protection of susceptible populations by the implementation of screening programs in high-risk patients should be established.

Conflict of interest

The author declares no conflict of interest.

Author details

Hande Berk Cam
Antalya Training and Research Hospital, Clinical Microbiology and Infectious Diseases Clinic, Antalya, Turkey

*Address all correspondence to: handeberk@hotmail.com

References

[1] Chlamydia: Genital and Ocular Infections; Infertility; Atypical Pneumonia - ClinicalKey [Internet]. [cited 2022 Nov 1]. Available from: https://www.clinicalkey.com/#!/content/book/3-s2.0-B9780702072000000345

[2] Geisler WM. Diseases Caused by Chlamydiae [Internet]. Twentieth ed. Goldman's Cecil Medicine. Elsevier Inc.; 2012. pp. 150-156. DOI: 10.1016/B978-0-323-53266-2.00302-7

[3] Sandoz KM, Rockey DD. Antibiotic resistance in Chlamydiae. Future Microbiology. 2010;**5**(9):1427-1442

[4] WHO. Web Annex D: Evidence Profiles and Evidence-to-Decision Frameworks. 2016. Available from: http://apps.who.int/iris/bitstream/handle/10665/246165/9789241549714-webannexD-eng.pdf?sequence=5

[5] Chlamydial Infections - STI Treatment Guidelines [Internet]. [cited 2022 Nov 1]. Available from: https://www.cdc.gov/std/treatment-guidelines/chlamydia.htm

[6] Mestrovic T, Ljubin-Sternak S. Molecular mechanisms of *Chlamydia trachomatis* resistance to antimicrobial drugs. Frontiers in Bioscience - Landmark. 2018;**23**(4):656-670

[7] Hammerschlag MR, Kohlhoff SA. Treatment of chlamydial infections. Expert Opinion on Pharmacotherapy. 2012;**13**(4):545-552

[8] Suchland RJ, Geisler WM, Stamm WE. Methodologies and cell lines used for antimicrobial susceptibility testing of *chlamydia* spp. Antimicrobial Agents and Chemotherapy. 2003;**47**(2):636-642 [Internet]. Available from: https://journals.asm.org/doi/abs/10.1128/AAC.47.2.636-642.2003

[9] Borel N, Leonard C, Slade J, Schoborg RV. Chlamydial antibiotic resistance and treatment failure in veterinary and human medicine. Current Clinical Microbiology Reports. 2016;**3**(1):10-18

[10] Lenart J, Andersen AA, Rockey DD. Growth and development of tetracycline-resistant chlamydia suis. Antimicrobial Agents and Chemotherapy. 2001;**45**(8):2198-2203

[11] Hogan RJ, Mathews SA, Mukhopadhyay S, Summersgill JT, Timms P. Chlamydial persistence: Beyond the biphasic paradigm. Infection and Immunity. 2004;**72**(4):1843-1855 [Internet]. Available from: https://journals.asm.org/doi/10.1128/IAI.72.4.1843-1855.2004

[12] Pandey N, Cascella M. Beta Lactam Antibiotics. Antibiotic Discovery and Development. 2022;**9781461414001**:79-117. [Internet] [cited 2022 Nov 14]. Available from: https://www.ncbi.nlm.nih.gov/books/NBK545311/

[13] Darville T. Chlamydia infections. In: Infectious Diseases of the Fetus and Newborn Infant. Philadelphia: Elsevier; 2006. pp. 385-392. [Internet] [cited 2022 Nov 17]. Available from: https://linkinghub.elsevier.com/retrieve/pii/B072160537050013X

[14] Wyrick PB. *Chlamydia trachomatis* persistence In vitro: An overview. The Journal of Infectious Diseases. 2010;**201**(S2):88-95 [Internet]. Available from: https://academic.oup.com/jid/article-lookup/doi/10.1086/652394

[15] Wyrick PB, Knight ST. Pre-exposure of infected human endometrial

epithelial cells to penicillin in vitro renders *Chlamydia trachomatis* refractory to azithromycin. The Journal of Antimicrobial Chemotherapy. 2004;**54**(1):79-85

[16] Kutlin A, Roblin PM, Hammerschlag MR. In vitro activities of azithromycin and ofloxacin against chlamydia pneumoniae in a continuous-infection model. Antimicrobial Agents and Chemotherapy. 1999;**43**(9):2268-2272

[17] Reveneau N, Crane DD, Fischer E, Caldwell HD. Bactericidal activity of first-choice antibiotics against gamma interferon-induced persistent infection of human epithelial cells by *Chlamydia trachomatis*. Antimicrobial Agents and Chemotherapy. 2005;**49**(5):1787-1793

[18] Tien V, Punjabi C, Holubar MK. Antimicrobial resistance in sexually transmitted infections. Journal of Travel Medicine. 2020;**27**(1):1-11

[19] Binet R, Maurelli AT. Frequency of development and associated physiological cost of azithromycin resistance in *chlamydia psittaci* 6BC and *C. trachomatis* L2. Antimicrobial Agents and Chemotherapy. 2007;**51**(12):4267-4275 [Internet]. Available from: https://journals.asm.org/doi/abs/10.1128/AAC.00962-07

[20] Antibiotic Resistance [Internet]. [cited 2022 Nov 19]. Available from: https://www.who.int/news-room/fact-sheets/detail/antibiotic-resistance

[21] Benamri I, Azzouzi M, Sanak K, Moussa A, Radouani F. An overview of genes and mutations associated with Chlamydiae species' resistance to antibiotics. Annals of Clinical Microbiology and Antimicrobials. 2021;**20**(1):1-11. [Internet]. DOI: 10.1186/s12941-021-00465-4

[22] O'Neill CE, Seth-Smith HMB, Van Der Pol B, Harris SR, Thomson NR, Cutcliffe LT, et al. *Chlamydia trachomatis* clinical isolates identified as tetracycline resistant do not exhibit resistance in vitro: Whole-genome sequencing reveals a mutation in porB but no evidence for tetracycline resistance genes. Microbiology (Reading, England). 2013;**159**(Pt 4):748-756

[23] Dinos GP. The macrolide antibiotic renaissance. British Journal of Pharmacology. 2017;**174**(18):2967-2983 [Internet]. Available from: https://bpspubs.onlinelibrary.wiley.com/doi/abs/10.1111/bph.13936

[24] Hooper DC. Emerging mechanisms of fluoroquinolone resistance. Emerging Infectious Diseases. 2001;**7**(2):337-341

[25] Aldred KJ, Kerns RJ, Osheroff N. Mechanism of quinolone action and resistance. Biochemistry. 2014;**53**(10):1565-1574

[26] Kutlin A, Kohlhoff S, Roblin P, Hammerschlag MR, Riska P. Emergence of resistance to rifampin and rifalazil in Chlamydophila pneumoniae and *Chlamydia trachomatis*. Antimicrobial Agents and Chemotherapy. 2005;**49**(3):903-907

[27] DeMars R, Weinfurter J, Guex E, Lin J, Potucek Y. Lateral gene transfer In vitro in the intracellular pathogen *Chlamydia trachomatis*. Journal of Bacteriology. 2007;**189**(3):991-1003 [Internet]. Available from: https://journals.asm.org/doi/abs/10.1128/JB.00845-06

[28] Burton MJ. Trachoma: An overview. British Medical Bulletin. 2007;**84**(1):99-116

[29] Balasopoulou A, Kokkinos P, Pagoulatos D, Plotas P, Makri OE, Georgakopoulos CD, et al. Symposium

recent advances and challenges in the management of retinoblastoma globe - saving treatments. BMC Ophthalmology. 2017;**17**(1):1 [Internet]. Available from: http://www.ncbi.nlm.nih.gov/pubmed/28331284%0Ahttp://www.pubmedcentral.nih.gov/articlerender.fcgi?artid=PMC5354527%5Cnhttp://bmcpsychiatry.biomedcentral.com/articles/10.1186/1471-244X-11-49%5Cnhttp://bmcophthalmol.biomedcentral.com/articles/10.1186/s12886

[30] Sarier M, Demir M, Turgut H, Hizel A, Emek M, Kukul E, et al. New approach to microscopy of gram-stained urethral smear: The kissing slide method. Sexually Transmitted Diseases. 2020;**47**(10):712-715

[31] Juliana NCA, Omar AM, Pleijster J, Aftab F, Uijldert NB, Ali SM, et al. The natural course of *Chlamydia trachomatis*, neisseria gonorrhoeae, trichomonas vaginalis, and mycoplasma genitalium in pregnant and post-delivery women in Pemba island, Tanzania. Microorganisms. 2021;**9**(6):1180

[32] Centers for Disease Control and Prevention. Chlamydia Detailed Fact Sheet. 2022. pp. 1-7. Available from: https://www.cdc.gov/std/chlamydia/stdfact-chlamydia-detailed.htm#:~:text=Estimates show that 1 in,14-24 years has chlamydia.&text=Disparities persist among racial and,six times that of Whites.&text=Chlamydia is also common among MSM

[33] Rours GIJG, Duijts L, Moll HA, Arends LR, de Groot R, Jaddoe VW, et al. *Chlamydia trachomatis* infection during pregnancy associated with preterm delivery: A population-based prospective cohort study. European Journal of Epidemiology. 2011;**26**(6):493-502

[34] Carter JD, Inman RD. Chlamydia-induced reactive arthritis: Hidden in plain sight? Best Practice & Research Clinical Rheumatology. 2011;**25**(3):359-374

[35] Fleming DT, Wasserheit JN. From epidemiological synergy to public health policy and practice: The contribution of other sexually transmitted diseases to sexual transmission of HIV infection. Sexually Transmitted Infections. 1999;**75**(1):3-17

[36] Trachoma [Internet]. [cited 2022 Nov 20]. Available from: https://www.who.int/news-room/fact-sheets/detail/trachoma

[37] Trachoma | MSF Medical Guidelines [Internet]. [cited 2023 Jan 13]. Available from: https://medicalguidelines.msf.org/en/viewport/CG/english/trachoma-16689733.html

[38] Evans JR, Solomon AW, Kumar R, Perez Á, Singh BP, Srivastava RM, et al. Antibiotics for trachoma. Cochrane Database of Systematic Reviews [Internet]. 2019 Sep 25 [cited 2022 Nov 20];(9). Available from: https://doi.wiley.com/10.1002/14651858.CD001860.pub4

[39] Tian L, Wang NL. Trachoma control: The SAFE strategy. International Journal of Ophthalmology. 2018;**11**(12):1887-1888

[40] World Health Organization. WHO alliance for the global elimination of trachoma by 2020: Progress report, 2019. Weekly Epidemiological Record. 2020;**95**(30):349-360 [Internet]. Available from: https://pesquisa.bvsalud.org/portal/resource/en/mdl-20203426091

[41] Schachter J, Grossman M, Sweet RL, Holt J, Jordan C, Bishop E. Prospective study of perinatal transmission of *Chlamydia trachomatis*. Journal of the American Medical Association. 1986;**255**(24):3374-3377

[42] Rours IGIJG, Hammerschlag MR, Ott A, De Faber TJTHN, Verbrugh HA, de Groot R, et al. *Chlamydia trachomatis* as a cause of neonatal conjunctivitis in Dutch infants. Pediatrics. 2008;**121**(2): e321-e326

[43] Workowski KA, Bachmann LH, Chan PA, Johnston CM, Muzny CA, Park I, et al. Sexually transmitted infections treatment guidelines, 2021. MMWR Recommendations and Reports. 2021;**70**(4):1-187 [Internet] [cited 2022 Nov 28]. Available from: https://www.cdc.gov/mmwr/volumes/70/rr/rr7004a1.htm

[44] Zikic A, Schünemann H, Wi T, Lincetto O, Broutet N, Santesso N. Treatment of neonatal chlamydial conjunctivitis: A systematic review and meta-analysis. Journal of the Pediatric Infectious Diseases Society. 2018;7(3):e107-e115

[45] Niforatos JD, Rothman RE. Sexually transmitted infections treatment guidelines, 2021. Annals of Emergency Medicine. 2022;**80**(1):68-70

[46] Heggie AD. Topical Sulfacetamide vs Oral erythromycin for neonatal chlamydial conjunctivitis. Archives of Pediatrics & Adolescent Medicine. 1985;**139**(6):564 [Internet]. Available from: http://archpedi.jamanetwork.com/article.aspx?doi=10.1001/archpedi.1985.02140080034027

[47] Hammerschlag MR. Chlamydial and gonococcal infections in infants and children. Clinical Infectious Diseases. 2011;**53**(suppl_3):S99-S102 [Internet]. Available from: http://academic.oup.com/cid/article/53/suppl_3/S99/312712/Chlamydial-and-Gonococcal-Infections-in-Infants

[48] Lee WJA, Chen CC. Adult inclusion conjunctivitis diagnosed by polymerase chain reaction and Giemsa stain. IDCases. Netherlands. 2022;**27**:e01367

[49] Sarıer M. Prevalence of Polymicrobial infection in urethritis. Journal of Urological Surgery. 2019;**6**(3):180-183

[50] Sarıer M, Duman İ, Göktaş Ş. Demirorcid.org M, Kukul E. results of multiplex polymerase chain reaction assay to identify urethritis pathogens. Journal of Urological Surgery. 2017;**4**(1):18-22

[51] Recommendations for the laboratory-based detection of Chlamydia trachomatis and Neisseria gonorrhoeae--2014. MMWR Recommendations and reports: Morbidity and mortality weekly report. Recommendations and reports. 2014;**63**(RR-02):1-19

[52] Sarier M, Sepin N, Duman I, Demir M, Hizel A, Göktaş Ş, et al. Microscopy of gram-stained urethral smear in the diagnosis of urethritis: Which threshold value should be selected? Andrologia. 2018;**50**(10):1-4

[53] World Health Organization (WHO). Guidelines for the Management of Symptomatic Sexually Transmitted Infections [Internet]. 2021. p. 216. Available from: https://pubmed.ncbi.nlm.nih.gov/34370424/

[54] Kong FYS, Tabrizi SN, Fairley CK, Vodstrcil LA, Huston WM, Chen M, et al. The efficacy of azithromycin and doxycycline for the treatment of rectal chlamydia infection: A systematic review and meta-analysis. Journal of Antimicrobial Chemotherapy. 2014;**70**(5):1290-1297

[55] Páez-Canro C, Alzate JP, Gonzalez LM, Rubio-Romero JA, Lethaby A, Gaitan HG. Antibiotics for treating urogenital *Chlamydia trachomatis* infection in men and non-pregnant women. Cochrane Database of Systematic Reviews. [Internet]. 2019 Jan 25 [cited 2022 Nov 28];**2019**(3).

Available from: http://doi.wiley.com/10.1002/14651858.CD010871.pub2

[56] Lau A, Kong FYS, Fairley CK, Templeton DJ, Amin J, Phillips S, et al. Azithromycin or doxycycline for asymptomatic rectal *Chlamydia trachomatis*. The New England Journal of Medicine. 2021;**384**(25):2418-2427

[57] Dombrowski JC, Wierzbicki MR, Newman LM, Powell JA, Miller A, Dithmer D, et al. Doxycycline versus azithromycin for the treatment of rectal chlamydia in men who have sex with men: A randomized controlled trial. Clinical Infectious Diseases : an Official Publication of the Infectious Diseases Society of America. 2021;**73**(5):824-831

[58] Khosropour CM, Dombrowski JC, Barbee LA, Manhart LE, Golden MR. Comparing azithromycin and doxycycline for the treatment of rectal chlamydial infection: A retrospective cohort study. Sexually Transmitted Diseases. 2014;**41**(2):79-85

[59] Dukers-Muijrers NHTM, Wolffs PFG, De Vries H, Götz HM, Heijman T, Bruisten S, et al. Treatment effectiveness of azithromycin and doxycycline in uncomplicated rectal and vaginal *Chlamydia trachomatis* infections in women: A multicenter observational study (FemCure). Clinical Infectious Diseases. 2019;**69**(11):1946-1954. [Internet]. DOI: 10.1093/cid/ciz050

[60] Manavi K, Hettiarachchi N, Hodson J. Comparison of doxycycline with azithromycin in treatment of pharyngeal chlamydia infection. International journal of STD & AIDS. 2016;**27**(14):1303-1308

[61] Dukers-Muijrers NHTM, Schachter J, van Liere GAFS, Wolffs PFG, Hoebe CJPA. What is needed to guide testing for anorectal and pharyngeal *Chlamydia trachomatis* and *Neisseria gonorrhoeae* in women and men? Evidence and opinion. BMC Infectious Diseases. [Internet] 2015;**15**(1):533. DOI: 10.1186/s12879-015-1280-6

[62] Kent CK, Chaw JK, Wong W, Liska S, Gibson S, Hubbard G, et al. Prevalence of rectal, urethral, and pharyngeal chlamydia and gonorrhea detected in 2 clinical settings among men who have sex with men: San Francisco, California, 2003. Clinical Infectious Diseases: an Official Publication of the Infectious Diseases Society of America. 2005;**41**(1):67-74

[63] Bradley MG, Hobson D, Lee N, Tait IA, Rees E. Chlamydial infections of the urethra in women. Genitourinary Medicine. 1985;**61**(6):371-375

[64] Sarier M, Kukul E. Classification of non-gonococcal urethritis: A review. International Urology and Nephrology. 2019;**51**(6):901-907. [Internet]. DOI: 10.1007/s11255-019-02140-2

[65] Urethritis and Cervicitis - STI Treatment Guidelines [Internet]. [cited 2022 Nov 27]. Available from: https://www.cdc.gov/std/treatment-guidelines/urethritis-and-cervicitis.htm

[66] Moi H, Blee K, Horner PJ. Management of non-gonococcal urethritis. BMC Infectious Diseases. 2015;**15**:294

[67] Marcus JL, Kohn RP, Barry PM, Philip SS, Bernstein KT. *Chlamydia trachomatis* and *Neisseria gonorrhoeae* transmission from the female oropharynx to the male urethra. Sexually Transmitted Diseases. 2011;**38**(5):372-373

[68] Bernstein KT, Stephens SC, Barry PM, Kohn R, Philip SS, Liska S, et al. *Chlamydia trachomatis* and *Neisseria gonorrhoeae* transmission from the oropharynx to the urethra among men

who have sex with men. Clinical Infectious Diseases: an Official Publication of the Infectious Diseases Society of America. 2009;**49**(12):1793-1797

[69] Trojian TH, Lishnak TS, Heiman D. Epididymitis and orchitis: An overview. American Family Physician. 2009;**79**(7):583-587

[70] Scieux C, Barnes R, Bianchi A, Casin I, Morel P, Perol Y. Lymphogranuloma Venereum: 27 cases in Paris. The Journal of Infectious Diseases. 1989;**160**(4):662-668. [Internet]. DOI: 10.1093/infdis/160.4.662

[71] Koper NE, van der Sande MA, Gotz HM, Koedijk FD, on behalf of the Dutch STI clinics C. Lymphogranuloma venereum among men who have sex with men in the Netherlands: Regional differences in testing rates lead to underestimation of the incidence, 2006-2012. Eurosurveillance [Internet]. Aug 2013;**18**(34):2006-2012. Available from: https://www.eurosurveillance.org/content/10.2807/1560-7917.ES2013.18.34.20561

[72] Kohlhoff SA, Hammerschlag MR. Treatment of chlamydial infections: 2014 update. Expert Opinion on Pharmacotherapy. 2015;**16**(2):205-212

[73] Nwokolo NC, Dragovic B, Patel S, Tong CW, Barker G, Radcliffe K. 2015 UK national guideline for the management of infection with *Chlamydia trachomatis*. International Journal of STD and AIDS. 2016;**27**(4):251-267

[74] Chlamydia and LGV guide: Treatment and follow-up - Canada.ca [Internet]. [cited 2022 Dec 5]. Available from: https://www.canada.ca/en/public-health/services/infectious-diseases/sexual-health-sexually-transmitted-infections/canadian-guidelines/chlamydia-lgv/treatment-follow-up.html

[75] James G. H. Dinulos. Sexually transmitted bacterial infections. Habif's Clinical Dermatology. 2020;**1**:376-412

[76] Fan H, Gilbert R, O'Callaghan F, Li L. Associations between macrolide antibiotics prescribing during pregnancy and adverse child outcomes in the UK: Population based cohort study. BMJ (Clinical research ed). 2020;**368**:m331

[77] Op de Coul ELM, Peek D, van Weert YWM, Morré SA, Rours I, Hukkelhoven C, et al. *Chlamydia trachomatis*, *Neisseria gonorrhoea*, and *Trichomonas vaginalis* infections among pregnant women and male partners in Dutch midwifery practices: Prevalence, risk factors, and perinatal outcomes. Reproductive Health. 2021;**18**(1):132. [Internet]. DOI: 10.1186/s12978-021-01179-8

[78] Beem MO, Saxon E, Tipple MA. Treatment of chlamydial pneumonia of infancy. Pediatrics. 1979;**63**(2):198-203

[79] Kvien TK, Gaston JSH, Bardin T, Butrimiene I, Dijkmans BAC, Leirisalo-Repo M, et al. Three month treatment of reactive arthritis with azithromycin: A EULAR double blind, placebo controlled study. Annals of the Rheumatic Diseases. 2004;**63**(9):1113-1119

[80] Yli-Kerttula T, Luukkainen R, Yli-Kerttula U, Möttönen T, Hakola M, Korpela M, et al. Effect of a three month course of ciprofloxacin on the late prognosis of reactive arthritis. Annals of the Rheumatic Diseases. 2003;**62**(9):880-884

[81] *Chlamydia pneumoniae*: Clinical Features and Complications | CDC [Internet]. [cited 2022 Dec 7]. Available from: https://www.cdc.gov/pneumonia/atypical/cpneumoniae/hcp/clinical.html

[82] Marchello C, Dale AP, Thai TN, Han DS, Ebell MH. Prevalence of atypical

pathogens in patients with cough and community-acquired pneumonia: A meta-analysis. The Annals of Family Medicine. 2016;**14**(6):552 LP-552566 [Internet]. Available from: http://www.annfammed.org/content/14/6/552.abstract

[83] Shibli F, Chazan B, Nitzan O, Flatau E, Edelstein H, Blondheim O, et al. Etiology of community-acquired pneumonia in hospitalized patients in northern Israel. The Israel Medical Association journal : IMAJ. 2010;**12**(8):477-482

[84] Metlay JP, Waterer GW, Long AC, Anzueto A, Brozek J, Crothers K, et al. Diagnosis and treatment of adults with community-acquired pneumonia. American Journal of Respiratory and Critical Care Medicine. 2019;**200**(7):E45-E67

[85] Shim JY. Current perspectives on atypical pneumonia in children. Clin Exp Pediatr. 2020;**63**(12):469-476. [Internet]. DOI: 10.3345/cep.2019.00360

[86] Harris JA, Kolokathis A, Campbell M, Cassell GH, Hammerschlag MR. Safety and efficacy of azithromycin in the treatment of community-acquired pneumonia in children. The Pediatric Infectious Disease Journal. 1998;**17**(10):865-871

[87] Roblin PM, Hammerschlag MR. Microbiologic efficacy of azithromycin and susceptibilities to azithromycin of isolates of chlamydia pneumoniae from adults and children with community-acquired pneumonia. Antimicrobial Agents and Chemotherapy. 1998;**42**(1):194-196

[88] Block S, Hedrick J, Hammerschlag MR, Cassell GH, Craft JC. Mycoplasma pneumoniae and chlamydia pneumoniae in pediatric community-acquired pneumonia: Comparative efficacy and safety of clarithromycin vs. erythromycin ethylsuccinate. The Pediatric Infectious Disease Journal. 1995;**14**(6):471-477

[89] Hammerschlag MR, Roblin PM. Microbiologic efficacy of moxifloxacin for the treatment of community-acquired pneumonia due to chlamydia pneumoniae. International Journal of Antimicrobial Agents. 2000;**15**(2):149-152

[90] Hammerschlag MR, Roblin PM. Microbiological efficacy of levofloxacin for treatment of community-acquired pneumonia due to chlamydia pneumoniae. Antimicrobial Agents and Chemotherapy. United States. 2000;**44**:1409

[91] Roblin PM, Montalban G, Hammerschlag MR. Susceptibilities to clarithromycin and erythromycin of isolates of chlamydia pneumoniae from children with pneumonia. Antimicrobial Agents and Chemotherapy. 1994;**38**(7):1588-1589

[92] el Moussaoui R, de Borgie CAJM, van den Broek P, Hustinx WN, Bresser P, van den Berk GEL, et al. Effectiveness of discontinuing antibiotic treatment after three days versus eight days in mild to moderate-severe community acquired pneumonia: Randomised, double blind study. BMJ (Clinical research ed). 2006;**332**(7554):1355

[93] Tansarli GS, Eleftherios M. Systematic Review and Meta-analysis of the Efficacy of Short-Course Antibiotic Treatments for Community-Acquired Pneumonia in Adults. Antimicrobial Agents and Chemotherapy [Internet]. 27 Aug 2018;**62**(9):e00635-e00618. DOI: 10.1128/AAC.00635-18

[94] Same RG, Amoah J, Hsu AJ, Hersh AL, Sklansky DJ, Cosgrove SE, et al. The Association of Antibiotic Duration with successful treatment of

community-acquired pneumonia in children. Journal of the Pediatric Infectious Diseases Society. 2021;**10**(3):267-273

[95] NICE. Summary of Antimicrobial Prescribing Guidance - Managing Common Infections. 2019;(February):1-23. Available from: https://www.nice.org.uk/about/what-we-do/our-programmes/nice-guidance/antimicrobial-prescribing-guidelines

[96] Lee RA, Centor RM, Humphrey LL, Jokela JA, Andrews R, Qaseem A, et al. Appropriate Use of Short-Course Antibiotics in Common Infections: Best Practice Advice From the American College of Physicians. Annals of Internal Medicine [Internet]. 2021;**174**(6):822-827. DOI: 10.7326/M20-7355

[97] Bradley JS, Byington CL, Shah SS, Alverson B, Carter ER, Harrison C, et al. The management of community-acquired pneumonia in infants and children older than 3 months of age: Clinical practice guidelines by the Pediatric Infectious Diseases Society and the Infectious Diseases Society of America. Clinical infectious diseases: an official publication of the Infectious Diseases Society of America. 2011;**53**(7):e25-e76

[98] Porritt RA, Crother TR. Chlamydia pneumoniae infection and inflammatory diseases. Forum on Immunopathological Diseases and Therapeutics. 2016;**7**(3-4): 237-254 [Internet]. Available from: http://www.dl.begellhouse.com/journals/1a654bf03faf67ac,6deddb8911c6adff,516cae7d4008babc.html

[99] Psittacosis: Clinical Disease Specifics | CDC [Internet]. [cited 2023 Jan 13]. Available from: https://www.cdc.gov/pneumonia/atypical/psittacosis/hcp/disease-specifics.html

[100] Psittacosis - GOV.UK [Internet]. [cited 2023 Jan 13]. Available from: https://www.gov.uk/guidance/psittacosis

[101] Hogerwerf L, DE Gier B, Baan B, VAN DER Hoek W. Chlamydia psittaci (psittacosis) as a cause of community-acquired pneumonia: A systematic review and meta-analysis. Epidemiology and infection. 2017;**145**(15):3096-3105

[102] Surg AM. Psittacosis: Clinical features and complications. CDC. 2022;**31**(April 2013):2-3 Available from: https://www.cdc.gov/pneumonia/atypical/psittacosis/hcp/clinical-features-complications.html

[103] Yin Q, Li Y, Pan H, Hui T, Yu Z, Wu H, et al. Atypical pneumonia caused by chlamydia psittaci during the COVID-19 pandemic. International Journal of Infectious Diseases: IJID : Official Publication of the International Society for Infectious Diseases. 2022;**122**:622-627

[104] Liu J, Gao Y. Tigecycline in the treatment of severe pneumonia caused by chlamydia psittaci: A case report and literature review. Frontiers in Medicine. 2022;**9**(November):1-10

[105] Psittacosis: Clinical Diagnosis, Treatment, and Prevention | CDC [Internet]. [cited 2023 Jan 13]. Available from: https://www.cdc.gov/pneumonia/atypical/psittacosis/hcp/diagnosis-treatment-prevention.html

[106] Psittacosis - StatPearls - NCBI Bookshelf [Internet]. [cited 2022 Dec 13]. Available from: https://www.ncbi.nlm.nih.gov/books/NBK538305/

[107] Mi H, Li H, Yu J. Psittacosis. Radiology of Infectious Diseases. 2022;**2**:207-212 [Internet] [cited 2022 Dec 13]. Available from: https://www.ncbi.nlm.nih.gov/books/NBK538305/

Chapter 8

Persistence in *Chlamydia*

Ramón Scharbaai-Vázquez, Francisco J. López Font and Félix A. Zayas Rodríguez

Abstract

Chlamydia spp. are important causes of acute and persistent/chronic infections. All *Chlamydia spp.* display a unique biphasic developmental cycle alternating between an infectious elementary body (EB) and a replicative form, the reticulate body (RB), followed by the multiplication of RBs by binary fission and progressive differentiation back into EBs. During its intracellular life, *Chlamydia* employs multiple mechanisms to ensure its persistence inside the host. These include evasion of diverse innate immune responses, modulation of host cell structure and endocytosis, inhibition of apoptosis, activation of pro-signaling pathways, and conversion to enlarged, non-replicative but viable "aberrant bodies" (ABs). Early research described several systems for Chlamydial persistence with a significant number of variables that make a direct comparison of results difficult. Now, emerging tools for genetic manipulations in *Chlamydia* and advances in global microarray, transcriptomics, and proteomics have opened new and exciting opportunities to understand the persistent state of *Chlamydia* and link the immune and molecular events of persistence with the pathogenesis of recurrent and chronic Chlamydial infections. This chapter reviews our current understanding and advances in the molecular biology of *Chlamydia* persistence.

Keywords: *Chlamydia* persistence, elementary bodies (EBs), reticulate bodies (RBs), aberrant bodies (ABs), inclusion, inhibition of apoptosis, non-coding RNAs, pro-survival pathways, genome-scale analyses, interference innate immune system

1. Introduction

1.1 Overview of Chlamydial persistence

Persistence is the ability of bacteria to remain viable in the host for a prolonged period of time. Bacteria have evolved several strategies by which subpopulations can survive conditions that are lethal for most members of bacterial populations. Well-known examples are the formation of endospores in Bacillales and Clostridiales orders, the formation of exospores in Actinomycetales, the presence of "persister" cells occurring in most bacteria, and the formation of viable but nonculturable cells [1]. All the survival stages are characterized by partial or complete inhibition of metabolism and cell division. Common to all of these survival states is the ability of the "persister" cells to resume their developmental stage under favorable conditions [1].

In the context of *Chlamydia*, persistence or Chlamydial stress response is the reversible inhibition of cell division that interrupts the pathogen's developmental cycle in the presence of unfavorable growth conditions [2]. Chlamydial persistence *in vitro* is characterized by the presence of a "viable but non-cultivable growth stage resulting in a long-term relationship with the infected cell" [3]. Persistence is an important cause of recurrent Chlamydial disease characterized by chronic inflammation and tissue damage in epithelial cells. This chapter will discuss the recent developments in our understanding of *Chlamydia* persistence, focusing on past and current insights that have been obtained into the molecular and immunological basis of this stage of *Chlamydia* development.

2. The Chlamydial developmental life cycle

Chlamydiae are gram-negative obligate intracellular pathogens characterized by their biphasic life cycle [4–6]. *Chlamydiae* primarily infect mucosal epithelial cells and alternate between two morphologic forms. The first, known as the elementary body (EB), is the infectious form that attaches to the cell membrane of a host cell. Shortly after interacting with host cell membrane receptors, the bacterial ligands induce endocytosis of the pathogenic EB, leading to the creation of an EB-containing vacuole known as the inclusion [4]. Once inside the cell, the EB within the inclusion takes around 6–8 hours to transform into the second morphologic subtype, known as the reticulate body (RB). The RB modifies the inclusion's membrane to prevent its degradation, while also prompting migration of the inclusion toward the microtubule-organization center (MTOC) to facilitate movement toward nutrient-rich areas within the host cell (e.g., periphery of the Golgi apparatus) [4].

Due to the parasitic nature of *Chlamydiae,* these pathogens not only rely on essential nutrients from the host cell but also require several metabolic enzymes, which are subsequently hijacked from the host. Thus, approximately 8–16 hours after infection, the mid-cycle begins, where the RB produces effectors that facilitate the looting of nutrients and enzymatic hijacking [2, 4]. Finally, after 24 hours of replication and growth, RBs can revert to EBs via an asynchronous process that allows them to exit the host cell (e.g., cell lysis or extrusion). *Chlamydiae* can also transform into a third morphologic subtype under certain conditions. When *Chlamydiae* experience physiologic stressors, RBs can transform into abnormally large bacteria known as an aberrant body (AB) [4]. ABs are characterized by their non-infectious "hibernating" state, allowing them to re-enter the normal biphasic life cycle once the underlying stressor subsides to continue producing infectious EBs [4].

3. Overview of *Chlamydia* pathogenesis

3.1 Acute infections

Chlamydia species cause widespread infections in humans. *Chlamydia trachomatis* serovars A–C are the leading cause of non-congenital trachoma and are the major cause of blindness and visual impairment in developing nations [7, 8]. *C. trachomatis* serovars D–K are considered the world's most common sexually transmitted pathogen causing disease in the genital tract and in men, are the primary cause of non-gonococcal urethritis [7, 9]. Following vertical transmission through an infected birth canal, *C. trachomatis* serovars D–K cause neonatal conjunctivitis and pneumonia. Respiratory infection with *C. pneumoniae* causes an average of 10% of community-acquired pneumonia cases and 5% of bronchitis and sinusitis cases. In addition, avian strains of *C. psittaci* have long been known to cause zoonotic respiratory illness in humans [10]. The *C. trachomatis* lymphogranuloma venereum (LGV) biovar (serovars L1–L3) causes invasive urogenital or anorectal infection [11].

3.2 Persistent and chronic Chlamydial infections

C. trachomatis serovars D–K are responsible for about 15–40% of ascending upper genital tract infections leading to serious complications in women, such as salpingitis, pelvic inflammatory disease, ectopic pregnancy, epididymitis in men, and infertility in women and men [8]. *C. trachomatis* originating from the genital tract is also associated with reactive arthritis, which develops in 1-3% of patients after genital Chlamydial infection [9]. *C. pneumoniae*, which can also disseminate from the site of the initial infection, is linked to several chronic diseases, including asthma, atherosclerosis, arthritis, cardiovascular disease, and even late-onset Alzheimer's disease [12]. In addition, unresolved respiratory *C. pneumoniae* infection may contribute to the pathogenesis of chronic inflammatory lung diseases, such as asthma and chronic obstructive pulmonary disease [12]. Further, *C. trachomatis* impedes human papillomavirus (HPV)-induced mechanisms that maintain cellular and genomic integrity, and it may be linked to cervical cancer [13].

Clinical conditions associated with inapparent *Chlamydial* infections include asymptomatic urethritis in male individuals and cervicitis in female individuals, and silent pelvic inflammatory disease in female individuals [3, 14]. The clinical significance of persistent infection is associated with the reactivation of infection after weeks or months in individuals treated with antibiotics, and negative culture results for individuals with strong serological titers and epidemiological associations [3].

4. Structural elements contributing to persistent infection in *Chlamydia*

4.1 The Chlamydial inclusion

In *Chlamydia*, a large part of the intracellular survival strategy involves the formation of a unique membrane-bound vacuole called an inclusion. The inclusion represents the ideal "protected niche" that ensures *Chlamydia* its survival by evading the endolysosomal pathway and the innate immune responses of the cell and favoring its growth by modulating host cell processes. Active transcription and translation within the lumen of the inclusion are required for the transition from the non-replicative ER to the replicative, morphologically larger RB. Concomitantly, the nascent *Chlamydia*-containing inclusions traffic along microtubules from the cell periphery to the microtubule organizing center (MTOC), where the inclusion resides for the duration of the life cycle [15].

The inclusion membrane (IM) serves as the means by which the bacterium communicates with the host cell. A notable component of the IM is the *Chlamydia*-specific Type III secretion (T3SS) effector transmembrane Inclusion membrane proteins (Incs) [16], Reviewed in [17]. Bioinformatic studies have estimated that *C. trachomatis* encodes 50–100 putative Incs proteins, which represent approximately 6% of the coding capacity of the organism [18]. At least, three classes of Incs have been identified during the Chlamydial developmental cycle: early-cycle Incs (highest mRNA levels between ~2 and 6 h post-infection); mid-cycle Incs (highest mRNA levels between 6 and 20 h post-infection); and late-cycle Incs (highest mRNA levels after ~20 h post-infection) [19]. The activity of some of these Incs proteins is important to ensure the *Chlamydia* long-term survival through the acquisition of nutrients, avoidance of fusion of the inclusion with lysosomes, stability of the inclusion membrane, and modulation of host cell death. For instance, *C. trachomatis* CpoS (*Chlamydia* promoter of Survival), Inclusion membrane C and CT383 have been reported to inhibit host cell death processes in *Chlamydia*-infected cells by controlling inclusion membrane stability [20, 21]. In addition, some Chlamydial Incs interfere with the innate host immune signaling [22]. Recent studies using conditional Incs mutants in *C. trachomatis* and *Chlamydia muridarum* has identified Incs as a key effector in the transition from infectious (EB) to replicative (RB) during the early stages of *Chlamydia* development in vivo [23]. Although only a few Incs have been characterized to date, the role of many Incs remains largely unknown.

4.1.1 Role of actin in the inclusion maturation

After the invasion, *Chlamydia* continues to manipulate the host cytoskeleton by assembling and maintaining an actin-rich cage around the Chlamydial inclusion [24]. One of the components of the actin cage (F-actin ring) provides structural rigidity and stability to the mature inclusion, as demonstrated by its resistance to nonionic detergents and the antimitotic agent nocodazole [25]. Intermediate filaments have also been shown to contribute to the stability and function of the inclusion cage by providing additional rigidity. Once the invasion is complete, actin is recruited via a RhoA/ROCK-mediated actin contraction signal pathway to the maturing inclusion alongside the intermediate filaments and septins, providing dynamic structural reinforcement to *Chlamydia's* replicative niche [25]. Other studies suggest that the actin-ring cage formation may depend upon the de novo, unbranched polymerization of actin at inclusions [26]. The two proposed models of actin cage suggest that mechanism of cage assembly changes with the maturation of the inclusion. While the precise mechanism of F-actin synthesis and regulation within the actin cage is somewhat unclear, further study will give an insight into the dynamics of the inclusion vacuole during the Chlamydial persistent stage.

4.2 Aberrant bodies

Under non-bacteriocidal stress conditions, *Chlamydia* responds by markedly arresting RB division and differentiates into an atypical morphology referred to as aberrant body (AB) [3]. ABs are capable of remaining viable within the inclusion vacuole for extended period of time. Aberrant bodies were first described in 1993 on *Chlamydia* cultured on McCoy cells and incubated in Eagle's minimal essential medium lacking all 13 amino acids [27]. *Chlamydia* AB formation is also induced *in vitro* by antibiotics (beta-lactam antibiotics, fosfomycin, novobiocin, fosmidomycin, and *Azithromycin*) [28–33]), depletion of essential nutrients (i.e., iron, amino acids, and glucose), heat shock, coinfection with Herpes Simplex virus [27, 34–39], infection of monocytes and macrophages [40–42], cytokines (Interferon-gamma and IFN-γ) [43], and a number of other pressures [44, 45]. AB in certain Chlamydial species is also induced by treatment with LPC-011 (LPC), a potent inhibitor of the zinc-dependent cytoplasmic deacetylase LpxC, which catalyzed the first step in the Chlamydial lipooligosaccharide (LOS) biosynthesis pathway [46]. When the stress stimulus is removed, cell division in the ABs resumes, allowing *Chlamydia* to complete the developmental cycle. ABs have been classically distinguished by their enlarged size (2–10 mm; for reference, the EB is ≤0.5 μm and the RB is ~1 μm), the inhibition of cell division, and the inhibition of EB production [3]. However, a recent study using immunolabeling has shown that bacterial cell enlargement is not a prerequisite for persistence in *C. trachomatis* [2]. In addition, aberrant *Chlamydia* exhibits differences in the capacity to synthesize the cell wall polymer peptidoglycan in the presence of different aberrance-inducing conditions [2]. Moreover, some AB inducers halt the peptidoglycan biosynthesis pathway early enough to prevent the synthesis and release of the peptidoglycan component, muramyl tripeptide. These immunostimulatory components are ligands that activate the intracellular NOD1/NF-κB-mediated IL-8 inflammatory immune response to Chlamydial infections, and the prevention of this signaling pathway by a subset of persistent forms of *Chlamydia* inhibiting PG synthesis may confer an immunoevasive advantage during aberrancy [2]. In addition, ABs incorporate Incs effector proteins at various stages of the Chlamydial AB formation which suggests that persistent forms of *Chlamydia* exhibit differences in their abilities to undergo homotypic fusion and induce actin cage formation [2].

In addition to differences in the AB physiology, other studies have found that the transcriptional and translational responses of *Chlamydiae* differ according to the persistence-inducing stimuli [Reviewed in [47]]. For instance, different models of AB induction *in vitro* and *in vivo* data using *Chlamydia*-infected tissues revealed differences in the relative levels of expression in the major outer membrane protein (MOMP), Chlamydial heat shock protein 60 (cHSP60), and the three groEL genes (encoding cHSP60 homologs) [48–50]. Other studies analyzed the patterns of expression in genes related to cell division and chromosome replication in the *Chlamydia* ABs. These studies analyzed expression of genes encoding products predicted to function in DNA replication (polA, dnaA, and mutS), chromosome partitioning (parB and minD), and cell division (ftsK and ftsW) in various *in vitro* AB inducible systems and *in vivo* [51, 52]. These studies demonstrated mixed data in the expression patterns of the chromosome segregation gene, ftsK, and septum-peptidoglycan biosynthetic protein, ftsW. Similarly, DNA replication gene expression profiles were varied in the microarray study of IFN-exposed *C. trachomatis*, with some genes upregulated (dnaB, topA, and xerC) and others downregulated (dnaA-2, dnlJ, and ihfA) [51]. The varied data regarding cell division and DNA replication gene expression during persistence may indicate that RBs show different morphological alterations during the establishment of persistence.

Several studies on AB-inducible systems have reported variations in expression of genes involved in energy metabolism *in vitro* and *in vivo* [48]. Genes encoding enzymes belonging to glycolysis (pyk, gap, and pgk) and the pentose phosphate pathway (gnd and tal) were found to be selectively downregulated *in vitro* and *in vivo* relative to genes encoding enzymes in the tricarboxylic acid cycle (mdhC and fumC) [48]. The microarray expression data for genes encoding tricarboxylic acid cycle enzymes in IFN-induced persistence of *C. trachomatis* were mixed. Genes encoding 2-oxoglutarate dehydrogenase (sucA, sucB-1, and sucB-2) and succinate thiokinase (sucC and sucD) were downregulated. In contrast, genes encoding other enzymes in the cycle were either upregulated (fumC and sdhB) or unchanged (mdhC, sdhA, and sdhC) [48].

Electron microscopic visualization in chronically diseased tissues shows similar morphologically aberrant forms resembling those observed *in vitro*, though the viability of these particles is uncertain. The presence of viable but atypical *Chlamydiae in vivo* is suggested by the detection of enlarged, pleomorphic RB within infected human-derived samples such as fibroblasts and macrophages in synovial membrane samples from patients with *C. trachomatis*-associated reactive arthritis or Reiter's syndrome [53], macrophages in aortic valve samples from patients with degenerative aortic valve stenosis [54], and prostatic secretion samples from patients with chronic Chlamydial prostatitis [55]. Moreover, Chlamydial inclusions were found in the luminal epithelium of the oviducts of mice experimentally inoculated with the mouse pneumonitis (MoPn) biovar of *C. trachomatis* [56]. Aberrant bodies are not exclusive of human *Chlamydia*e, as members of the zoonotic Chlamydiales and "*Chlamydia*-related bacteria" also exhibit the persistent AB phenotype under several experimental conditions *in vitro* and *in vivo* [57–59].

5. Immunological basis of *Chlamydia* persistence

Chlamydia employs several mechanisms to interfere with the host innate immune response to persist within the host cell.

5.1 Modulation of proinflammatory signaling pathways

The epithelial cells of the urethra or vagina/endocervix represent the first contact and innate immune barrier against *Chlamydia*. The cells can recognize the pathogen through pattern recognition receptors (PRRs) such as Toll-like receptors (TLRs), nucleotide-binding oligomerization domain (NOD)-like receptors or cyclic guanosine monophosphate (GMP)-adenosine monophosphate (AMP) (cGAMP) synthase (cGAS), which induces the production of proinflammatory cytokines via nuclear factor-κB (NF-κB) or activator protein 1 (AP-1) signaling [Reviewed in 61]. The stimulation of cGAS by *Chlamydia spp*. DNA leads to the dimerization and activation of the IFN regulatory factor 3 (IRF3), which then translocates into the nucleus and promotes the transcription of type I IFN and IFN-inducible genes [60].

The NFκB pathway may be modulated by several different Chlamydial proteins and mechanisms, all of which can interfere with NFκB-mediated gene transcription and regulation. Some of these mechanisms include: (1) blocking the degradation of the NF-κB retention factor, IκBα via *C. trachomatis* deubiquitination (DUB) proteins ChlaDub1 and ChlaDub2 [61], (2) preventing the nuclear translocation of NF-κB, thus stopping or dampening NF-κB transcription, (3) sequestration of the NF-κB activator 1 (Act1) upon binding of the *C. pneumonia*-specific inclusion membrane protein (Inc) CP0236 [22], and (4) suppression of NF-κB signaling by *Chlamydia* secreted proteases (the tail-specific protease of *C. trachomatis*, CT441, and Chlamydial protease-like activity factor, CPAF) [62].

5.2 Interference with proinflammatory cytokines

Inflammation participates significantly not only in host defenses against *Chlamydia spp*., but it also contributes to the pathophysiology of infection. *Chlamydia*-infected host cells produce a number of cytokines and chemokines, including CXC-chemokine ligand 1 (CXCL1), CXCL8 (also known as interleukin-8, IL-8), TNF-α, and IL-1β and cause activation of various inflammasome pathways, including the NLRP3/ASC inflammasome [60]. These proinflammatory mediators recruit immune cells to the site of infection and cause local inflammation and tissue damage. *Chlamydia* employs several mechanisms to interfere with inflammation, promoting Chlamydial persistence. For instance, the *C. trachomatis* inclusion membrane protein CpoS can inhibit host inflammasome responses [20]. Another mechanism is the overexpression of the anti-inflammatory cytokine IL-10 [63]. This *in vitro* study was confirmed by findings of an increased *in vivo* expression of IL-10 in the semen and serum of patients infected with *C. trachomatis* [64]. *Chlamydia* CPAF contributes to the anti-inflammatory state required for persistence by inhibiting the IL-1ß-dependent secretion of IL-8 through cleavage of the transcription factor p65/RelA [65]. CPAF is also involved in the inhibition of the complement activation by cleavage of the complement factors B and C3 and attenuating the production of proinflammatory cytokines [66].

5.3 IFN-γ-induced persistence

IFN-γ is the major component of the innate immune response against *Chlamydia* and is the factor that has received the most research attention as a Chlamydial inducer of persistence [41, 43, 44, 67]. Various mechanisms of IFN-γ-induced persistence have been proposed. IFN-γ activates the catabolic depletion of L-tryptophan (Trp) via indoleamine-2,3-dioxygenase (IDO), the enzyme that degrades tryptophan. Since tryptophan is an essential amino acid for *C. trachomatis*, the presence of this enzyme induces a tryptophan starvation that inhibits the growth of Chlamydial RBs [41, 43]. IFN-γ is also involved in the inhibition of the transcription factor and proto-oncogene c-Myc, the key regulator of host cell metabolism and a central regulator of *Chlamydia* persistence [67].

5.4 Autophagy: mediated resistance

Autophagy is a physiological degradation process that occurs within the lysosomes of most cell types. Its main functions are to maintain cellular homeostasis and selectively remove intracellular bacteria or viruses. In *C. trachomatis*, Guanylate-binding proteins (GBPs) and the immunity-related GTPases (IRGs) such as GBP1, GBP2, Irga6, and Irgd, which can induce lysis and infection clearance by autophagy, were found to accumulate in the *Chlamydial* inclusions [68, 69], suggesting a role for these proteins in the autophagy-mediated resistance to *C. trachomatis* infection.

5.5 Interaction with innate immune cells

5.5.1 Macrophages (Mϕ)

Macrophages (Mϕ), unlike epithelial cells, are not a hospitable niche for Chlamydial intracellular replication. Mϕs migrate to Chlamydial infection sites, phagocytose bacteria, produce proinflammatory cytokines, and destroy *C. trachomatis* with host cell autophagy [69, 70]. Also, studies have demonstrated that Mϕ autophagy can enhance antigen presentation to T-cells [69]. Furthermore, IFN-γ has been shown to enhance both autophagy and upregulation of MHC class II molecules in Mϕ [71]. Several mechanisms of *Chlamydia spp*. persistence in macrophages have been described: (1) living as aberrant RBs; (2) interaction with organelles to acquire sufficient nutrients [72, 73]; (3) modulation of inflammatory cytokines such as TNF-α, IFN-γ, and ILs, to escape eradication via apoptosis or autophagy [74]; and (4) the production of adhesion molecules such as the intercellular cell adhesion molecule-1

(ICAM-1), to increase macrophage adherence, thus facilitating the migration of EBs to their preferred sites of replication [75].

Mϕs are involved in the engulfment and transient persistence of the Chlamydial extrusions [76]. Upon release from infected epithelial cells, *Chlamydia*-containing extrusions are engulfed by macrophages. Migration of these macrophages, followed by eventual escape of *Chlamydia* from them, can result in the dissemination of infectious *C. trachomatis* to more distant sites, for example, away from inflammatory foci surrounding the primary site of infection, to draining lymph nodes or to new hosts [76].

5.5.2 Monocytes and dendritic cells (DC)

Monocytes are responsible for spreading *C. trachomatis* throughout the body, while dendritic cells (DCs) play an important role in mediating immune response against bacterial infection. The *C. trachomatis* serovars Ba, D, and L2 can productively infect human peripheral blood monocytes and monocyte-derived DCs in a comparable manner [77]. *Chlamydia* Serovars Ba and D are able to persist on monocytes, while they degrade within DC's [77]. The mechanism of persistence within monocytes is not known.

6. Molecular basis of Chlamydial persistence

During the persistent state, *Chlamydiae* can activate pro-survival pathways and inhibit apoptosis to ensure long-term survival inside the cells. Extensive research has established a strong correlation between inhibition of host cell apoptosis and persistent *C. trachomatis* infection.

6.1 Inhibition of apoptosis

Apoptosis is an active process of cellular death induced by both extrinsic (death receptor signaling) and intrinsic (mitochondrial) pathways in response to variety of physiological and stress stimuli. Host cell death has long been recognized as the final stage of the *Chlamydia* infection cycle, enabling the release of EBs and spreads of infection. However, *Chlamydia* must protect the host cell from succumbing to stress-induced death before the Chlamydial developmental cycle is complete. The ability of *Chlamydiae* to induce host-cell apoptosis under some circumstances and actively inhibit apoptosis to complete their obligate intracellular growth has been extensively studied for decades ([78]; reviewed in Ref. [79]). *C. trachomatis* inhibits specifically the mitochondrial pathway, while signals that originate at death receptors and bypass mitochondria are not blocked [80]. Apoptosis inhibition in *Chlamydia* is observed in a variety of cell lines and primary cells from diverse origins, including epithelial cells, fibroblasts, endothelial cells, monocytes, and lymphoid cells, and not only during active but also during persistent infection [78].

6.1.1 Interaction with mitochondria

Mitochondria play a central role in energy (ATP) metabolism via oxidative phosphorylation, biosynthesis of macromolecules, and cell death regulation. Within the host cell, the mitochondria constitute the primary target for *C. trachomatis*. Its high demand for metabolites during its inclusion phase induces massive stress in the host cell, eventually leading to the induction of apoptotic cell death as a cell autonomous defense mechanism. Accumulating evidence suggests that *Chlamydia* can manipulate the mitochondrial morphology to promote their own replication or to escape from host immune responses (Reviewed in Ref. [81]). Altered mitochondrial dynamics of fusion and fission allow *Chlamydia* to maintain the cycle of reproduction and growth. *Chlamydia* suppresses mitochondrial fission and promotes mitochondrial fusion in the host cell via lowering ROS generation, inhibiting the tumor suppressor protein P53 transcription, increasing P53 protein ubiquitination levels, and inhibiting the dynamin-related protein 1(DRP1) oligomerization [81, 82]. Another study provided evidence that *Chlamydia* promotes intracellular survival by inducing mitochondrial elongation during the early phase of infection via phosphorylated fission mediator protein Drp1 followed by a fragmentation phase at the late stages of infection [83].

6.2 Modulation of Bcl-2 family pro-apoptotic proteins

The Bcl-2 family proteins and caspase-3 are critical regulatory proteins in cell apoptosis. Members of the Bcl-2 family can regulate the mitochondrial outer membrane permeability and control cell apoptosis by activating the caspase-3-mediated pathway [84]. Bcl-2 family can be divided into anti-apoptotic proteins (such as Bcl-2 and BclxL) and proapoptotic proteins (such as Bax and Bak). The ratio of anti-apoptotic to proapoptotic proteins is involved in the determination of cellular fate. Activated Bax/Bak induces the formation of oligomers that form pores in the mitochondrial outer membrane. These pores are channels for proapoptotic factors such as cytochrome c to translocate to the cytoplasm. The result is twofold: the loss of cytochrome c from mitochondria disables energy production, and cytosolic cytochrome c instigates a proteolytic cascade that dismantles the cell [85].

Various mechanisms of interference with pro-apoptotic BCL-2 family proteins have been described in *Chlamydia:* (1) sequestration of the BCL-2-associated agonist of cell death (BAD) to the inclusion membrane via the host-cell adapter 14-3-3β-binding, (2) prevention of cytochrome c release from the mitochondria by *Chlamydia*-dependent anti-apoptotic factors, (3) upregulation of the expression of genes that encode the myeloid leukemia cell differentiation protein (Mcl-1), an anti-apoptotic member of the BCL-2 family, and (4) upregulation of BCL-2-associated athanogene 1 (BAG1), aBCL-2 binding protein, via RAF/MEK/ERK signaling pathway [60, 79]. Recent data provided strong evidence that *Chlamydial* apoptosis inhibition in infected human cells occurs during the activation of Bax and Bak, and the Chlamydial porin OmpA can interfere with Bak activation [86].

Chlamydial plasmid-encoded secreted protein PGP3 also contributes to apoptosis inhibition by regulating expression levels of Bax and Bcl-2 and activation of caspase-3. Anti-apoptotic activity of PGP3 involves ERK activation via upregulation of caspase DJ-1 protein [87] and phosphorylation and nuclear entry of MDM2, and p53 degradation via activation of the PI3K/AKY signaling pathway [88].

6.3 Inactivation of pro-apoptosis factors by kinases

Kinases regulate host cell processes by phosphorylation of their target proteins and are fundamental for suppressing host cell apoptosis. A key subset of host proteins sequestered by *Chlamydia* during its survival and development within the inclusion include an assortment of host kinase signaling networks vital for many Chlamydial processes, including entry, nutrient acquisition, and suppression of host cell apoptosis (Reviewed in Ref. [89]).

The mitogen-activated protein-MAP kinase/extracellular signal-regulated kinase (MEK/ERK) and Phosphatidylinositol-3-kinase (PI3K) signaling pathways are among the most prominent kinase signaling networks utilized by *Chlamydia* in activating pro-survival mechanisms [89]. MEK/ERK signaling and P13K pathways are activated immediately after entry upon binding to host receptor tyrosine kinases. Phosphorylation of the *Chlamydial* TarP activates the MEK/ERK signaling through interaction with SRC homology 2 domain-containing transforming protein C1 (SHC1). ERK activation and upregulation of the BCL-2 family member MCL-1 are involved in the anti-apoptotic state by activating the PI3K pathway [89]. Activation of the PI3K pathway results in the phosphorylation and activation of the serine/threonine kinase (Akt) cell survival cascade. The PI13K/Akt complex maintains the BCL-2-associated agonist of cell death (BAD) in a phosphorylated state as it is sequestered by the host-cell adapter 14-3-3ß protein at the inclusion vacuole [90]. Depletion of AKT through short-interfering RNA reverses the resistance to apoptosis of *C. trachomatis*-infected cells. Other kinases (PKCδ, GSK3ß) interact with the inclusion by binding to diacylglycerol-enriched membranes and activating pro-apoptotic signals via different mechanisms [89].

Other pro-survival signaling pathway activated by *Chlamydia* is the Wnt/β-catenin signaling through the interaction of *Chlamydia* with fibroblast growth factor receptor (FGFR) or the receptor tyrosine kinases (RTKs) and the ephrin receptor A2 (EPHA2) [79].

6.4 Inhibition of apoptosis by non-coding RNA's

Non-coding RNAs (ncRNAs) are a novel type of short RNAs that regulate gene expression at multiple levels via various mechanisms, thus influencing development, differentiation, and metabolism [91]. One type of ncRNAs, long non-coding RNA (lncRNAs) regulates gene expression and function, either positively or negatively, by interacting with DNA, RNA, and proteins and also modulate transcriptional, post-transcriptional, and post-translational processes [91].

Chlamydia trachomatis expresses distinct patterns of ncRNAs during normal development [92]. Expression of many ncRNAs is altered during growth stress stimuli that induce persistent growth, particularly IFN-γ and carbenicillin [92]. Recent findings provided evidence that lncRNAs are involved in regulating apoptosis pathways in *Chlamydia* [93, 94]. The anti-apoptotic activity of the lncRNAs includes modulation of the DNA replication and apoptosis of host cells via Wnt/β-catenin pathway [93] or downregulation of the Bcl-2/Bax ratio with a marked release of cytochrome c, resulting in a significantly elevated level of caspase-3 activation [94]. One of the Chlamydial targeted lncRNA (MIAT) was involved in regulating Chlamydial development during the persistent infection [94]. The discovery of non-coding circular RNAs (circRNAs) has opened the possibility of the role of these rare RNAs in *Chlamydia* persistence.

7. Molecular tools to study *Chlamydia* persistence

Historically, genetic manipulation of *Chlamydia* has been a challenge to scientists because of its obligate intracellular lifestyle, biphasic developmental cycle, and limited metabolic activity of EBs during persistence. On the other hand, scientists have presumed *Chlamydia spp.* to deliver over 100 proteins through its T3SS that interfere with normal host cell processes to promote invasion, intracellular replication, inclusion formation, and dissemination [17]. Bioinformatics has identified several *C. trachomatis* effector proteins (Reviewed in Ref. [95]), yet the biological role in persistence remains to be elucidated.

In the context of Chlamydial persistence, the two intracellular morphological forms (RB and AB) have features that render them more suitable than the infectious EB for genetic manipulation. Unlike the rigid cell-walled EB, the RBs slow levels of peptidoglycan in its cell wall, which could facilitate the uptake of DNA [96]. RBs also undergo cell division and express DNA repair enzymes that mediate the chromosomal integration of DNA by homologous recombination during division. Thus, RBs are likely to be naturally competent for transformation. However, one challenge in the genetic manipulation of the Chlamydial RBs in persistence studies is the fact that transformation within infected cells requires exogenous DNA to traverse through several other lipid bilayers (the host plasma membrane and the inclusion membrane) before encountering the RB outer and inner membranes and eventually the chromosome [96].

7.1 Molecular manipulation of *Chlamydia*

With the recent advances in the molecular genetic manipulation of *Chlamydia,* it is now possible to perform targeted gene inactivation, whole-genome sequencing to identify mutations, and plasmid transformation to generate fluorescent reporter strains to identify proteins involved in the pathogenesis of *Chlamydia* [96]. On the other hand, the ability to express exogenous proteins, epitope tags, and fluorescent and other reporter proteins in *Chlamydia* has expanded the repertoire of possible technologies to study the *Chlamydia*–host interface [97]. High-resolution microscopy has complemented the advances in genetic and biochemical approaches [96].

Molecular manipulation in *Chlamydia* takes advantage of the sequencing of the first *Chlamydiae* genome [98]. *C. trachomatis* can insert exogenous DNA into its genome because it encodes an intact DNA recombination machinery that facilitates the development of a stable transformation system of *Chlamydia* with recombinant DNA [99]. This transformation system has enabled the construction of a series of shuttle vectors for gene inactivation by targeted gene knockouts with versatile multiple-cloning sites (MCS), fluorescent protein reporters, inducible promoters, and new selectable markers. Strategies to mediate targeted genetic modifications, such as gene disruptions and gene replacements, include the Targeting Induced Local Lesions in Genomes (TILLING) technology and TargeTron, based on the transient transformation of *Chlamydia* with a plasmid that encodes an altered group-II intron (Reviewed in Ref. [100]). The recent development of a Fluorescence-reported allelic exchange mutagenesis (FRAEM) using the suicide vector pSUmC has allowed the generation of null mutation strains via the complete deletion of chromosomal genes in *C. trachomatis* [101].

7.2 Genome-scale analyses

7.2.1 Transcriptomics

High-throughput analysis of protein-encoding mRNA (transcriptomic approaches) has explored the differential expression of genes at different stages of the Chlamydial infectious cycle, allowing the identification of previously unrecognized early Chlamydial gene expression and complex host cell responses [102–104]. However, such bulk-cell approaches can potentially miss cell-cell variability or cells that contribute to overlapping phenotypic characteristics, potentially masking critical biological heterogeneity as irrelevant signals from non-participating cells that can skew the average [105].

Single-cell RNA sequencing (scRNA-seq) is an alternative to bulk cell populations as it can analyze RNA molecules in individual cells with high resolution and on a genomic scale [105]. The construction of a pilot dataset, applying scRNA-Seq to *C. trachomatis* infected and mock-infected epithelial cells (HEp-2) has allowed the differential expression of genes involved with cell cycle regulation, innate immune responses, cytoskeletal components, lipid biosynthesis, and cellular stress at early times of infection [105].

7.2.2 Whole-proteome microarrays

Proteome microarray is a novel alternative to gene expression profiling by microarrays for studying *Chlamydia*–host interaction. Proteins expressed on microarrays display antigenic epitopes, thereby providing an efficient method for immunoprofiling patients and allowing *de novo* identification of disease-related serum antibodies. The technology takes advantage of the recent construction of a whole-proteome microarray using on-chip protein expression of the *C. trachomatis* 895 proteins [106]. Comparison of antibody reactivity patterns allowed the identification of new antigens recognized by known *C. trachomatis* seropositive samples and antigens reacting only with samples from cervical cancer patients [106]. More recently, the whole *C. trachomatis* screening identified antibody patterns associated with pelvic inflammatory disease (PID), tubal factor infertility, chronic pelvic pain (CPP), and ectopic pregnancy that results from a Chlamydial persistent infection [106, 107]. Although protein microarrays have been used in the field of clinical diagnosis for *de novo* identification of antibodies associated with general infection and disease-related serum antibodies, the technique can easily be adapted to the identification of antigen biomarkers of *Chlamydia* persistence.

7.3 In vitro cell systems

The 2D *in vitro* cell-culture models have been the most widely used models for studying the dynamics of Chlamydial persistence, including its virulence factors and molecular and cellular pathways. The findings of altered morphological forms of *C. psittaci* in infected mouse fibroblasts (L cells) constituted the first *in vitro* model of *Chlamydial* persistence [108]. Since then, the induction of persistent *C. trachomatis* has been studied extensively using different *in vitro* cell lines (Reviewed in Ref. [3]). The different *in vitro* persistence systems have revealed altered *Chlamydial* growth characteristics, for example, enlarged pleomorphic inclusions with a loss of infectivity and cell division. These changes are generally reversible upon removal of the growth inhibitory factor. One advantage of these systems is that they can be used under highly controlled experimental conditions; however, they fail to mimic the complex and dynamically changing structure of *in vivo* human host tissues.

Three-dimensional (3D) cell-culture models based on primary cells are acquiring great importance as a new and robust platform for studying complex biological processes and might be a promising alternative in *C. trachomatis* pathogenetic studies

(Reviewed in [109]). The 3D "organoid" models mimic the microenvironment that *C. trachomatis* encounters in the host tissue, allowing a deeper understanding of host–pathogen interactions by promoting direct cell-to-cell contact, interacting with cells of the extracellular matrix and allowing *in vivo* exchange of soluble factors. In addition, 3D cell culture models retain the cellular structural integrity resembling the *in vivo* parental tissue than the 2D cell culture models.

The recent development of Female Reproductive Tract (FRT) Organoid technology is opening up new possibilities to investigate the mechanisms of *Chlamydia* disease in the FRT [Reviewed in 113]. Human and mouse-derived primary cervical epithelial three-dimensional (3D) organoids resembling the *in vivo* FTR native tissue architecture offer a unique possibility to elucidate the dynamics and impact of different infections and co-infections in pathogenesis and carcinogenesis [110]. One advantage of using FTR organoids is that they can be propagated and expanded long term under their optimal culture conditions ($\geq$6 months), thus providing the ideal model to study persistence in *Chlamydia*. For instance, in a human ectocervical organoid model, co-infection with Human papillomavirus (HPV)16 E6E7 slowed down the *C. trachomatis* developmental life cycle by inhibiting the redifferentiation of RBs into EBs, thus inducing persistence [111].

8. Animal models

Extending the *in vitro* observations of Chlamydial persistence to an animal infection model has remained challenging. The first and only animal model to study *Chlamydia* persistence was reported a decade ago [112]. The study showed that amoxicillin could induce persistence in BALB/c mice infected intravaginally with the murine pathogen *C. muridarum*, a close relative of *C. trachomatis*. Another relevant observation is that amoxicillin-induced persistence resulted in increased failure of subsequent treatment with the first-choice antiChlamydial antibiotic azithromycin [112]. Interestingly, a murine model of naturally chronic nonhuman Chlamydial infection has been recently developed [113].

Other animal models to study *Chlamydia* genital tract pathogenesis, including guinea pig, nonhuman primate, pig, rat, and the rabbit, have been developed (Reviewed in Ref. [114]). However, none of the animal models perfectly mimics the anatomy, histology, and endocrinology of the human reproductive system or the pathogenesis and immune responses occurring during a chronic human genital *C. trachomatis* infection [114]. In addition, the use of animal models possesses important ethical issues [114].

9. Concluding remarks

Chlamydia's ability to manipulate the host cell biology, evade immunity, and undergo morphological aberrant conformations allows these successful intracellular pathogens to enter a persistent state. Persistence has been studied for decades by observing the ability of *Chlamydia* to survive for long periods of time in cell culture in response to stress stimuli. The stress responses that lead to persistence in *Chlamydia* comprise complex regulatory networks that control the expression of multiple genes to inhibit apoptosis and activate pro-signaling pathways and immunomodulation. The transcriptional response of *Chlamydia* differs according to the persistence-inducing stimuli, suggesting differences in the host cell response. On the other hand, isolated *in vitro* studies indicate common pathways that are down- or upregulated in a similar way by different stress conditions, which may interact and crosstalk between these regulons. Thus, an understanding of the morphological features, as well as the regulatory mechanisms and functional redundancies in pathways involved in persistence, is very critical for the design of novel anti-Chlamydial strategies.

Methodological advances in *Chlamydial* gene mutagenesis and DNA transformation, deep sequencing technologies, and the implementation of high-throughput genome-scale analysis and improvement in *in vitro* cell systems have opened new opportunities in our understanding of persistence. The genes encoding critical functional proteins are potential drug targets for treating persistent *C. trachomatis* infections. Understanding the gene-level changes that take place for *Chlamydia* to enter persistence could help researchers develop strategies to block these changes from occurring, making the organism more vulnerable to antibiotics and circumventing chronic Chlamydial infections.

Acknowledgements

We thank Dr. Estela S. Estape for her critical reading of the manuscript and the San Juan Bautista School of Medicine for its institutional support.

Conflict of interest

The authors declare no conflict of interest.

Author details

Ramón Scharbaai-Vázquez*, Francisco J. López Font and Félix A. Zayas Rodríguez
School of Medicine, San Juan Bautista School of Medicine, Caguas, Puerto Rico

*Address all correspondence to: rscharbaai@sanjuanbautista.edu

References

[1] Eisenreich W, Rudel T, Heesemann J, Goebel W. Persistence of intracellular bacterial pathogens-with a focus on the metabolic perspective. Frontiers in Cellular and Infection Microbiology. 2021;**10**:615450. DOI: 10.3389/fcimb.2020.615450

[2] Brockett MR, Liechti GW. Persistence alters the interaction between *Chlamydia trachomatis* and its host cell. Infection and Immunity. 2021;**89**(8):e0068520. DOI: 10.1128/IAI.00685-20

[3] Wyrick PB. *Chlamydia trachomatis* persistence *in vitro*: An overview. The Journal of Infectious Diseases. 2010;**201**(Suppl. 2):S88-S95. DOI: 10.1086/652394

[4] Elwell C, Mirrashidi K, Engel J. *Chlamydia* cell biology and pathogenesis. Nature Reviews. Microbiology. 2016;**14**(6): 385-400. DOI: 10.1038/nrmicro.2016.30

[5] Helble JD, Starnbach MN. T cell responses to *Chlamydia*. Pathogens and Disease. 2021;**79**(4):ftab014. DOI: 10.1093/femspd/ftab014

[6] Gitsels A, Sanders N, Vanrompay D. Chlamydial infection from outside to inside. Frontiers in Microbiology. 2019;**10**:2329. DOI: 10.3389/fmicb.2019.02329

[7] Mandell GL, Bennett JE, Dolin R, editors. Mandell, Douglas, and Bennett's Principles and Practice of Infectious Diseases. 7th ed. Vol. 2. Churchill Livingstone/Elsevier; 2010

[8] Rank RG. In vivo Chlamydial infection. In: Tan M, Bavoil PM, editors. Intracellular Pathogens, I: Chlamydiales. Washington, DC, USA: ASM Press; 2012. pp. 285-310

[9] de Barbeyrac BB. Genital *Chlamydia trachomatis* infections. Clinical Microbiology and Infection. 2009;**15**(1):4-10

[10] Ravichandran K, Anbazhagan S, Karthik K, Angappan M, Dhayananth B. A comprehensive review on avian chlamydiosis: A neglected zoonotic disease. Tropical Animal Health and Production. 2021;**53**(4):414. DOI: 10.1007/s11250-021-02859-0

[11] De Vrieze NH, de Vries HJ. Lymphogranuloma venereum among men who have sex with men. An epidemiological and clinical review. Expert Review of Anti-Infective Therapy. 2014;**12**:697-704

[12] Leonard CA, Borel N. Chronic Chlamydial diseases: From atherosclerosis to urogenital infections. Current Clinical Microbiology. 2014;**Rpt 1**:61-72. DOI: 10.1007/s40588-014-0005-8

[13] Yang X, Siddique A, Khan AA, Wang Q, Malik A, Jan AT, et al. *Chlamydia trachomatis* infection: Their potential implication in the Etiology of cervical cancer. Journal of Cancer. 2021;**12**(16):4891-4900. DOI: 10.7150/jca.58582

[14] Lan J, Melgers I, Meijer M, Walboomers JM, Roosendal R, Burger C, et al. Prevalence and serovar distribution of asymptomatic cervical *Chlamydia trachomatis* infection as determined by highly sensitive PCR. Journal of Clinical Microbiology. 1995;**33**:3194-3197

[15] Wesolowski J, Paumet F. Taking control: Reorganization of the host cytoskeleton by *Chlamydia*. F1000Res. 2017;**6**:2058. DOI: 10.12688/f1000research.12316.1

[16] Bannantine JP, Rockey DD, Hackstadt T. Tandem genes of *Chlamydia psittaci* that encode proteins localized to the inclusion membrane. Molecular Microbiology. 1998;**28**(5):1017-1026. DOI: 10.1046/j.1365-2958.1998.00867. x

[17] Bugalhão JN, Mota LJ. The multiple functions of the numerous *Chlamydia trachomatis* secreted proteins: The tip of the iceberg. Microbial Cell. 2019;**6**(9):414-449. DOI: 10.15698/mic2019.09.691

[18] Dehoux P, Flores R, Dauga C, Zhong G, Subtil A. Multi-genome identification and characterization of *Chlamydiae*-specific type III secretion substrates: The Inc proteins. BMC Genomics. 2011;**12**:109

[19] Shaw EI, Dooley CA, Fischer ER, Scidmore MA, Fields KA, Hackstadt T. Three temporal classes of gene expression during the *Chlamydia trachomatis* developmental cycle. Molecular Microbiology. 2000;**37**(4):913-925. DOI: 10.1046/j.1365-2958.2000.02057. x

[20] Sixt BS, Bastidas RJ, Finethy R, Baxter RM, Carpenter VK, Kroemer G, et al. The *Chlamydia trachomatis* inclusion membrane protein CpoS counteracts STING-mediated cellular surveillance and suicide programs. Cell Host & Microbe. 2017;**21**:113-121. DOI: 10.1016/j.chom.2016.12.002

[21] Weber MM, Lam JL, Dooley CA, Noriea NF, Hansen BT, Hoyt FH, et al. Absence of specific Chlamydia trachomatis inclusion membrane proteins triggers premature inclusion membrane lysis and host cell death. Cell Reports. 2017;**19**(7):1406-1417

[22] Wolf K, Plano GV, Fields KA. A protein secreted by the respiratory pathogen Chlamydia pneumoniae impairs IL-17 signalling via interaction with human Act1. Cellular Microbiology. 2009;**11**:769-779. DOI: 10.1111/j.1462-5822.2009. 01290.x

[23] Cortina ME, Bishop RC, DeVasure BA, Coppens I, Derré I. The inclusion membrane protein IncS is critical for initiation of the Chlamydia intracellular developmental cycle. PLoS Pathogens. 2022;**18**(9):e1010818. DOI: 10.1371/journal.ppat.1010818

[24] Caven L, Carabeo RA. Pathogenic puppetry: Manipulation of the host actin cytoskeleton by *Chlamydia trachomatis*. International Journal of Molecular Sciences. 2020;**21**(1):90

[25] Kumar Y, Valdivia RH. Actin and intermediate filaments stabilize the *Chlamydia trachomatis* vacuole by forming dynamic structural scaffolds. Cell Host & Microbe. 2008;**4**:159-169

[26] Chin E, Kirker K, Zuck M, James G, Hybiske K. Actin recruitment to the *Chlamydia* inclusion is spatiotemporally regulated by a mechanism that requires host and bacterial factors. PLoS One. 2012;**7**:e46949

[27] Coles AM, Reynolds DJ, Harper A, Devitt A, Pearce JH. Low-nutrient induction of abnormal Chlamydial development: A novel component of Chlamydial pathogenesis? FEMS Microbiol. Letter. 1993;**106**:193-200

[28] Matsumoto A, Manire GP. Electron microscopic observations on the effects of penicillin on the morphology of *Chlamydia psittaci*. Journal of Bacteriology. 1970;**101**:278-285

[29] Kintner J, Lajoie D, Hall J, Whittimore J, Schoborg RV. Commonly prescribed beta-lactam antibiotics induce C. trachomatis persistence/stress in culture at physiologically relevant

concentrations. Frontiers in Cellular and Infection Microbiology. 2014;**4**:44. DOI: 10.3389/fcimb.2014.00044

[30] Pilhofer M, Aistleitner K, Biboy J, et al. Discovery of Chlamydial peptidoglycan reveals bacteria with murein sacculi but without FtsZ. Nature Communications. 2013;**4**:2856. DOI: DOI/10.1038/ncomms3856

[31] Scherler A, Jacquier N, Kebbi-Beghdadi C, Greub G. Diverse stress-inducing treatments cause distinct aberrant body morphologies in the Chlamydia-related bacterium, *Waddlia chondrophila*. Microorganisms. 2020;**8**(1):89. DOI: 10.3390/microorganisms8010089

[32] Slade JA, Brockett M, Singh R, Liechti GW, Maurelli AT. Fosmidomycin, an inhibitor of isoprenoid synthesis, induces persistence in *Chlamydia* by inhibiting peptidoglycan assembly. PLoS Pathogens. 2019;**15**(10):e1008078. DOI: 10.1371/journal. ppat.1008078

[33] Xue Y, Zheng H, Mai Z, et al. An in vitro model of azithromycin-induced persistent Chlamydia trachomatis infection. FEMS Microbiology Letters. 2017;**364**(14):10.1093/femsle/fnx145. DOI: 10.1093/femsle/fnx145

[34] Tamura A, Manire GP. Effect of penicillin on the multiplication of meningopneumonitis organisms (*Chlamydia psittaci*). Journal of Bacteriology. 1968;**96**:875-880

[35] Wiedeman JA, Kaul R, Heuer LS, Thao NN, Pinkerton KE, Wenman WM. Tobacco smoke induces a persistent, but recoverable state in *Chlamydia pneumoniae* infection of human endothelial cells. Microbial Pathogenesis. 2005;**39**:197-204. DOI: 10.1016/j.micpath.2005.09.001

[36] Huston WM, Theodoropoulos C, Mathews SA, Timms P. *Chlamydia trachomatis* responds to heat shock, penicillin induced persistence, and IFN-gamma persistence by altering levels of the extracytoplasmic stress response protease HtrA. BMC Microbiology. 2008;**8**:190. DOI: 10.1186/1471-2180-8-190

[37] Raulston JE. Response of *Chlamydia trachomatis* serovar E to iron restriction in vitro and evidence for iron-regulated Chlamydial proteins. Infection and Immunity. 1997;**65**:4539-4547

[38] Kahane S, Friedman MG. Reversibility of heat shock in Chlamydia trachomatis. FEMS Microbiology Letters. 1992;**76**:25-30

[39] Deka S, Vanover J, Dessus-Babus S, Whittimore J, Howett MK, Wyrick PB, et al. *Chlamydia trachomatis* enters a viable but non-cultivable (persistent) state within herpes simplex virus type 2 (HSV-2) co-infected host cells. Cellular Microbiology. 2006;**8**:149-162

[40] Koehler L, Nettelnbreker E, Hudson AP, Ott N, Gerard HC, Branigan PJ, et al. Ultrastructural and molecular analyses of the persistence of *Chlamydia trachomatis* (serovar K) in human monocytes. Microbial Pathogenesis. 1997;**22**:133-142

[41] Nettelnbreker E, Zeidler H, Bartels H, Dreses-Werringloer U, Daubener W, Holtmann H, et al. Studies of persistent infection by *Chlamydia trachomatis* serovar K in TPA-differentiated U937 cells and the role of IFN-gamma. Journal of Medical Microbiology. 1998;**47**:141-149

[42] Gracey E, Lin A, Akram A, Chiu B, Inman RD. Intracellular survival and persistence of *Chlamydia muridarum* is determined by macrophage polarization. PLoS One. 2013;**8**:e69421

[43] Beatty WL, Byrne GI, Morrison RP. Morphologic and antigenic

characterization of interferon gamma-mediated persistent *Chlamydia trachomatis* infection *in vitro*. Proceedings of the National Academy of Sciences of the United States of America. 1993;**90**:3998-4002

[44] Beatty WL, Belanger TA, Desai AA, Morrison RP, Byrne GI. Tryptophan depletion as a mechanism of gamma interferon-mediated Chlamydial persistence. Infection and Immunity. 1994;**62**:3705-3711

[45] Borel N, Dumrese C, Ziegler U, Schifferli A, Kaiser C, Pospischil A. Mixed infections with *Chlamydia* and porcine epidemic diarrhea virus—A new *in vitro* model of Chlamydial persistence. BMC Microbiology. 2010;**10**:201

[46] Cram ED, Rockey DD, Dolan BP. *Chlamydia spp*. development is differentially altered by treatment with the LpxC inhibitor LPC-011. BMC Microbiology. 2017;**17**(1):98. DOI: 10.1186/s12866-017-0992-8

[47] Hogan RJ, Mathews SA, Mukhopadhyay S, Summersgill JT, Timms P. Chlamydial persistence: Beyond the biphasic paradigm. Infection and Immunity. 2004;**72**(4):1843-1855. DOI: 10.1128/IAI.72.4.1843-1855.2004

[48] Gérard HC, Freise J, Wang Z, Roberts G, Rudy D, Krauβ-Opatz B, et al. *Chlamydia trachomatis* genes whose products are related to energy metabolism are expressed differentially in active vs. persistent infection. Microbes and Infection. 2002;**4**:13-22

[49] Belland RJ, Nelson DE, Virok D, Crane DD, Hogan D, Sturdevant D, et al. Transcriptome analysis of Chlamydial growth during IFN-γ-mediated persistence and reactivation. Proceedings of the National Academy of Sciences of the United States of America. 2003;**100**:15971-15976

[50] Gérard HC, Whittum-Hudson JA, Schumacher HR, Hudson AP. Differential expression of three *Chlamydia trachomatis* hsp60-encoding genes in active vs. persistent infections. Microbial Pathogenesis. 2004;**36**:35-39

[51] Byrne GI, Ouellette SP, Wang Z, Rao JP, Lu L, Beatty WL, et al. *Chlamydia pneumoniae* expresses genes required for DNA replication but not cytokinesis during persistent infection of HEp-2 cells. Infection and Immunity. 2001;**69**:5423-5429

[52] Gérard HC, Krauβe-Opatz B, Wang Z, Rudy D, Rao JP, Zeidler H, et al. Expression of *Chlamydia trachomatis* genes encoding products required for DNA synthesis and cell division during active versus persistent infection. Molecular Microbiology. 2001;**41**:731-741

[53] Nanagara R, Li F, Beutler A, Hudson A, Schumacher HR. Alteration of *Chlamydia trachomatis* biologic behavior in synovial membranes: Suppression of surface antigen production in reactive arthritis and Reiter's syndrome. Arthritis and Rheumatism. 1995;**38**:1410-1417

[54] Skowasch D, Yeghiazaryan K, Schrempf S, Golubnitschaja O, Welsch U, Preusse CJ, et al. Persistence of *Chlamydia pneumoniae* in degenerative aortic valve stenosis indicated by heat shock protein 60 homologues. The Journal of Heart Valve Disease. 2003;**12**:68-75

[55] Mazzoli S, Bani D, Salvi A, Ramacciotti I, Romeo C, Bani T. *In vivo* evidence of *Chlamydia trachomatis* miniature reticulary bodies (MRB) as persistence markers in patients with chronic Chlamydial prostatitis.

Proceedings of European Society for Chlamydia Research. 2000;**4**:40

[56] Phillips DM, Swenson CE, Schachter J. Ultrastructure of *Chlamydia trachomatis* infection of the mouse oviduct. Journal of Ultrastructure Research. 1984;**88**:244-256

[57] Kebbi-Beghdadi C, Cisse O, Greub G. Permissivity of Vero cells, human pneumocytes and human endometrial cells to *Waddlia chondrophila*. Microbes and Infection. 2011;**13**:566-574

[58] De Barsy M, Bottinelli L, Greub G. Antibiotic susceptibility of *Estrella lausannensis*, a potential emerging pathogen. Microbes and Infection. 2014;**16**:746-754

[59] Vouga M, Baud D, Greub G. *Simkania negevensis*, an example of the diversity of the antimicrobial susceptibility pattern among Chlamydiales. Antimicrobial Agents and Chemotherapy. 2017;**61**(8):e00638-17. DOI: 10.1128/AAC.00638-17

[60] Chen H, Wen Y, Li Z. Clear victory for *Chlamydia*: The subversion of host innate immunity. Frontiers in Microbiology. 2019;**10**:1412. DOI: 10.3389/fmicb.2019.01412

[61] Le Negrate G, Krieg A, Faustin B, Loeffler M, Godzik A, Krajewski S, et al. ChlaDub1 of *Chlamydia trachomatis* suppresses NF-kappaB activation and inhibits I kappa B alpha ubiquitination and degradation. Cellular Microbiology. 2008;**10**:1879-1892

[62] Lad SP, Li J, da Silva Correia J, Pan Q, Gadwal S, Ulevitch RJ, et al. Cleavage of p65/RelA of the NF-kappaB pathway by *Chlamydia*. Proceedings of the National Academy of Sciences of the United States of America. 2007;**104**:2933-2938. DOI: 10.1073

[63] Azenabor AA, York J. *Chlamydia trachomatis* evokes a relative anti-inflammatory response in a free Ca2+ dependent manner in human macrophages. Comparative Immunology, Microbiology and Infectious Diseases. 2010;**33**:513-528. DOI: 10.1016/j.cimid.2009.09.002

[64] Hakimi H, Zare-Bidaki M, Zainodini N, Assar S, Arababadi MK. Significant roles played by IL-10 in *Chlamydia infections*. Inflammation. 2014;**37**:818-823. DOI: 10.1007/s10753-013-9801-1

[65] Christian J, Vier J, Paschen SA, Hacker G. Cleavage of the NF-kappaB family protein p65/RelA by the Chlamydial protease-like activity factor (CPAF) impairs proinflammatory signaling in cells infected with *Chlamydiae*. The Journal of Biological Chemistry. 2010;**285**:41320-41327. DOI: 10.1074/jbc.M110.152280

[66] Yang Z, Tang L, Zhou Z, Zhong G. Neutralizing antiChlamydial activity of complement by *Chlamydia*-secreted protease CPAF. Microbes and Infection. 2016;**18**:669-674. DOI: 10.1016/j.micinf.2016.07.002

[67] Vollmuth N, Schlicker L, Guo Y, Hovhannisyan P, Janaki-Raman S, Kurmasheva N, et al. c-Myc plays a key role in IFN-γ-induced persistence of *Chlamydia trachomatis*. eLife. 2022;**11**:e76721. DOI: 10.7554/eLife.76721

[68] Al-Zeer MA, Al-Younes HM, Braun PR, Zerrahn J, Meyer TF. IFN-gamma-inducible Irga6 mediates host resistance against *Chlamydia trachomatis* via autophagy. PLoS One. 2009;**4**:e4588

[69] Yasir M, Pachikara ND, Bao X, Pan Z, Fan H. Regulation of Chlamydial infection by host autophagy and vacuolar ATPase-bearing organelles. Infection and Immunity. 2011;**79**:4019-4028

[70] Vasilevsky S, Greub G, Nardelli-Haefliger D, Baud D. Genital *Chlamydia trachomatis*: Understanding the roles of innate and adaptive immunity in vaccine research. Clinical Microbiology Reviews. 2014;**27**(2):346-370. DOI: 10.1128/CMR.00105-13

[71] Cao H, Wolff RG, Meltzer MS, Crawford RM. Differential regulation of class II MHC determinants on macrophages by IFN-gamma and IL-4. Journal of Immunology. 1989;**143**:3524-3531

[72] Paradkar PN, De Domenico I, Durchfort N, Zohn I, Kaplan J, Ward DM. Iron depletion limits intracellular bacterial growth in macrophages. Blood. 2008;**112**:866-874. DOI: 10.1182/blood-2007-12-126854

[73] Sun HS, Eng EW, Jeganathan S, Sin AT, Patel PC, Gracey E, et al. *Chlamydia trachomatis* vacuole maturation in infected macrophages. Journal of Leukocyte Biology. 2012;**92**:815-827. DOI: 10.1189/jlb.0711336

[74] Jendro MC, Fingerle F, Deutsch T, Liese A, Kohler L, Kuipers JG, et al. *Chlamydia trachomatis*-infected macrophages induce apoptosis of activated T cells by secretion of tumor necrosis factor-alpha in vitro. Medical Microbiology and Immunology. 2004;**193**:45-52. DOI: 10.1007/s00430-003-0182-1

[75] Yeung ATY, Hale C, Lee AH, Gill EE, Bushell W, Parry-Smith D, et al. Exploiting induced pluripotent stem cell-derived macrophages to unravel host factors influencing *Chlamydia trachomatis* pathogenesis. Nature Communications. 2017;**8**:15013. DOI: 10.1038/ncomms15013

[76] Zuck M, Ellis T, Venida A, Hybiske K. Extrusions are phagocytosed and promote *Chlamydia* survival within macrophages. Cellular Microbiology. 2017;**19**(4):e12683-95. DOI: 10.1111/cmi.12683

[77] Datta B, Njau F, Thalmann J, Haller H, Wagner AD. Differential infection outcome of *Chlamydia trachomatis* in human blood monocytes and monocyte-derived dendritic cells. BMC Microbiology. 2014;**14**:209. DOI: 10.1186/s12866-014-0209-3

[78] Fan T, Lu H, Hu H, Shi L, McClarty GA, Nance DM, et al. Inhibition of apoptosis in *Chlamydia*-infected cells: Blockade of mitochondrial cytochrome c release and caspase activation. The Journal of Experimental Medicine. 1998;**187**:487-496

[79] Sixt BS. Host cell death during infection with *Chlamydia*: A double-edged sword. FEMS Microbiology Reviews. 2021;**45**(1):fuaa043. DOI: 10.1093/femsre/fuaa043

[80] Vaux DL, Strasser A. The molecular biology of apoptosis. Proceedings of the National Academy of Sciences of the United States of America. 1996;**93**:2239-2244

[81] Chowdhury SR, Rudel T. *Chlamydia* and mitochondria—An unfragmented relationship. Microbial Cell. 2017;**4**(7):233-235. DOI: 10.15698/mic2017.07.582

[82] Yang Y, Lei W, Zhao L, Wen Y, Li Z. Insights into mitochondrial dynamics in Chlamydial infection. Frontiers in Cellular and Infection Microbiology.

2022;**12**:835181. DOI: 10.3389/fcimb.2022.835181

[83] Kurihara Y, Itoh R, Shimizu A, Walenna NF, Chou B, Ishii K, et al. *Chlamydia trachomatis* targets mitochondrial dynamics to promote intracellular survival and proliferation. Cellular Microbiology. 2019;**21**(1):e12962. DOI: 10.1111/cmi.12962

[84] Kale J, Osterlund E, Andrews D. BCL-2 family proteins: Changing partners in the dance towards death. Cell Death and Differentiation. 2018;**25**:65-80. DOI: /10.1038/cdd.2017.186

[85] Liu X, Kim CN, Yang J, Jemmerson R, Wang X. Induction of apoptotic program in cell-free extracts: Requirement for dATP and cytochrome C. Cell. 1996;**86**:147-157

[86] Waguia Kontchou C, Gentle IE, Weber A, et al. *Chlamydia trachomatis* inhibits apoptosis in infected cells by targeting the pro-apoptotic proteins Bax and Bak. Cell Death and Differentiation. 2022;**29**:2046-2059. DOI: /10.1038/s41418-022-00995-0

[87] Luo F, Shu M, Gong S, Wen Y, He B, Su S, et al. Antiapoptotic activity of *Chlamydia trachomatis* Pgp3 protein involves activation of the ERK1/2 pathway mediated by upregulation of DJ-1 protein. Pathogens and Disease. 2019;**77**(9):ftaa003. DOI: 10.1093/femspd/ftaa003

[88] Zou Y, Lei W, Su S, Bu J, Zhu S, Huang Q, et al. Chlamydia trachomatis plasmid-encoded protein Pgp3 inhibits apoptosis via the PI3K-AKT-mediated MDM2-p53 axis. Molecular and Cellular Biochemistry. 2019;**452**(1-2):167-176. DOI: 10.1007/s11010-018-3422-9

[89] Sah P, Lutter EI. Hijacking and use of host kinases by *Chlamydiae*. Pathogens. 2020;**9**(12):1034. DOI: 10.3390/pathogens9121034

[90] Verbeke P, Welter-Stahl L, Ying S, Hansen J, Hacker G, Darville T, et al. Recruitment of BAD by the *Chlamydia trachomatis* vacuole correlates with host-cell survival. PLoS Pathogens. 2006;**2**:e45. DOI: 10.1371/journal.ppat.0020045

[91] Qin T, Li J, Zhang KQ. Structure, regulation, and function of linear and circular long non-coding RNAs. Frontiers in Genetics. 2020;**11**:150. DOI: 10.3389/fgene.2020.00150

[92] AbdelRahman YM, Rose LA, Belland RJ. Developmental expression of non-coding RNAs in *Chlamydia trachomatis* during normal and persistent growth. Nucleic Acids Research. 2011;**39**(5):1843-1854. DOI: /10.1093/nar/gkq1065

[93] Wen Y, Luo F, Zhao L, Su S, Lei W, Liu Y, et al. Long non-coding RNA FGD5-AS1 induced by *Chlamydia trachomatis* infection inhibits apoptosis via Wnt/β-catenin Signaling pathway. Frontiers in Cellular and Infection Microbiology. 2021;**11**:701352. DOI: 10.3389/fcimb.2021.701352

[94] Luo F, Wen Y, Zhao L, Su S, Zhao Y, Lei W, et al. *Chlamydia trachomatis* induces lncRNA MIAT upregulation to regulate mitochondria-mediated host cell apoptosis and Chlamydial development. Journal of Cellular and Molecular Medicine. 2022;**26**(1):163-177. DOI: 10.1111/jcmm.17069

[95] Andersen SE, Bulman LM, Steiert B, Faris R, Weber MM. Got mutants? How advances in Chlamydial genetics have furthered the study of effector proteins. Pathogens and Disease. 2021;**79**(2):ftaa078. DOI: 10.1093/femspd/ftaa078

[96] Bastidas RJ, Valdivia RH. Emancipating *Chlamydia*: Advances in the genetic manipulation of a recalcitrant intracellular pathogen. Microbiology and Molecular Biology Reviews. 2016;**80**(2):411-427. DOI: 10.1128/MMBR.00071-15

[97] Dolat L, Valdivia RH. A renewed tool kit to explore *Chlamydia* pathogenesis: From molecular genetics to new infection models. F1000Research. 2019;**8**:935. DOI: 10.12688/f1000research.18832.1

[98] Stephens RS, Kalman S, Lammel C, Fan J, Marathe R, Aravind L, et al. Genome sequence of an obligate intracellular pathogen of humans: *Chlamydia trachomatis*. Science. 1998;**282**:754-759. DOI: 10.1126/science.282.5389.754

[99] Wang Y, Kahane S, Cutcliffe LT, Skilton RJ, Lambden PR, Clarke IN. Development of a transformation system for *Chlamydia trachomatis*: Restoration of glycogen biosynthesis by acquisition of a plasmid shuttle vector. PLoS Pathogens. 2011;7:e1002258. DOI: 10.1371/journal.ppat.1002258

[100] Rahnama M, Fields KA. Transformation of *Chlamydia*: Current approaches and impact on our understanding of Chlamydial infection biology. Microbes and Infection. 2018;**20**(7-8):445-450. DOI: 10.1016/j.micinf.2018.01.002

[101] Wolf K, Rahnama M, Fields KA. Genetic manipulation of *Chlamydia trachomatis*: Chromosomal deletions. Methods in Molecular Biology. 2019;**2042**:151-164. DOI: 10.1007/978-1-4939-9694-0_11

[102] Albrecht M, Sharma CM, Dittrich MT, Muller T, Reinhardt R, Vogel J, et al. The transcriptional landscape of *Chlamydia pneumoniae*. Genome Biology. 2011;**12**:R98. DOI: 10.1186/gb-2011-12-10-r98

[103] Porcella SF, Carlson JH, Sturdevant DE, Sturdevant GL, Kanakabandi K, Virtaneva K, et al. Transcriptional profiling of human epithelial cells infected with plasmid-bearing and plasmid-deficient *Chlamydia trachomatis*. Infection and Immunity. 2015;**83**:534-543. DOI: 10.1128/IAI.02764-14

[104] Humphrys MS, Creasy T, Sun Y, Shetty AC, Chibucos MC, Drabek EF, et al. Simultaneous transcriptional profiling of bacteria and their host cells. PLoS One. 2013;**8**:e80597. DOI: 10.1371/journal.pone.0080597

[105] Hayward RJ, Marsh JW, Humphrys MS, Huston WM, Myers GSA. Early transcriptional landscapes of *Chlamydia trachomatis*-infected epithelial cells at single cell resolution. Frontiers in Cellular and Infection Microbiology. 2019;**9**:392. DOI: 10.3389/fcimb.2019.00392

[106] Hufnagel K, Lueong S, Willhauck-Fleckenstein M, et al. Immunoprofiling of *Chlamydia trachomatis* using whole-proteome microarrays generated by on-chip in situ expression. Scientific Reports. 2018;**8**:7503. DOI: 10.1038/s41598-018-25918-3

[107] Hufnagel K, Hoenderboom B, Harmel C, Rohland JK, van Benthem BHB, Morré SA, et al. *Chlamydia trachomatis* whole-proteome microarray analysis of the Netherlands Chlamydia cohort study. Microorganisms. 2019;**7**(12):703. DOI: 10.3390/microorganisms7120703

[108] Moulder JW, Levy NJ, Schulman LP. Persistent infection of mouse fibroblasts

(L cells) with *Chlamydia psittaci*: Evidence for a cryptic Chlamydial form. Infection and Immunity. 1980;**30**(3):874-883. DOI: 10.1128/iai.30.3.874-883.1980

[109] Filardo S, Di Pietro M, Sessa R. Better *In vitro* tools for exploring *Chlamydia trachomatis* pathogenesis. Life (Basel). 2022;**12**(7):1065. DOI: 10.3390/life12071065

[110] Chumduri C, Turco MY. Organoids of the female reproductive tract. Journal of Molecular Medicine (Berlin, Germany). 2021;**99**(4):531-553. DOI: 10.1007/s00109-020-02028-0 Epub 2021 Feb 13

[111] Koster S, Gurumurthy RK, Kumar N, et al. Modelling *Chlamydia* and HPV co-infection in patient-derived ectocervix organoids reveals distinct cellular reprogramming. Nature Communications. 2022;**13**:1030. DOI: 10.1038/s41467-022-28569-1

[112] Phillips-Campbell R, Kintner J, Schoborg RV. Induction of the *Chlamydia muridarum* stress/persistence response increases azithromycin treatment failure in a murine model of infection. Antimicrobial Agents and Chemotherapy. 2014;**58**(3):1782-1784. DOI: 10.1128/AAC.02097-13

[113] Del Río L, Murcia A, Buendía AJ, Álvarez D, Ortega N, Navarro JA, et al. Development of an *in vivo* model of *Chlamydia abortus* chronic infection in mice overexpressing IL-10. Veterinary Microbiology. 2018;**213**:28-34. DOI: 10.1016/j.vetmic.2017.11.009

[114] De Clercq E, Kalmar I, Vanrompay D. Animal models for studying female genital tract infection with *Chlamydia trachomatis*. Infection and Immunity. 2013;**81**(9):3060-3067. DOI: 10.1128/IAI.00357-13

Section 3

Multidisciplinary Approach to Chlamydial Infection

Chapter 9

Chlamydia and the Gastrointestinal System

Erhan Alkan

Abstract

Chlamydiae are intracellular, gram-negative, and prokaryotic microorganisms. Capable of causing disease in many mammalian and avian species, there are three types that cause disease in humans: *Chlamydia trachomatis*, *Chlamydia pneumoniae*, and *Chlamydia psittaci*. Among the chlamydia species, *C. trachomatis* is the most studied and encountered type because it is a leading cause of trachoma and sexually transmitted diseases. *C. trachomatis*, a known pathogen of the genital tract, can also be routinely detected in the human gastrointestinal tract. It can infect the enteroendocrine cells of the gastrointestinal tract. The best-known manner for *C. trachomatis* to enter the gastrointestinal tract is through oral and anal sex. Most of them are dormant, without causing any infection in the infected person. Chlamydia proctitis is the most well-known disease caused by *C. trachomatis* in the gastrointestinal tract. In this section, we evaluated the often-overlooked *Chlamydia* and the gastrointestinal system findings within the gastroenterology practice, the diseases it causes, and the treatments for these diseases.

Keywords: chlamydia, gastrointestinal system, oropharyngitis, proctitis, Chlamydia trachomatis

1. Introduction

Among the diseases caused by chlamydia, trachoma is the most widely known. The earliest known information about trachoma is found in Egyptian papyrus and Ancient Chinese inscriptions [1–3]. Intracytoplasmic inclusion bodies of *Chlamydia trachomatis* were first demonstrated by the researchers Halberstaedter and Von Prowazek [4]. In 1907, Halberstaedter and Von Prowazek applied a sample from a patient with trachoma to the conjunctiva of a monkey and, after the infection emerged, were able to show the intracytoplasmic inclusion bodies by staining the mucopurulent exudate sample with Giemsa. They defined these bodies as protozoa and named them Chlamidozoa [5]. The role of *C. trachomatis* in genital infections was evidenced by the same researchers in 1909 when they showed inclusion bodies in the conjunctival cells of babies with non-gonococcal ophthalmia neonatorum, in the cervical epithelial cells of the mothers of babies, and in the urethral epithelial cells of male patients with non-gonococcal urethritis. In 1910, Lindner showed how the mother and father of a baby with inclusion conjunctivitis showed inclusion bodies in the mother's cervical and father's urethral specimens [5]. Lymphogranuloma venereum (LGV) was first described in the late 1700s [3] and was reported by Durand, Nicolas, and Favre in 1913. Gamma and Favre showed inclusion bodies in the cytoplasm of mononuclear cells in an infected lymph node in 1924 [5]. Psittacosis was first described in humans by Ritter in 1879. Later, outbreaks were reported in many European countries. In the 1950s, attention was drawn to contamination, especially from poultry [3]. *Chlamydia pneumonia* was first isolated in 1965 during trachoma vaccine studies in Taiwan. It was later isolated from throat cultures of children with pharyngitis in the United States in 1983 [3, 6]. *C. trachomatis* was produced in the yolk sac of embryonated eggs by T'ang et al. in 1957 and isolated from cell culture by Gordon and Quan in 1965. In 1970, the microimmunofluorescence technique started being used in diagnosis, and Direct Fluorescent Antibody (DFA) and Enzyme Immunoassay (EIA) tests were developed in the 1980s [3, 7]. After the 1990s, polymerase chain reaction (PCR), ligase chain reaction (LCR), and nucleic acid amplification tests (NAAT) have been used in diagnosis [8, 9].

Chlamydiae are gram-negative, cocci-shaped, immobile, and obligate intracellular microorganisms that cause many diseases in humans. Although they have many enzymes and limited metabolic activities, they have been studied among viruses for many years due to their lack of mechanisms for providing metabolic energy and their inability to generate their own energy (Adenosine Triphosphate). However, they are distinguished from viruses by the fact that they contain both DNA and RNA, reproduce by dividing in the middle, have a similar cell wall structure to gram-negative bacteria, have ribosomes, have various enzymes that provide metabolic activity, and are sensitive to various antibiotics [1]. Unlike other bacteria, chlamydia has a biphasic life cycle. During their life cycles, they appear in two forms, which are called elementary bodies and reticular bodies, with different metabolic activity characteristics, sizes, and morphological appearances. Elementary body is the infective form that is resistant to environmental conditions and is not metabolically active. Reticular body, on the other hand, is the metabolically active form that has no infective properties but has the ability to proliferate within the host cell. Because chlamydia are compulsory intracellular parasites, they cannot be grown in artificial media [10]. They require live cell environments for their reproduction [2].

Chlamydias belong to the *Chlamydiaceae* family, which is under the order Chlamydiales. In the taxonomic classification according to their phenotypic characteristics, there are four species in the genus *Chlamydia*, namely *C. trachomatis*, *C. psittaci*, *C. pneumoniae*, and *C. pecorum*. Among these four species, only *C. pecorum* does not cause disease in humans [5]. Apart from this classification, two different genera were proposed based on 16S rRNA and 23S rRNA sequence analyses. There are three species within the genus *Chlamydia*, *C. trachomatis*, *C. suis*, and *Chlamydia muridarum*, and six species within the genus *Chlamydophila*, *C. pneumonia*, *C. psittaci*, *C. pecorum*, *C. felis*, *Chlamydophila caviae*, and *C. abortus*. However, since this classification is not accepted by many researchers, both classifications are used in the literature today [1, 8, 11, 12]. There are three biovars within the species *C. trachomatis*. These are Trachoma biovar associated with oculogenital diseases, Lymphogranuloma biovar, and rat pneumonia causative biovar. Wang and Grayston determined 15 serotypes according to antigenic structures in trachoma and LGV agents [13]. Three of these serotypes (L1–3) determined by the microimmunofluorescence method were associated with LGV, and the other 12 were associated with oculogenital diseases. The rat pneumonia-causing agent does not infect humans [8, 13, 14]. The L1, L2, and L3 serotypes of *C. trachomatis* are associated with Lymphogranuloma venereum (LGV) and are sexually transmitted. The A, B, Ba, and C serotypes cause endemic trachoma and are transmitted by hand-eye contact and flies. The D, E, F, G, H, I, J, and K serotypes cause inclusion conjunctivitis, nongonococcal urethritis, cervicitis, salpingitis, proctitis, epididymitis, neonatal pneumonia, and conjunctivitis and are transmitted sexually, perinatally, and by hand-eye contact. Today, *C. trachomatis* is one of the most important causes of sexually transmitted diseases [15]. *C. trachomatis* usually infects epithelial cells lining the mucous membranes. These are columnar cells in the cervix, cells of the urethra, rectum, conjunctiva, and cells of the newborn's respiratory system [16]. *C. trachomatis* is the cardinal pathogen of non-gonococcal urethritis [17]. Sexually transmitted *C. trachomatis* infection can sometimes be asymptomatic [18]. In this case, accurate and early diagnosis is important since patients will continue to transmit the infection [19]. Undiagnosed and untreated *C. trachomatis* infections cause diseases such as pelvic inflammatory disease and may result in ectopic pregnancy and tubal infertility. It has also been reported that *C. trachomatis* infections seen during pregnancy may be associated with pregnancy complications such as postpartum endometritis, premature rupture of membranes, premature birth, stillbirth, and low birthweight. *C. trachomatis* is also one of the important causes of reactive arthritis [8].

Cytological examination, cell culture, antigen determination, DFA, EIA, and NAAT are used in the diagnosis of *C. trachomatis*. The sensitivity of the cell culture method varies from 50 to 85%. For DFA and EIA, the sensitivity is given as 45.5–85% and 52–84.4%, respectively. Various studies have shown that the sensitivity for NAAT is from 80 to 100%. The specificity of all tests varies from 90 to 100% [20].

2. Gastrointestinal chlamydial infections in humans

York and Baker reported for the first time in cattle that *Chlamydia* was present in the gastrointestinal (GI) tract but did not cause a pathological response [21]. Later, Storz and Thornley reported that sheep have low levels of complement-fixing antibodies despite being infected. Antibody levels were found to be high in some sheep with positive fecal isolation but were observed as returning to low levels in the follow-up [22]. Cordy, Storz, and Dungworth stated that the presence of chlamydia in the intestine does not create a resistance against parenteral and respiratory tract infections [23–25]. Perry and Hughes observed that genital chlamydial infection may be somewhat protective against respiratory tract infections, but it does not prevent infection in the GI tract [26]. The reason why chlamydial GI infection could not be eliminated is the inability of the gastrointestinal tract to produce an adequate immune response. However, there are also data showing that oral infection is a potent immunization. Oral infection with live chlamydia has been shown to elicit a strong systemic immune response and a partial protective response in the genital area in both rat and guinea pig models [27, 28]. Nichols et al. showed that oral infection may be somewhat protective against conjunctival infection in the guinea pig [29]. Although these data suggest that GI chlamydial infection may trigger immunity, this immune response is insufficient. The absence of pathological findings may also indicate the complete absence of a local host response to chlamydial GI infection. In addition to the lack of pathology seen at various times after oral infection with *C. muridarum*, Igietsme et al. were unable to detect expression of VCAM-1 associated with the inflammatory response after oral infection and did not observe an increase in the number and density of intraepithelial lymphocytes. Hyperplasia of Peyer's patches was the only finding for a local immune response [30, 31]. Yeruv L et al. examined whether a local and systemic response developed as a result of *C. muridarum* gastrointestinal infection in rats. They showed that IgG was produced at a level similar to the serum IgG level that occurs in chlamydia genital infection and remained high during the 75-day observation period, while anti-chlamydia IgA appeared in the intestine 2–3 weeks after the infection, peaking on the 50th day and decreasing on the 75th day [32]. Since it has been determined that the natural site of infection for chlamydia in many animal hosts is the gastrointestinal tract, it comes to mind that the natural site of infection in humans is the gastrointestinal tract as well. Apart from direct infection with anal intercourse, there are indications that both men and women can be infected orally. There is evidence that chlamydia can pass through the stomach and small intestine and settle in the large intestine after oral infection of rats [32]. Dunlop et al. found that both cervical and rectal cultures were positive in 5 (13.2%) of 38 women who had intercourse with men with ocular chlamydial infection or urethritis [33, 34]. Rectal cultures were also positive in 7 of 11 women with ocular infection only, and rectum and cervix were infected simultaneously in 6 of them. LGV serotypes were not found in rectal isolated cases. For this reason, it was thought that the rectum also serves as a reservoir, same as the genital tract, for chlamydial infection in women [34]. It has been shown by Jones et al. that men and women can be orally infected. They took pharyngeal samples from 706 heterosexual men and 686 women and rectal samples from 1223 women at risk for chlamydia infection. *C. trachomatis* was isolated in the pharynx of 3.7% of men and 3.2% of women. *C. trachomatis* was also isolated in the rectal culture of 5.2% of women at risk. However, they could not find a statistical relationship between positive rectal isolation and anal intercourse [35]. A strong correlation was found between positive genital and rectal cultures. While 11% of genital culture-positive women were positive in the rectum, rectal swab was positive in only 2.7% of genital culture-negative women. Positive rectal cultures having been detected in homosexual men were not surprising. Stamm et al. found a positive rectal culture in 33 of 155 heterosexual women with STDs. A high percentage of these women were having anal intercourse. However, 16 of 29 asymptomatic women with positive rectal cultures did not report anal intercourse [36]. Another source of information on persistent gastrointestinal chlamydia infection comes from studies on neonates exposed to chlamydia infection at birth. A 5-year prospective study by Schachter et al. followed 131 infants born to mothers infected with chlamydia. Inclusion conjunctivitis was confirmed by culture in 18% of infants and chlamydial pneumonia in 16%. Serological response was present in 60% of the infants. Interestingly, asymptomatic rectal and vaginal infections were detected in 14% of infants at risk. Conjunctival infections were detected in the first 22 days of life, while rectal cultures were positive after 2–3 months, and vaginal cultures after 70–154 days. This suggested that the vaginal infection was due to possible fecal contamination. A high titer IgM increase was also detected in positive rectal cultures [37].

3. Chlamydial oropharyngitis–tonsillitis

C. trachomatis can be transmitted after oral sex. Many patients with *C. trachomatis* in the oropharyngeal region are asymptomatic. Rarely, it can cause oropharyngitis and tonsillitis. In this case, it can lead to symptoms such as sore throat, difficulty swallowing, and fever. Swab samples taken from this region are used for diagnosis. NAATs are one of the most sensitive tests used in the examination of samples and are recommended for use in diagnosing *C. trachomatis*. Its specificity and sensitivity are quite high [38]. Although the clinical significance of oropharyngeal *C. trachomatis* infection is unclear and oropharyngeal sampling is not routinely recommended during screening for chlamydia infection, existing evidence has shown that oropharyngeal chlamydia infection can be transmitted sexually to the genital areas [39]. Therefore, if *C. trachomatis* is detected in the oropharyngeal sample, the patient should be treated with azithromycin and doxycycline. There is not enough clinical information to compare the efficacy of antimicrobials in oropharyngeal *C. trachomatis* infection. In a double-blind randomized controlled study, no significant difference was found in terms of treatment success of urogenital *C. trachomatis* infection in men and women between the use of a delayed release 200 mg doxycycline tablet for 7 days and a 100 mg doxycycline tablet twice a day for 7 days, although gastrointestinal side effects were less in the group that received a single dose of 200 mg. On the other hand, the cost of a single-dose 200 mg tablet is higher [40].

4. Rectal *C. trachomatis* infection

C. trachomatis is the most common bacterial sexually transmitted infection in the world. There were an estimated 4 million cases of chlamydia in the United States in 2018 [41]. This has made it the most frequently reported condition nationally. Despite public health chlamydia control programs, its frequency has increased over the past 20 years [42]. Chlamydial infections are more common in young women (<25 years), especially Black, Hispanic, and Native American women, and homosexual men [43]. *C. trachomatis* infects epithelial cells of the oropharynx, genitourinary tract, and gastrointestinal tract. The rectum is increasingly recognized as a common anatomical site of *C. trachomatis* infection in humans. *C. trachomatis* is a common cause of symptomatic proctitis and proctocolitis, especially in homosexual men [8]. While 10–15% of homosexual men who apply to sexual health clinics have a positive rectal chlamydia test, this rate is 8–9% in cisgender women. Despite the high prevalence of rectal chlamydial infections, there is a lack of knowledge about the biological, epidemiological, and clinical aspects of these infections. Asymptomatic rectal carriage of *C. trachomatis* can occur in infants and adults. 85% of rectal *C. trachomatis* infections are asymptomatic. However, rectal infection is known to cause proctitis. Infection with the L1, L2, and L3 serotypes of *C. trachomatis* can cause lymphogranuloma venorum syndrome. The most common clinical manifestation of rectal LGV is proctocolitis, while urogenital LGV is inguinal and femoral painful and tender lymphadenopathies [44]. Despite the prevalence of L serotype *C. trachomatis* among homosexual men, 25–50% of these infections are asymptomatic [45]. Although there is a high prevalence of chlamydia among women in sexual health clinics, this has no clinical significance. It is not clear whether rectal *C. trachomatis* is auto-inoculated from the rectum to the genital tract, and if so, how often. Such auto-inoculation has been demonstrated in animal models [32, 46]. However, this auto-inoculation has not been proven in humans. Along with that, in several epidemiological studies, it has been emphasized that undiagnosed or inadequately treated rectal *C. trachomatis* infection may be the source of recurrent urogenital chlamydia infection in women [47, 48]. Rectal *C. trachomatis* has been described in many ways. The primary means of acquiring rectal *C. trachomatis* among homosexual men are through receptive anal sex. Apart from this, there are several articles showing that oral-anal sex, use of sex toys, fingering, and use of saliva as a lubricant may lead to rectal *C. trachomatis* acquisition [49, 50].

Considering that the prevalence of rectal chlamydia in women is similar between those who report and do not report anal sex, it is unlikely that anal sex is the primary route of acquiring of rectal *C. trachomatis* in women [51]. Considering the anatomical proximity of the vagina and anus, toilet hygiene practices, and the positive rectal *C. trachomatis* test in most (70%) women with urogenital *C. trachomatis*, many women can get rectal chlamydia from urogenital *C. trachomatis* infection. There are articles showing that up to 87% of rectal *C. trachomatis* infections in women are acquired from urogenital infections [52]. Several researchers have suggested that oral ingestion of *C. trachomatis* infection (through penile-oral sex) may lead to rectal chlamydia. In this case, in order for *C. trachomatis* to colonize and infect the large intestine, it must survive passing through the upper gastrointestinal tract. This has been demonstrated in animal models [30, 53, 54]. In humans, this has not been demonstrated experimentally, although is supported by some epidemiological evidence [55, 56]. We have stated that asymptomatic rectal carriage of *C. trachomatis* can be seen in infants and adults. However, we also emphasize that *C. trachomatis* is a common cause of symptomatic proctitis and proctocolitis [8]. Both LGV serotypes and D to K serotypes can cause these clinical presentations. The severity and prevalence of the infection also vary accordingly. Infection with agents other than LGV serotypes usually occurs by direct inoculation of the agent during anal intercourse. It remains as a limited superficial inflammation in the rectum. Its main symptoms include anal itching and mucus rectal discharge. LGV serotypes, on the other hand, come to the infection site by lymphatic spread and cause ulcers, granulomas, and cryptic abscesses in the rectum and colon mucosa. They cause symptoms such as rectal pain, tenesmus, rectal bleeding, and fever. Perirectal abscesses, rectovesical fistulas, strictures due to fibrous tissue formation in the intestinal wall, and lymphoid tissue accumulation similar to hemorrhoids due to obstruction of lymphatic drainage may occur in untreated individuals, and the infection may be confused with inflammatory bowel diseases [8]. Methods used in diagnosis include cytological examination, isolation in cell culture, antigen determination, serological examinations, and molecular methods in which nucleic acid of the agent is detected [8, 57, 58]. NAATs are one of the most sensitive tests used in the examination of samples [59, 60] and are recommended for use in diagnosing chlamydia infection [38]. *C. trachomatis* culture has been generally abandoned. Since there is no significant difference in the outcome between the samples taken by the clinician and the samples taken by the patient themself, the patient's sampling themself can be used for rectal chlamydia infection detection [61, 62]. In chlamydia screening by NAAT, especially in cases where it is difficult to reach the clinician, the patient's own samples can be an alternative to the samples taken by the clinician.

4.1 Treatment

Treating people infected with *C. trachomatis* and their partners is of great importance in preventing reproductive health-related complications, stopping the transmission of the disease to individuals, and preventing re-infection. Doxycycline and azithromycin are the most commonly used drugs for the treatment of rectal chlamydia. Before 2020, the treatment guidelines for sexually transmitted infections recommended azithromycin 1 g orally as a single dose or doxycycline 100 mg orally 2x1 for 7 days for the treatment of rectal chlamydia infection. As alternative treatments, erythromycin base 500 mg orally 4x1 for 7 days or erythromycin 800 mg orally for 4x1 7 days or levofloxacin 500 mg orally 1x1 for 7 days or ofloxacin 300 mg 2x1 for 7 days can be used. Many clinicians prefer to use azithromycin because of the ease of use of single-dose therapy and the possibility of treatment under direct supervision. In the gonorrhea treatment guideline, which was renewed in 2020, it is recommended to use doxycycline for treatment in cases where rectal chlamydial infection is not excluded. In the sexually transmitted diseases guide published in 2021, doxycycline was presented as a revised recommendation as the treatment of choice for chlamydia treatment [44, 63]. Recommendations for the treatment of rectal chlamydia have long been derived from studies of urogenital chlamydia. However, in some observational studies, it has been shown that azithromycin is less effective than doxycycline, and the difference in effectiveness in the rectum is greater than in the urogenital region [64, 65]. Two randomized controlled trials have recently been published on the treatment of rectal chlamydia among homosexual men. These studies compared azithromycin with doxycycline. While microbiological cure was achieved at a rate of 74–76% in the azithromycin group, this rate was found to be 97–100% in the doxycycline group [48, 66]. Results showing that doxycycline is superior to azithromycin in the treatment of rectal chlamydia in cisgender women have been suggested [67]. In light of this information, doxycycline treatment may be the first choice in the treatment of rectal chlamydia. In patient groups where treatment compliance may be low, direct single dose azithromycin may be preferred for treatment. If possible, it can be ensured that the patient is taking the drug under the supervision of the physician. Again, in cases where 7-day treatment with doxycycline will be given, the first dose can be given immediately and under the supervision of a physician. In order to minimize the transmission of the disease to sexual partners, it should be recommended that the patient abstain from sexual activity for the next 7 days if they received a single dose of treatment, and if they received 7 days of treatment, to abstain during the treatment and until the symptoms completely regress. To minimize the risk of re-infection, it is important for people with multiple sexual partners to avoid intercourse until all partners have completed their treatment.

4.2 Sexual partner management during treatment

All partners who have had sexual intercourse with the patient up to 60 days before the onset of symptoms of the disease should be tested for chlamydia infection. Although the frequency of intercourse and the time elapsed since the last intercourse affect the risk of transmission of the disease, the last sexual intercourse partner (even if more than 60 days have passed since the last sexual intercourse) must be treated. In cases where the partners cannot reach the doctor and medical services directly, sending the prescription or the drugs themselves to the patient's partner can also be considered as an option. It has been shown that such practices significantly reduce the risk of persistent or recurrent infections [68–70]. In homosexual individuals, since chlamydial infection is likely to be accompanied by other sexually transmitted diseases (especially undiagnosed HIV infection), partners should be thoroughly evaluated by a physician before being treated. Suggesting that patients come with their partners during follow-up visits may also make partner treatment more effective. To prevent re-infection, patients' partners should be advised to abstain from sexual intercourse until the disease is completely cured (within 7 days after a single dose treatment or until the end of treatment in 7 days of treatment) and until the symptoms have completely receded.

4.3 Post-treatment follow-up

Re-testing 3–4 weeks after the end of treatment is not recommended except in cases where there is doubt about the patient's compliance with treatment, when symptoms persist, or when re-infection is suspected. Performing the NAAT test earlier than 3 weeks after the end of the treatment may lead to false positive results since non-viable microorganisms can still be found in the body. Therefore, in cases where recovery is uncertain and retesting is required, at least 3 weeks should have passed since the first treatment before the test [38, 71].

5. Conclusion

C. trachomatis is the most common bacterial sexually transmitted infection in the world. It can cause significant health problems in both men and women. *C. trachomatis*, a known pathogen of the genital tract, can also be routinely detected in the human GI tract. Its entry into the GI tract has risen due to increased oral-anal sex. Most remain dormant in infected people. Chlamydia proctitis is the most well-known disease caused by *C. trachomatis* in the GI tract. Rarely, it can cause oropharyngitis and tonsillitis. Due to these infections, the frequency of which is increasing day by day, and the possibility of patients to apply to gastroenterology outpatient clinics is also increasing. It is important to consider this situation, which is often overlooked in gastroenterology practice.

Author details

Erhan Alkan
Department of Gastroenterology, Medicalpark Hospital, Antalya, Turkey

*Address all correspondence to: dr.erhan@hotmail.com

References

[1] Ertem E. Klamidyaların Genel Özellikleri, Chlamydia trachomatis. In: Topçu AW, Söyletir G, Doğanay M, editors. Enfeksiyon Hastalıkları ve Mikrobiyolojisi (s.1945-1964). İstanbul: Nobel Tıp Kitabevleri Ltd. Şti; 2008

[2] Mabey DCW, Solomon AW, Foster A. Trachoma. Lancet. 2003;**362**:223-229

[3] Schachter J. Chlamydial infections. The Western Journal of Medicine. 1990;**153**:523-534

[4] McGregor JA, French JI. Chlamydia trachomatis infection during pregnancy. American Journal of Obstetrics and Gynecology. 1991;**164**(6):1782-1789

[5] Schachter J. In: Holmes KK, Sparling PF, Mardh PA, Lemon MS, editors. Biology of *Chlamydia trachomatis*, Sexually Transmitted Diseases (s.391-405). Third ed. New York: McGraw-Hill; 1999

[6] Mardh, P., Domeika, M. (1994), Pneumonia and Allied Conditions Caused by *Chlamydia psittaci* and *Chlamydia pneumoniae*

[7] Barnes RC. Laboratory diagnosis of human chlamydial infections. Clinical Microbiology Reviews. 1989;**2**(2):119-136

[8] Stamm WE, Jones RB, Batteiger BE. Introduction to chlamydial diseases and chlamydia trachomatis. In: Mandell GL, Benett JE, Dolin R, editors. Mandell, Douglas and Benett's Principles and Practice of Infectious Diseases. 6th. ed. Philadelphia: Churcill Livingstone; 2005. pp. 2236-2268

[9] Schachter J. DFA, EIA, PCR, LCR and other technologies: What tests should be used for diagnosis of chlamydia infections? Immunological Investigations. 1997;**26**(1&2):157-161

[10] Sarier M, Duman İ, Göktaş Ş, Demir M, Kukul E. Results of multiplex polymerase chain reaction assay to identify urethritis pathogens. Journal of Urological Surgery. 2017;**1**:18-22. DOI: 10.4274/jus.1328

[11] Brooks GF, Butel JS, Ornston LN. Chlamydiae. In: Jawetz E, Melnick JL, Adelberg EA, editors. Jawetz, Melnick & Adelberg's Medical Microbiology. Twentieth ed. Prentice-Hall International Inc.; 1995. pp. 294-302

[12] Everett KDE, Bush RM, Andersen AA. Emended description of the order Chlamydiales, proposal of Parachlamydiaceae fam. Nov. and Simkaniaceae fam. Nov., each containing one monotypic genus, revised taxonomy of the family Chlamydiaceae, including a new genus and five new species, and standards for the identification of organisms. International Journal of Systematic Bacteriology. 1999;**49**:415-440

[13] Holmes KK. The chlamydia epidemic. JAMA. 1981;**245**(17):1718-1723

[14] Guaschino S, De Seta F. Update on chlamydia trachomatis. The New England Journal of Medicine. 2000;**900**:293-300

[15] Sarier M, Sepin N, Duman I, et al. Microscopy of gram-stained urethral smear in the diagnosis of urethritis: Which threshold value should be selected? Andrologia. 2018:e13143. DOI: 10.1111/and.13143

[16] Kelly KA. Cellular immunity and chlamydia genital infection: Induction,

recruitment and effector mechanisms. International Reviews of Immunology. 2003;**22**:3-41

[17] Sarier M, Kukul E. Classification of non-gonococcal urethritis: A review. International Urology and Nephrology. 2019;**51**(6):901-907. DOI: 10.1007/s11255-019-02140-2

[18] Sarier M, Demir M, Turgut H, et al. New approach to microscopy of gram-stained urethral smear: The kissing slide method. Sexually Transmitted Diseases. 2020;**47**(10):712-715. DOI: 10.1097/OLQ.0000000000001228

[19] Sarier M, Sepin N, Emek M, et al. Evaluating the utility of the a.F. genital system test for pathogen diagnosis in acute male urethritis. Andrologia. 2022;**54**(4):e14377. DOI: 10.1111/and.14377

[20] Watson EJ, Templeton A, Russell I, Paavonen J, Mardh PA, Stary A, et al. The accuracy and efficacy of screening tests for chlamydia trachomatis: A systematic review. Journal of Medical Microbiology. 2002;**51**:1021-1031

[21] York CJ, Baker JA. A new member of the psittacosislymphogranuloma group of viruses that causes infection in calves. The Journal of Experimental Medicine. 1951;**93**:587-604. DOI: 10.1084/jem.93.6.587

[22] Storz J, Thornley WR. Serological and etiological studies on the intestinal psittacosis-lymphogranuloma infection of sheep. Zentralblatt für Veterinärmedizin. Reihe B. 1966;**13**:14-24 (In German.)

[23] Dungworth DL, Cordy DR. The pathogenesis of ovine pneumonia. II. Isolation of virus from faeces; comparison of pneumonia caused by faecal, enzootic abortion and pneumonitis viruses. Journal of Comparative Pathology. 1962;**72**:71-79

[24] Storz J. Intestinal infections of ruminants. In: Storz J, editor. Chlamydia and Chlamydia-Induced Diseases. Springfield, IL: Charles C. Thomas; 1971. pp. 146-154

[25] Storz J. Superinfection of pregnant ewes latently infected with a psittacosis-lymphgranuloma agent. The Cornell Veterinarian. 1963;**53**:469-480

[26] Perry LL, Hughes S. Chlamydial colonization of multiple mucosae following infection by any mucosal route. Infection and Immunity. 1999;**67**:3686-3689

[27] Kelly KA, Robinson EA, Rank RG. Initial route of antigen administration alters the T-cell cytokine profile produced in response to the mouse pneumonitis biovar of chlamydia trachomatis following genital infection. Infection and Immunity. 1996;**64**:4976-4983

[28] Rank RG, Batteiger BE, Soderberg LSF. Immunization against chlamydial genital infection in Guinea pigs with UV-inactivated and viable chlamydiae administered by different routes. Infection and Immunity. 1990;**58**:2599-2605

[29] Nichols RL, Murray ES, Nisson PE. Use of enteric vaccines in protection against chlamydial infections of the genital tract and the eye of Guinea pigs. The Journal of Infectious Diseases. 1978;**138**:742-746. DOI: 10.1093/infdis/138.6.742

[30] Igietseme JU, Portis JL, Perry LL. Inflammation and clearance of chlamydia trachomatis in enteric and nonenteric mucosae. Infection and Immunity. 2001;**69**:1832-1840. DOI: 10.1128/IAI.69.3.1832-1840.2001

[31] Perry LL, Feilzer K, Portis JL, Caldwell HD. Distinct homing pathways direct T lymphocytes to the genital and intestinal mucosae in chlamydia-infected mice. Journal of Immunology. 1998;**160**:2905-2914

[32] Yeruva L, Spencer N, Bowlin AK, Wang Y, Rank RG. Chlamydial infection of the gastrointestinal tract: A reservoir for persistent infection. Pathogens and Disease. 2013;**68**:88-95. DOI: 10.1111/2049 -632X.12052

[33] Darougar S, Kinnison JR, Jones B. Chlamydial isolates from the rectum in association with chlamydial infection of the eye or genital tract. I. Laboratory aspects. In: Nichols RL, editor. Trachoma and Related Disorders. Princeton, NJ: Excerpta Medica; 1970. pp. 501-506

[34] Dunlop EMC, Hare MJ, Darougar S, Jones B. Chlamydial isolates from the rectum in association with chlamydial infection of the eye or genital tract. II. Clinical aspects. In: Nichols RL, editor. Trachoma and Related Disorders. Princeton, NJ: Excerpta Medica; 1970. pp. 507-512

[35] Jones RB, Rabinovitch RA, Katz BP, Batteiger BE, Quinn TS, Terho P, et al. Chlamydia trachomatis in the pharynx and rectum of heterosexual patients at risk for genital infection. Annals of Internal Medicine. 1985;**102**:757-762. DOI: 10.7326/0003-4819-102-6-757

[36] Stamm W, Quinn ETC, Mkrtichian E, Wang SP, Schuffler MD, Holmes KK. Chlamydia trachomatis proctitis. In: Mardh P-A, Holmes K, Oriel JD, Piot P, Schachter J, editors. Chlamydial Infections. Amsterdam, Netherlands: Elsevier Biomedical Press; 1982. pp. 111-114

[37] Schachter J, Grossman M, Sweet RL, Holt J, Jordan C, Bishop E. Prospective study of perinatal transmission of chlamydia trachomatis. JAMA. 1986;**255**:3374-3377. DOI: 10.1001/jama.1986.03370240044034

[38] Centers for Disease Control and Prevention. Recommendations for the laboratory-based detection of *Chlamydia trachomatis* and *Neisseria gonorrhoeae*—2014. MMWR - Recommendations and Reports. 2014;**63**:1-19

[39] Marcus JL, Kohn RP, Barry PM, et al. Chlamydia trachomatis and Neisseria gonorrhoeae transmission from the female oropharynx to the male urethra. Sexually Transmitted Diseases. 2011;**38**:372-373

[40] Geisler WM, Koltun WD, Abdelsayed N, et al. Safety and efficacy of WC2031 versus vibramycin for the treatment of uncomplicated urogenital chlamydia trachomatis infection: A randomized, double-blind, double-dummy, active-controlled, multicenter trial. Clinical Infectious Diseases. 2012;**55**:82-88

[41] World Health Organization. Sexually Transmitted Infections (STIs). 2016. Available from: https://www.who.int/newsroom/fact-sheets/detail/sexually-transmitted-infections-(stis). Updated 14 June 2019. [Accessed: September 17, 2020]

[42] Kreisel KM, Weston EJ, St Cyr SB, Spicknall IH. Estimates of the prevalence and incidence of chlamydia and gonorrhea among US men and women, 2018. Sexually Transmitted Diseases. 2021;**48**(4):222-231

[43] Centers for Disease Control and Prevention. Sexually Transmitted Disease Surveillance 2018. Atlanta, Georgia: US Department of Health and Human Services; 2019

[44] Workowski KA, Bachmann LH, Chan PA, et al. Sexually transmitted infections treatment guidelines, 2021. MMWR - Recommendations and Reports. 2021;**70**(4):1-187

[45] De Vrieze NH, van Rooijen M, Schim van der Loeff MF, de Vries HJ. Anorectal and inguinal lymphogranuloma venereum among men who have sex with men in Amsterdam, the Netherlands: Trends over time, symptomatology and concurrent infections. Sexually Transmitted Infections. 2013;**89**(7):548-552

[46] Craig AP, Kong FY, Yeruva L, et al. Is it time to switch to doxycycline from azithromycin for treating genital chlamydial infections in women? Modelling the impact of autoinoculation from the gastrointestinal tract to the genital tract. BMC Infectious Diseases. 2015;**15**:200

[47] Whittington WL, Kent C, Kissinger P, et al. Determinants of persistent and recurrent chlamydia trachomatis infection in young women: Results of a multicenter cohort study. Sexually Transmitted Diseases. 2001;**28**(2):117-123

[48] Dombrowski JC, Wierzbicki MR, Newman LM, et al. Doxycycline versus azithromycin for the treatment of rectal chlamydia in men who have sex with men. Clinical Infectious Diseases. 2021;**2**:19. DOI: 10.1093/cid/ciab153

[49] Cornelisse VJ, Fairley CK, Read TRH, et al. Associations between anorectal chlamydia and Oroanal sex or saliva use as a lubricant for anal sex: A cross-sectional survey. Sexually Transmitted Diseases. 2018;**45**(8):506-510

[50] Heiligenberg M, Rijnders B, Schim van der Loeff MF, et al. High prevalence of sexually transmitted infections in HIV-infected men during routine outpatient visits in the Netherlands. Sexually Transmitted Diseases. 2012;**39**(1):8-15

[51] Lau A, Kong FYS, Huston W, et al. Factors associated with anorectal chlamydia trachomatis or Neisseria gonorrhoeae test positivity in women: A systematic review and meta-analysis. Sexually Transmitted Infections. 2019;**95**(5):361-367

[52] Heijne JCM, van Liere G, Hoebe C, et al. What explains anorectal chlamydia infection in women? Implications of a mathematical model for test and treatment strategies. Sexually Transmitted Infections. 2017;**93**(4):270-275

[53] Rank RG, Yeruva L. An alternative scenario to explain rectal positivity in chlamydia-infected individuals. Clinical Infectious Diseases. 2015;**60**(10):1585-1586

[54] Zhu C, Lin H, Tang L, et al. Oral chlamydia vaccination induces transmucosal protection in the airway. Vaccine. 2018;**36**(16):2061-2068

[55] Batteiger TA, Jordan SJ, Toh E, et al. Detection of rectal chlamydia trachomatis in heterosexual men who report cunnilingus. Sexually Transmitted Diseases. 2019;**46**(7):440-445

[56] Khosropour CM, Soge OO, Suchland R, et al. Recurrent/intermittent vaginal and rectal chlamydial infection following treatment: A prospective cohort study among female sexually transmitted disease clinic patients. Journal of Infectious Diseases. 2019;**220**(3):476-483

[57] Essig A. Chlamydia and Chlamydophila; manual of clinical microbiology. In: Murray PR, Baron EJ,

Jorgensen JH, Landry ML, Pfaller MA, editors. 9th ed. Washington, DC: ASM Press; 2007. pp. 1021-1035

[58] Sarier M, Sepin N, Guler H, et al. Prevalence of sexually transmitted disease in asymptomatic renal transplant recipients. Experimental and Clinical Transplantation. 2018;(1). DOI: 10.6002/ect.2017.0232

[59] Sarier M. Polymerase chain reaction assay in acute urethritis. Andrologia. 2019;**51**(8):e13366. DOI: 10.1111/and.13366), 10.1111/and.13366)

[60] Sarier M. Prevalence of Polymicrobial infection in urethritis. Journal of Urological Surgery. 2019;**6**(3):180-183. DOI: 10.4274/jus.galenos.2019.2405

[61] Sexton ME, Baker JJ, Nakagawa K, et al. How reliable is self-testing for gonorrhea and chlamydia among men who have sex with men? The Journal of Family Practice. 2013;**62**:70-78

[62] Dodge B, Van Der Pol B, Reece M, et al. Rectal self-sampling in non-clinical venues for detection of sexually transmissible infections among behaviourally bisexual men. Sexual Health. 2012;**9**:190-191

[63] St Cyr S, Barbee L, Workowski KA, et al. Update to CDC's treatment guidelines for gonococcal infection, 2020. MMWR. Morbidity and Mortality Weekly Report. 2020;**69**(50):1911-1916

[64] Khosropour CM, Dombrowski JC, Barbee LA, et al. Comparing azithromycin and doxycycline for the treatment of rectal chlamydial infection: A retrospective cohort study. Sexually Transmitted Diseases. 2014;**41**(2):79-85

[65] Kong FY, Tabrizi SN, Fairley CK, et al. The efficacy of azithromycin and doxycycline for the treatment of rectal chlamydia infection: A systematic review and meta-analysis. The Journal of Antimicrobial Chemotherapy. 2015;**70**(5):1290-1297

[66] Lau A, Kong FYS, Fairley CK, et al. Azithromycin or doxycycline for asymptomatic rectal chlamydia trachomatis. The New England Journal of Medicine. 2021;**384**(25):2418-2427

[67] Dukers-Muijrers N, Wolffs PFG, De Vries H, et al. Treatment effectiveness of azithromycin and doxycycline in uncomplicated rectal and vaginal chlamydia trachomatis infections in women: A multicenter observational study (FemCure). Clinical Infectious Diseases. 2019;**69**(11):1946-1954

[68] Golden MR, Whittington WL, Handsfield HH, et al. Effect of expedited treatment of sex partners on recurrent or persistent gonorrhea or chlamydial infection. The New England Journal of Medicine. 2005;**352**:676-685

[69] Schillinger JA, Kissinger P, Calvet H, et al. Patient-delivered partner treatment with azithromycin to prevent repeated chlamydia trachomatis infection among women: A randomized, controlled trial. Sexually Transmitted Diseases. 2003;**30**:49-56

[70] Kissinger P, Mohammed H, Richardson-Alston G, et al. Patient-delivered partner treatment for male urethritis: A randomized, controlled trial. Clinical Infectious Diseases. 2005;**41**:623-629

[71] Renault CA, Israelski DM, Levy V, et al. Time to clearance of chlamydia trachomatis ribosomal RNA in women treated for chlamydial infection. Sexual Health. 2011;**8**:69-73

Chapter 10

Chlamydial Eye Infections

Seçil Özdemir Şahin

Abstract

Chlamydiae are obligate intracellular bacteria causing mucosal infections. The leading agent *Chlamydia trachomatis* causes three clinical features in eyes: trachoma, neonatal, and adult inclusion conjunctivitis. A rare chlamydial conjunctivitis form called Lymphogranuloma Venereum conjunctivitis can be venereally transmitted. Seldomly *Chlamydia psittaci* and *Chlamydia pneumonia* may cause follicular conjunctivitis. Trachoma, the most sight-threatening chlamydial eye infection, lead to approximately 6 million blindness worldwide. Classical trachoma is characterized by chronic follicular keratoconjunctivitis, conjunctival scarring, and pannus formation. According to WHO at least two of the following should be present for clinical trachoma diagnosis: Superior tarsal follicles, limbal follicles or Herbert Pits, typical conjunctival scarring and vascular pannus. These should also be supported by laboratory findings such as organismal isolation and humoral or local antibody detection. The treatment consists of the personal acute sporadic trachoma treatment, the eradication of the disease, and complication management. For acute personnel treatment, systemical and topical forms of Tetracycline, Doxycycline, or Erythromycin are used. For the eradication of the disease, oral Azithromycin is a well-tolerated antibiotic. The management of the complications consists of surgical interventions for scars. In spite of developing hygiene standards and control programs, trachoma is still a major cause of infectious blindness.

Keywords: chlamydia, conjunctivitis, trachoma, inclusion, pannus, blindness

1. Introduction

The Chlamydiae, lacking cytochromes, unable to synthesize ATP, and are therefore obligate intracellular microorganism. By including both DNA and RNA, reproduction by binary fission, and being sensitive to antibiotics, they are classified as bacteria. Chlamydiae are gram negative and symbionts of diverse organisms ranging from human beings to amoebae. This family comprises 11 species that are pathogenic to humans or animals [1].

Some species that are originally animal pathogens, such as the avian pathogen *Chlamydia psittaci*, can be transmitted to humans [1, 2].

The main agents that infect humans and cause the widest range of diseases are *Chlamydia trachomatis* and *Chlamydia pneumoniae* [2, 3].

Strains of *C. trachomatis* are divided into three biovars: trachoma biovar, genital tract biovar, and lympho granuloma venereum biovar. These biovars are further subtyped by 15 serovars. The trachoma biovar (serovars A–C) is the leading cause of preventable blindness in developing nations, whereas the genital tract biovar (serovars D–K) is the most prevalent sexually transmitted bacterium [3]. As an absolute sexually transmitted pathogen, *C. trachomatis* is isolated more in developed countries. It is one of the most common sexually translated microorganisms in the world [4].

It must be noted that *C. trachomatis infection* may be asymptomatic in both sexes. This makes it harder to diagnose and manage infection control. This microorganism is the most common acute urethritis cause in sexually active young population. In acute urethritis due to *C. trachomatis*, cardinal findings like urethral discharge, itching and dysuria are so mild or sometimes do not exist [5].

Although its prevalence varies geographically, it accounts for 20–50% of non-gonococcal urethritis cases and according to a study conducted in Turkiye, 84% of all urethritis cases are classified as nongonococcal [6].

C. trachomatis can cause epididymitis and male infertility in men.

The pathogen causes a wide range of diseases in women from acute cervicitis to pelvic inflammatory disease. The disease is usually asymptomatic, therefore, the patients unconsciously continue spreading the infection [7].

Another issue that makes the management of *C. trachomatis* infection harder is that it occurs most of the time as a coinfection with the other sexually transmitted pathogens [8]. Thus, early detection and management of *C. trachomatis* genital infections are very important [9].

For the time being, as culture and serological techniques are insufficient for diagnosis, with their high sensitivity and specificity, nucleic acid amplification tests like PCR are gold standard methods [10].

The World Health Organization estimated a prevalence of chlamydia at 4.2% (95% uncertainty interval: 3.7–4.7) worldwide among women aged 15–50 years in 2012. These figures correspond to approximately 131 million new cases of chlamydia annually (100–166 million). Ascending genitourinary infection may result in ectopic pregnancy, infertility, and chronic pelvic pain in some women [11].

The lymphogranuloma venereum biovar (serovars L1–L3) causes an invasive urogenital or anorectal infection.

Three Chlamydia species affect the eye by forming different types of conjunctivitis: *C. chlamydia*, *C. psittaci,* and *C. pneumonia*.

The ocular clinical manifestations of these three species are as follows [12]:

C. trachomatis: Trachoma, adult inclusion conjunctivitis, neonatal inclusion conjunctivitis, and lymphogranuloma venereum conjunctivitis.

C. psittaci: *C. psittaci* conjunctivitis.

C. pneumonia: *C. pneumonia* conjunctivitis.

C. trachomatis is the most frequent conjunctivitis causing one among all. Besides, it had been and still is, in endemic areas of the world causing trachoma and hereby blindness and low vision, which is a major problem of public health. Therefore *C. trachomatis* will be the prominent subject of this chapter.

2. *Chlamydia trachomatis* eye infections

2.1 Conjunctivitis due to *C. trachomatis*

C. trachomatis is divided into 15 serological subgroups (serovars) according to monoclonal antibody-based tests. These serovars are associated with many medical conditions such as:

A, B, Ba, and C: Trachoma is a serious eye disease that is endemic in certain regions of the world such as Asia and Africa, where close physical contact and poor hygiene conditions prevail. It is characterized by chronic follicular conjunctivitis and may cause visual damage.

D, E, F, G, H, I, J, and K: Sexual infections and neonatal infections due to eye contact with infected mother's cervix during the birth and adult eye infections in developed countries.

L1, L2, L3: Lymphogranuloma venereum (LGV), which correlates with genital ulcer disease in tropical areas.

C. trachomatis is spread by direct and indirect contact such as fomites, flies, bedding, towels, etc. Family and school are the main transmission environments for transmission. In healthy individuals, the immune system can cope with a single attack. However, in recurrent episodes of infection, it succumbs to the infection [13].

2.1.1 Trachoma

Trachoma is one of the oldest diseases known. Even in the twenty-seventh century BC in China and seventeenth century BC in Egypt, there are findings about the disease [12].

It had been the leading cause of blindness in history and still is the leading cause of blindness by an infectious agent worldwide.

Trachoma is a public health problem in 44 countries and is responsible for blinding or visually impairing 1.9 million people. Of all blindness worldwide, it causes about 1.4% [14].

The number of people at risk of trachoma has decreased by 91% from 1.5 billion in 2002 to about 137 million in 2020. Besides, the number of individuals requiring surgery has reduced by 68% from 7.6 million in 2002 to 2.5 million in 2019 [15].

Based on June 2022 data, 125 million people live in trachoma-endemic areas and are at risk of trachoma blindness.

Trachoma is hyperendemic in many of the poorest and most rural areas of Central and South America, Australia, Africa, Asia, and the Middle East. Overall, Africa remains the most affected continent and the one with the most intensive control efforts.

For this most sight-threatening neglected tropical disease, World Health Organization (WHO) adopted a strategy called SAFE in 1993.

Elimination programs in endemic countries are being implemented using this WHO-recommended SAFE strategy. It consists of:

- **S**urgery for the blinding phase treatment (trachomatous trichiasis);
- **A**ntibiotics to clear the infection, particularly mass drug administration of the antibiotic azithromycin, which is donated by the manufacturer to elimination programs, through the International Trachoma Initiative;
- **F**acial cleanliness; and
- **E**nvironmental improvement, particularly improving access to clean water and sanitation.

Most endemic countries have agreed to accelerate the implementation of this strategy to achieve elimination targets.

WHO's mandate is to provide leadership and coordinate the international efforts aiming to eliminate trachoma as a public health problem, and to report on progress toward that target.

In the year 1996, WHO launched the WHO Alliance for the Global Elimination of Trachoma by 2020. The Alliance is a partnership that supports the implementation of the SAFE strategy by the Member States, and the strengthening of national capacity through epidemiological surveys, project evaluation, monitoring, and resource mobilization.

The World Health Assembly adopted resolution WHA51.11 in 1998, targeting the global elimination of trachoma as a public health problem with 2020 as the target date. The neglected tropical diseases road map 2021–2030, endorsed by the World Health Assembly in 2020 through its decision 73(33), sets the date 2030 as the new target for global elimination [16].

2.1.1.1 Clinical features

The discomfort degree caused by ocular infection with *C. trachomatis* ranges from minimal to severe. Most of the infections are asymptomatic. Trachoma begins as a follicular conjunctivitis of the upper palpebral conjunctiva with associated limbal follicles. The incubation period is approximately one week. Other early findings include a mucopurulent discharge, conjunctival papillary hypertrophy, a superiorly based superficial corneal pannus (invasion of the vessels to the cornea), and a fine epithelial keratitis. Clinically, trachoma can be divided into its acute (active) and chronic or late-stage manifestations, but acute and chronic signs can occur at the same time in the same individual. As a result, the inflammation causes scarring and cicatrization of the cornea, conjunctiva, and eyelids.

The blinding complications of trachoma occur as a result of conjunctival connective tissue proliferation. Arlt's Line is the name given to a horizontal scar of the upper lid's pretarsal conjunctiva. Another sequel pathognomonic for trachoma, Herbert's pits are the delineated depressions that occur after cicatrization of the limbal follicles and the resultant clear spaces filled with epithelium. A homogenous clouding can be formed on the cornea as the superior pannus is regressed [17–19].

Resultants of conjunctival scarring, eyelid deformities as distichiasis, trichiasis, ectropion, and entropion may all occur. If sufficient transconjunctival scarring accumulates, contraction over the years will cause the upper lid to turn inward so that the eyelashes rub against the cornea and conjunctiva. This is named as trichiasis. If the whole lid edge is turned in, that condition is named as entropion. Scars around the bases of hair follicles can pull individual eyelashes into contact with the cornea, even entropion does not accompany. Corneal scarring, vascularization, ulceration, and even perforation resulting from these deformities can lead to visual acuity impairment and even blindness [20].

MacCallan developed a staging of the disease based on the conjunctival findings in 1908:

STAGE 1: Early lymphoid hyperplasia with immature follicle formation in the upper tarsal conjunctiva, diffuse punctate keratitis and early signs of pannus.
STAGE 2A: Mature upper tarsal follicles.
STAGE 2B: Fluoride inflammation due to pretarsal and limbal follicle enlargement and papillary hypertrophy and complicated pannus.

STAGE 3: Papillary hypertrophy regression, persistence of tarsal follicles, and onset of conjunctival scarring.
STAGE 4: No acute inflammation, scars replacing papillae and follicles, and regression of the pannus.

The WHO has developed a more practical grading system for trachoma, structured around diffuse inflammation, follicular conjunctivitis, trichiasis, tarsal scarring, and corneal opacification presence. The WHO simplified trachoma grading system is widely used for research and program monitoring purposes.

This system includes five signs:

- Trachomatous inflammation-follicular (TF): the presence of five or more follicles at least 0.5 mm in diameter in the central part of the upper tarsal conjunctiva;

- Trachomatous inflammation-intense (TI): pronounced inflammatory thickening of the upper tarsal conjunctiva obscuring more than half the normal deep tarsal vessels;

- Trachomatous scarring (TS): the presence of easily visible scars in the tarsal conjunctiva;

- Trachomatous trichiasis (TT): at least a single eyelash rub on the eyeball or evidence of recent removal of in-turned eyelashes;

- Corneal opacity (CO): easily visible corneal opacity over the pupil, so dense that at least part of the pupil margin is blurred when viewed through the opacity.

The presence or absence of each sign should be independently determined for each person examined. In the WHO system, the presence of TF and/or TI in one eye is necessary and sufficient to confer the diagnosis of acute trachoma [17, 21].

2.1.1.2 Laboratory diagnosis

Laboratory tests crucial for identifying *C. trachomatis* infections to confirm the diagnosis are [22]:

Giemsa staining of smears: The most common procedure worldwide for identificating *C. trachomatis* infection is microscopic evaluation of the cells with Giemsa stain. The easiest and earliest method of laboratory diagnosis was by direct indication of the Halberstaedter-Prowazek bodies with Giemsa staining of conjunctival smears. Although it may not be sensitive enough in patients with nonaggressive ocular disease, Giemsa stain detects the inclusions in most of the cases with follicular or papillar trachoma [12].

Antigen detection assays: The two tests available are Direct Fluorescent Antibody (DFA) and enzyme immunoassay (EIA). DFA with monoclonal antibodies is 90% sensitive and enzyme immunoassay (EIA) is believed to have a lower sensitivity. Both are used widely in routine.

Tissue Culture Isolation: Isolation of C. trachomatis in Hella cells or McCoy cells, etc., is the most specific method and is considered the "gold standard." However, sensitivity is low. C. trachomatis inclusions are detected either by Giemsa, Macchiavelli, or Gimenez staining or immunofluorescence assay after 48–72 h of incubation.

Serology: The most common tests are complement fixation and microimmunofluorescence tests. Infection by any serotype of C. trachomatis causes a crossreactive antibody reaction against all the serotypes. The antibodies persist for a long period; therefore, serology has a limited role in the diagnosis of acute chlamydial infections [23].

Nucleic acid amplification tests: The most commonly used tests are Polymerase Chain Reaction (PCR) assay and Ligase Chain Reaction (LCR) assay. Although they are the most sensitive and specific techniques for C. trachomatis detection, they are still not used for routine laboratory practices in poor countries due to the high cost and need for expertise [24].

2.1.1.3 Differential diagnosis

For the diagnosis of trachoma, although follicles are not pathognomonic, their presence in endemic areas should be a strong reason for suspicion. Pannus, conjunctival scarring, and trichiasis seen in these areas are almost always attributable to trachoma. Herbert's pits are pathognomonic for previous trachomatous inflammation.

The most common differential diagnosis are as follows:

- Bacterial conjunctivitis.
- Adult inclusion conjunctivitis.
- Viral conjunctivitis.
- Allergic conjunctivitis.

Toxic follicular conjunctivitis is secondary to topical medications or cosmetics.

In areas where trachoma is endemic, pannus, conjunctival scarring, and trichiasis are almost attributable to trachoma. Corneal opacity, however, has many possible etiologies [25].

2.1.1.4 Treatment

2.1.1.4.1 Personal (acute sporadic trachoma) treatment

Systemical

Trachoma treatment consists of a 3–4 week use of oral antibiotics. The most commonly used medications are tetracycline (tetracycline 1 g/day or doxycycline 100 mg/day) or oral erythromycin. Erythromycin is indicated for less side effects in children, breastfeeding women, and pregnant. The clinical response may take 9–18 weeks.

Topical

Topical tetracycline or erythromycin ointment is used at least twice a day for 5 days each for 6 months. Reusing topical medication is especially useful where the disease is endemic and reexposure is expected [26].

Treatment aiming the eradication of the disease

Through the provision of adequate water and hygiene facilities combined with education to promote facial cleanliness and the use of hygiene facilities, it was shown that only face-washing habits even reduced trachoma prevalence [27].

Reducing the fly population by 90%, causing less transmission with eye-seeking flies can reduce the active trachoma prevalence by 60% [28].

To clear ocular *C. trachomatis* infection in endemic fields, antibiotic treatment may be helpful. Oral azithromycin (1 g/day for adults, 20 mg/kg/day for children) as a single dose is used [29]. It is claimed that in endemic areas, instead of topical treatment, a single dose of oral azithromycin is enough [30, 31].

Azithromycin is well tolerated and systemic antibiotic and is also effective for extraocular infection [32]. Topical tetracycline treatment 3–4 x 1 for 6 weeks is claimed to be equal to a single dose of azithromycin [33].

Treatment of the complications

Individuals with trachomatous trichiasis and entropion are at risk of corneal opacification and vision loss. To prevent these features from developing, the abrasive action of lashes on the cornea must be stopped by surgical correction of the eyelid margin, with epilation perhaps as an acceptable short-term option. For long-term solution, operation procedures for bilamellar tarsal rotation and posterior lamellar tarsal rotation (or Trabut) are recommended by WHO [34–36].

2.1.2 Neonatal inclusion conjunctivitis

The most common type of neonatal conjunctivitis worldwide is inclusion conjunctivitis. Inclusion conjunctivitis is caused by *C. trachomatis* serotypes D-K, which form chronic follicular conjunctivitis. Even though chlamydial infection typically affects the sexually active population, it can be transmitted to newborns by their infected mother during delivery. Infants exposed to the agent from the mother's genital tract during delivery, develop chlamydial ophthalmia neonatorum. Approximately 30–50% of infants exposed at birth develop the disease. Neonatal chlamydial conjunctivitis occurs in 2–6% of all newborns [37, 38].

Neonatal chlamydial conjunctivitis is an acute infection of the conjunctiva that is characterized by edema and erythema of the eyelids, palpebral conjunctivae, and purulent eye secretion. It typically occurs 5–14 days after the birth, although it can present earlier. Usually, the infection has a mild and self-limiting course. However, severe diseases can occur. Corneal scarring secondary to peripheral corneal pannus and conjunctival scarring may occur [39, 40]. Laboratory procedures to identify *C. trachomatis* are necessary for diagnosis. One of the two most commonly used methods is Giemsa staining of the conjunctival swab. However, it has only 50–90% sensitivity and requires a trained technician for section evaluation. The other method is McCoy cell culture. It is very expensive and reaching the result takes 2–3 days. Fortunately, new laboratory techniques are available for diagnosis. The enzyme-linked immune assay test has a sensitivity of approximately 90% and a specificity of over 95% and gives results within 2 hours. Direct immunofluorescent monoclonal antibody staining of the conjunctival swab is probably the most useful stereological test and has a specificity of 77–90% with a sensitivity of over 95% for chlamydia. It can be read immediately. It can show diseases that other tests miss. DNA detection tests can also be used. These tests have 90% sensitivity and almost 100% specificity [41].

The therapy objective for neonatal chlamydial conjunctivitis includes both the regression of conjunctivitis and the eradication of respiratory colonization. Therefore topical treatment is insufficient. An oral erythromycin treatment of 50 mg/kg/day in four divided doses for 2 weeks is recommended. If a total recovery is not observed, a second regime of the therapy may be given. The oral treatment should be given to the mother and her sexual partner, with 500 mg tetracycline or 500 mg erythromycin four times a day for 7 days. If pregnancy or breastfeeding exists erythromycin should be chosen [42].

Ocular prophylaxis for newborns has been found to be ineffective in protecting against chlamydial conjunctivitis. Several developed countries have stopped ocular prophylaxis of newborns and replaced it with routine treatment and prenatal screening of pregnant with a sexually transmitted infection [43].

2.1.3 Adult inclusion conjunctivitis

As neonatal inclusion conjunctivitis, adult inclusion conjunctivitis occurs with *C. trachomatis* D-K serotypes. The transmission of the agent is by sexual or hand-eye contact. Epidemiology revolves around sexual contact. The mode of transmission is through orogenital activities and transmission of genital secretions from hand to eye. The incubation period is 4–12 days. Inclusion conjunctivitis is predicted to develop in one in 300 patients with vernal chlamydial infection. In addition, *C. trachomatis* is the most common cause of chronic follicular conjunctivitis and is responsible for 20% of acute conjunctivitis cases. Because the disease is difficult to distinguish from the clinical findings of early trachoma, the term "paratrachoma" has been used to describe the entire spectrum of the disease with venerally transmitted chlamydial infection [44, 45].

The severity of symptoms in patients with inclusion conjunctivitis is very extensive. Some patients present as acute and mucopurulent conjunctivitis but, most patients have mild symptoms lasting for weeks or months Keratitis may develop in the second week of onset. Corneal involvement consists of superficial punctate keratitis, small marginal and central infiltrates, subepithelial infiltrates, limbal swelling, and superior limbal pannus. The disease imitates acute atopic conjunctivitis or other infectious conjunctivitis because, the signs and symptoms are insidious and most patients have similar nonspecific complaints such as unilateral mucous secretion, hyperemic eyes, crusting of eyelashes, glued eyelids, swollen eyelids, photophobia, itching, lacrimation, foreign body sensation, irritation, and blurred vision [46].

Diagnostic tests for chlamydial keratoconjunctivitis include conjunctival cytological examination, inoculation of susceptible cell lines followed by observation of cytopathic effect or visualization using various chemical or immunological staining agents, eye tears for various antibodies, and detection of chlamydial antigens in conjunctival and corneal specimens. Although the sensitivity of Giemsa staining is low, it is costly and time-consuming, this traditional cytological investigation is still the "gold standard," as isolating an infectious agent is definitive and allows further characterization. The detection of *C. trachomatis* DNA from ocular smears using commercial PCR assays was shown to be as valid as using urogenital samples and reached 95.71% in sensitivity and 90.00% in specificity. Therefore, PCR tests may be a quick and ideal tool for detecting ocular *C. trachomatis* infection [47].

As the infection is not limited to conjunctiva, systemic antibiotic use is recommended. Moreover, the sexual consorts must also receive a full course of therapy. Simultaneous treatment of all sexual partners is important to prevent reinfection. The recommended treatment, given for 3 weeks, includes either oral doxycycline 100 mg twice a day, oral tetracycline 500 mg four times a day, or oral erythromycin 500 mg four times a day. Tetracycline should not be used in pregnant or lactating women [42].

2.2 Lymphogranuloma venereum conjunctivitis

Lymphogranuloma venereum conjunctivitis is a very rare chlamydial conjunctivitis caused by *C. trachomatis* serotypes L1, L2, and L3. These agents classically cause a venereal disease characterized by suppurative inguinal or femoral lymphadenopathy. Occasionally, there are extragenital manifestations of the disease including aseptic meningitis, hepatitis, and conjunctivitis. The first ocular manifestations are the redness and edema of the eyelids. Other ocular manifestations are follicular hypertrophy, hyperemia, chemosis, and large granulomas. Pannus formation and peripheral superficial keratitis may occur. In some cases, phlyctenular conjunctivitis is present too. Episcleritis, uveitis and optic neuritis are among other rare clinical conditions reported. A large preauricular lymph node may be palpable.

The laboratory diagnosis is based on the microscopic detection of inclusion bodies, macrophages, and monocytes in Giemsa-stained conjunctival smears.

For treatment, oral tetracycline, 500 mg four times a day, for 4 weeks or oral doxycycline, 100 mg two times a day, for 4 weeks is used.

3. Other chlamydial conjunctivitis

Other chlamydia subgroups that should be considered as causative agents of conjunctivitis are *C. psittaci* and *C. pneumoniae*.

C. psittaci is the causative agent of psittacosis, which is seen in people who have bird contact in their professional or private life. This infection may produce a wide spectrum of clinical manifestations, ranging from asymptomatic infection to severe systemic disease with severe pneumonia. The Association of *C. psittacine* with ocular adnexal lymphoma in humans has been reported.

C. psittaci is a cause of follicular conjunctivitis and epithelial keratitis. In cases with long-lasting follicular conjunctivitis with a story of close bird contact *C. psittaci* should be kept in consideration. The isolation of inclusion bodies in epithelial cells and the microorganism in tissue cultures are necessary for the diagnosis.

One of the most important differences between *C. psittaci* and *C. trachomatis* is the time required for treatment. While long-term treatments are required in *C. psittaci* eye infection, a single 1 g azithromycin dose is considered sufficient in *C. trachomatis* conjunctivitis. In *C. psittaci* conjunctivitis, oral tetracycline 500 mg four times a day or oral doxycycline 100 mg two times a day for 6 weeks should be used for treatment.

C. pneumoniae is a rare cause of chronic follicular conjunctivitis. For cases with long-lasting, resistant conjunctivitis, respiratory contact with cats having *C. pneumoniae* infection should be kept in mind. Limited documentation exists relating to *C. pneumoniae* seropositivity in cases of chronic follicular conjunctivitis. For clinicians treating patients presenting with chronic conjunctivitis unresponsive to conventional measures, obtaining serologic studies for *C. pneumoniae* may identify this association. Oral tetracycline 3–4 times a day is used for treatment [48].

4. Conclusions

Although the topic of this chapter was Chlamydial Eye Infections, the main issue was definitely trachoma. Being an ancient disease and a major blindness cause, *C. trachomatis* has been a great concern of medicine for centuries. As technological improvements gave us new possibilities to understand the nature of this blinding microorganism, the endemic fields have been reduced, but the WHO could not reach the goal of eliminating trachoma, yet. The SAFE strategy provides a targeted way to speed up the process of a general improvement in living conditions and hygiene that is needed to eliminate it in the most disadvantaged areas in the developing world. As increasing resources are brought to bear, the likelihood of eliminating blinding trachoma by 2030 becomes stronger.

Conflict of interest

The author has no conflict of interest to declare.

Author details

Seçil Özdemir Şahin
Medicalpark Antalya Hospital Complex Eye Clinic, Antalya, Turkiye

*Address all correspondence to: secilozdemir2003@yahoo.com

References

[1] Bachmann NL, Polkinghorne A, Timms P. *Chlamydia* genomics: Providing novel insights into chlamydial biology. Trends in Microbiology. 2014;**22**:464-472

[2] Mandell GL, Bennett JE, Dolin R. Mandell, Douglas, and Bennett's Principles and Practice of Infectious Diseases. 7th ed. Vol. 2. London: Churchill Livingstone/Elsevier; 2010

[3] Malhotra M, Sood S, Mukherjee A, Muralidhar S, Bala M. Genital *Chlamydia trachomatis*: An update. The Indian Journal of Medical Research. 2013;**138**:303-316

[4] Sarier M, Kukul E. Classification of non-gonococcal urethritis: A review. International Urology and Nephrology. Jun 2019;**51**(6):901-907. DOI: 10.1007/s11255-019-02140-2

[5] Sarier M, Demir M, Turgut H, et al. New approach to microscopy of gram-stained urethral smear: The kissing slide method. Sexually Transmitted Diseases. 2020;**47**(10):712-715. DOI: 10.1097/OLQ.0000000000001228

[6] Sarier M, Duman İ, Göktaş Ş, Demir M, Kukul E. Results of multiplex polymerase chain reaction assay to identify urethritis pathogens. Journal of Urological Surgery. 2017;**4**(1):18-22. DOI: 10.4274/jus.1328

[7] Sarier M, Sepin N, Emek M, et al. Evaluating the utility of the genital system test for pathogen diagnosis in acute male urethritis. Andrologia. 2022;**54**(4):e14377. DOI: 10.1111/and.14377

[8] Sarier M. Prevalence of polymicrobial infection in urethritis. Journal of Urological Surgery. 2019;**6**(3):180-183. DOI: 10.4274/jus.galenos.2019.2405

[9] Sarier M, Sepin N, Duman I, et al. Microscopy of Gram-stained urethral smear in the diagnosis of urethritis: Which threshold value should be selected? Andrologia. 2018;**2018**:e13143. DOI: 10.1111/and.13143

[10] Sarier M. Polymerase chain reaction assay in acute urethritis. Andrologia. 2019;**51**(8):e13366. DOI: 10.1111/and.13366

[11] Newman L, Rowley J, Vander Hoorn S, Wijesooriya NS, Unemo M, Low N, et al. Global estimates of the prevalence and incidence of four curable sexually transmitted infections in 2012 based on systematic review and global reporting. PLoS One. 2015;**10**(12):e0143304. DOI: 10.1371/journal.pone.0143304

[12] Özbal Y. In: Klamidyalar. Ustaçelebi Ş, editors. Temel ve Klinik Mikrobiyoloji. Güneş Kitabevi, Ankara, 1999: 706-714

[13] Lietman T, Brooks D, Moncada J, Schachter J, Dawson C, Dean D. Chronic follicular conjunctivitis associated with *Chlamydia psittaci* or *Chlamydia pneumoniae*. Clinical Infectious Diseases. 1998;**26**:1335-1340

[14] Global Burden of Disease. Seattle (WA): Institute for Health Metrics and Evaluation. Available from: http://www.healthdata.org/gbd

[15] WHO. Eliminating trachoma: WHO announces sustained progress with hundreds of millions of people no longer at risk of infection. In: Neglected Tropical Diseases [News Release]. Geneva: World Health Organization; 2019. Available from: https://www.who.int/neglected_diseases/news/

Trachoma-WHO-announces-sustained-progress/en/

[16] WHO. Report. 2022. Available from: http://www.who.int/publications/i/item/9789240010352

[17] Tylefors B, Dawson CR, Jones BR, et al. A symple system for the assessment of trachoma and its complications. Bulletin of the World Health Organization. 1987;**65**:477-483

[18] Dawson CR, Jones BR, Tarizzo M. Guide to Trachoma Control. Geneva: World Health Organisation; 1981. p. 56

[19] Dawson CR, Juster R, Marx R, et al. Limbal disease in trachoma and other ocular chlamydial infections: Risk factors for corneal vascularization. Eye. 1989;**3**:204-209

[20] Sandford-Smith J. Eye Diseases in Hot Climates. 3rd ed. London, United Kingdom: Butterworth Heinemann; 1997

[21] Burton MJ. Trachoma: An overview. British Medical Bulletin. 2007;**84**:99-116

[22] Mandell GL, Douglas GR, Bennett JE. Princibles and practice of infectious diseases. In: Bowie WR, Holmes KK, editors. *Chlamydia trachomatis* (Trachoma, Perinatal Infections, Lymphogranuloma Venereum and Other Genital Infections). New York: Churchill Livingstone Inc; 1990. pp. 1426-1444

[23] Treharne JD. *Chlamydia trachomatis*: Serological diagnosis. Infection. 1982;**10**(Suppl 1):S25-S31

[24] Schachter J, Moncada J, Dawson CR, Sheppard J, Courtright P, Said ME, et al. Nonculture methods for diagnosing chlamydial infection in patients with trachoma: A clue to the pathogenesis of the disease? The Journal of Infectious Diseases. 1988;**158**:1347-1352

[25] Solomon AW, Peeling RW, Foster A, Mabey DC. Diagnosis and assessment of trachoma. Clinical Microbiology Reviews. 2004;**17**:982-1011

[26] Dawson CR, Sheppard JD. Follicular conjunctivitis. In: Tasman W, Jaeger EA, editors. Duane's Clinical Ophthalmology. Vol. 4. Philadelphia: Lippincott; 1990. pp. 7-20

[27] West SK, Munoz B, Lynch M, et al. Impact of face washing on trachoma in Kongwa Tanzania. Lancet. 1994;**345**:155-158

[28] Emerson P, Lindsay SW, Walraven GE. Effect of fly control on trachoma and diarrhea. Lancet. 1999;**353**:1401-1403

[29] Tabbara KF, Abu-el-Asar, al-Omar O, et al. Single dose azithromycine in the treatment of trachoma. A controlled study. Ophthalmology. 1996;**103**:842

[30] Fraser-Hurt N, Bailey R, Cousens S, Mabey D, Faal H, Mabey D. Efficacy of oral azithromycin versus topical teracycline in mass treatment of endemic trachoma. Bulletin of the World Health Organization. 2001;**79**:632-640

[31] Dawson CR et al. A comparison of oral azithromycin with topical oxytetracycline/polymyxin for the treatment of trachoma in children. Clinical Infectious Diseases. 1997;**24**:363-368

[32] Schacter J, Wesr SK, Mabey D, et al. Azithromycin in control of trachoma. Lancet. 1999;**354**:630-635

[33] Bailey RL, Arullendran P, Whittle HC, Mabey DC. Randomised controlled trial of single dose azithromycin in treatment of trachoma. Lancet. 1993;**342**:453-456

[34] Rajak SN, Collin JRO, Burton MJ. Trachomatous trichiasis and its management in endemic countries. Survey of Ophthalmology. 2012;**57**:105-135

[35] Reacher M, Foster A, Huber J. Trichiasis Surgery for Trachoma— The Bilamellar Tarsal Rotation Procedure. Geneva: World Health Organization; 1993

[36] Reacher MH, Muñoz B, Alghassany A, Daar AS, Elbualy M, Taylor HR. A controlled trial of surgery for trachomatous trichiasis of the upper lid. Archives of Ophthalmology. 1992;**110**:667-674

[37] Chandler JW. Ophthalmia Neonatorum. In: Duane TD, Jaeger EA, editors. Duane's Clinical Ophthalmology. Vol. Vol 4. Philadelphia: Harper and Row; 1964. pp. 6.2-6.6

[38] Hammerschlag MR. Chlamydial and gonococcal infections in infants and children. Clinical Infectious Diseases. 2011;**53**:99-102

[39] Darville T. *Chlamydia trachomatis* infections in neonates and young children. Seminars in Pediatric Infectious Diseases. 2005;**16**:235-244

[40] Tylefors B, Negrel AD, Pararajasegaram R, Dadzie KY. Global data on blindness. Bulletin of the World Health Organization. 1995;**73**:115-121

[41] Rubinstein JB. Disorders of the conjunctiva and limbus. In: Yanoff M, Duker JS, editors. Ophthalmology. Mosby; 2004. Chap:5, 1.1-1.22

[42] Sanders LL, Harrison HR, Washington AE. Treatment of sexually transmitted chlamydial infections. Journal of the American Medical Association. 1986;**255**:1750-1756

[43] Darling EK, McDonald H. A meta-analysis of the efficacy of ocular prophylactic agents used for the prevention of gonococcal and chlamydial ophthalmia neonatorum. Journal of Midwifery & Women's Health. 2010;**55**:319-327

[44] Phillips JA. Chlamydia infections. Workplace Health & Safety. 2019;**67**(7):375-376. DOI: 10.1177/2165079919853590

[45] Tullo AB, Richmond SC, Esty PL. The presentation and incidence of paratrachoma in adults. The Journal of Hygiene. 1981;**87**:63-69

[46] Satpathy G, Behera HS, Ahmed NH. Chlamydial eye infections: Current perspectives. Indian Journal of Ophthalmology. 2017;**65**(2):97-102. DOI: 10.4103/ijo.IJO_870_16

[47] Pickering H, Holland MJ, Last AR, Burton MJ, Burr SE. Evaluation of a Chlamydia trachomatis-specific, commercial, real-time PCR for use with ocular swabs. Parasites Vectors. 2018;**11**(1):102. DOI: 10.1186/s13071-018-2686-y

[48] Tabbara K. Chlamydial conjunctivitis. In: Tabbara KF, Hyndiuk RA, editors. Infections of The Eye. 1986. pp. 421-436

Chapter 11

A Hidden Organism, Chlamydia in the Age of Atherosclerosis

Mehmet Besir Akpinar

Abstract

Atherosclerosis is a chronic inflammatory disease. It is still the leading cause of mortality and morbidity in the world. Inflammation in the vessels plays the most important role in the pathogenesis of atherosclerosis. Many studies have been emphasized that *Chlamydia pneumoniae* triggers inflammation in the vessels and associated with atherosclerosis. It is stated that most of the chlamydial infections are asymptomatic and around 40% of adult individuals are infected. Chlamydia has different subgroups. It was thought to be a virus due to its intracellular pathogenicity, but it was included in the bacteria genus because it contains DNA and RNA chromosomes and has enzymatic activity. Chlamidya can easily be transmitted through the respiratory tract and sexual transmission. Seroepidemiological and pathological studies of atherosclerotic plaques showed the presence of Chlamydia in the plaque. This section will provide relationship between Chlamydia and atherosclerosis on the recent researces and current information will be discussed.

Keywords: Chlamydia, atherosclerosis, inflammation, atheroma, coronary artery

1. Introduction

Cardiovascular diseases are the leading cause of morbidity and mortality in developed societies. The World Health Organization ranked coronary heart disease first and stroke fourth on its list of major life-threatening diseases. More than 40% of deaths from non-communicable diseases in the community are due to cardiovascular causes.

Cardiovascular disease can manifest in myriad ways, including heart attack, stroke, peripheral artery disease, organ ischemia and necrosis, and aortic and peripheral arterial aneurysms. The main pathogenetic mechanism underlying cardiovascular diseases is atherosclerosis. When evaluated in terms of cost and loss of labor, atherosclerosis is a malignant condition that requires enormous resource allocation and affects all aspects of humanity. Atherosclerosis is progressive and affects all arteries in the body to a varying extent. It is extremely common, occurring in almost all individuals in the population. The main factors associated with a higher rate of atherosclerosis are chronic inflammation, genetic predisposition, advanced age, male sex, hyperlipidemia, hypertension, smoking, diabetes, sedentary lifestyle, and obesity.

Studies conducted in different parts of the world have shown that atherosclerosis begins in childhood. Autopsy studies conducted in Japan demonstrated early atherosclerosis and fatty streaks in the aortas of 29% of infants younger than 12 months and in the coronary arteries of 3.1% of children aged 1–9 years [1]. Similarly, autopsy studies in the USA have shown that the prevalence of fatty streaks in the coronary arteries is 50% between the ages of 2 and 15 years and increases to 85% between the ages of 21 and 39 years. Atherosclerotic plaque formation, a more advanced form of fatty streaking, was observed in 8% of children aged 2–15 years and 69% of adults aged 26–39 years [2].

Atherosclerosis starts with endothelial dysfunction and progresses with subintimal thickening and smooth muscle cell proliferation. The process is characterized with medial thickening due to macrophage infiltration, scavenger cell accumulation, and plaque formation. Lipid deposition is a common vascular condition in which inflammatory and infective processes trigger each other.

Studies on atherosclerosis risk factors have shown that organic pathogenic microorganisms contribute to the inflammatory process. These include *Chlamydia pneumoniae, Helicobacter pylori*, influenza A virus, hepatitis C virus, cytomegalovirus, and HIV. Chronic inflammation induced by microorganisms can cause many chronic diseases, malignancies, autoimmune diseases, and inflammatory atherosclerosis [3, 4]. Some microorganisms have been directly linked to atherosclerotic disease because they can be isolated and cultured from plaques, whereas the presence of other organisms has been demonstrated by biochemical tests [5, 6]. Microorganisms influence the atherosclerosis process by triggering inflammation; inducing endothelial cell damage, macrophage-derived foam cell formation, and vascular smooth muscle cell proliferation; and stimulating the immune system at all of these stages.

Electron microscope images obtained from atheromatous plaques showed that their central nucleus consists of a lipid-rich structure containing lipid clusters, vesicles, and microorganisms mimicking the appearance of a lipid cluster [3]. In analyses of these microorganisms, *C. pneumoniae* is the causative bacteria most frequently associated with atherosclerosis.

This chapter examines the relationship between the atherosclerotic process and *C. pneumoniae* through a review of the relevant literature.

2. *Chlamydia pneumoniae*

The most important discovery related to the classification of *Chlamydia* was made by Moulder et al. in 1964. *Chlamydia* spp. were initially perceived as viruses because they were smaller than normal bacterial size and had life cycles in the host cell. However, they were included in the bacteria class because they have the ability to survive outside the cell. As such, they are defined as "compulsory intracellular bacteria" [3]. *Chlamydia* are generally larger than the average virus, but smaller than bacteria and human cells [3].

The genus *Chlamydia* is in the family Chlamydiaceae of the order Chlamydiales. Based on their antigenic structures, intracellular inclusions, and diseases they cause, the genus consists of four species: *C. pecorum*, *C. psittaci*, *C. trachomatis*, and *C. pneumoniae*. Except for *C. pecorum*, all can cause disease in humans. *C. trachomatis* is sexually transmitted and causes ocular trachoma, lymphogranuloma venerum, and neonatal infections. Infection is common in homosexuals [7]. *C. psittaci* causes a systemic disease often characterized by pneumonia. *C. psittaci* is also seen in birds and pets. Infection is common in occupational groups that come into contact with birds.

C. pneumoniae, previously known as TWAR, causes respiratory tract infections such as pneumonia, bronchitis, sinusitis, and pharyngitis [8]. It was first isolated from the conjunctival swab of a child with trachoma in Taiwan in 1965 and was named TW-183. The role of *C. pneumoniae* as a human pathogen was definitively determined in 1983 with the first respiratory tract isolate, named AR-39, obtained from a throat swab sample of a patient with pharyngitis in the USA. The name TWAR (TW+AR) comes from these first conjunctival and respiratory strains. In 1989, *C. pneumoniae* was identified as a unique species by electron microscopy morphological studies and DNA sequence analysis of TWAR [9]. Unlike *C. trachomatis*, *C. pneumoniae* is not sexually transmitted but is spread through respiratory secretions. Unlike *C. psittaci*, it does not cause disease in birds or animals. In addition to respiratory tract infections, *C. pneumoniae* is associated with atherosclerosis and cardiovascular diseases.

One in ten cases of community-acquired pneumonia is caused by *C. pneumoniae*, and studies have shown that the seroprevalence of *C. pneumonia* in adults is 80%. It has also been shown to cause diseases marked by chronic inflammatory processes, such as chronic obstructive pulmonary disease, asthma, lung cancer, Alzheimer's disease, arthritis, and atherosclerosis [10–15]. *Chlamydia* have a biphasic life cycle and are obligate intracellular bacteria. They are morphologically and structurally similar to gram-negative bacteria, with a three-layered, lipopolysaccharide-rich outer membrane. They require ATP from the host cell to develop and proliferate. *Chlamydia* were classified as bacteria because they contain both DNA and RNA, reproduce by division, have a cell membrane similar to gram-negative bacteria, and are susceptible to antibiotics [16].

Bacteria of the genus *Chlamydia* reproduce by forming incubation bodies in the cytoplasm of the cells they infect. The life cycle of *C. pneumoniae* is divided between two forms, the elementary body (EB) and reticulate body (RB). The EB form is metabolically inactive and is the extracellular form that is transmitted between hosts. It infects the respiratory tract through inhalation and attaches to the mucosal surfaces. The EB enters the host cell via endocytosis, where it transforms into the RB form. EBs are approximately 350 nanometers in diameter. After entering the host cell and becoming activated, they increase in size to a diameter of 800–1000 nm.

The RB form is metabolically active and exploits the host cell's metabolism. This transformation takes place within the first 24 hours after infection. It replicates within the host cell and then lyses that cell, spreading as newly formed EBs and propagating transmission. The RB form is protected from the endocytic-lysosomal degradation system of the host cell and can remain there for years. This feature enables it to persist in the body and cause a chronic inflammatory process [17, 18]. Its intracellular location enhances its ability to transform into a resistant and recurrent form [8, 19]. The bacteria infects the lung tissue and is taken up by monocytes and macrophages. However, instead of being eliminated they continue to thrive there and spread to the rest of the body via the circulation. *Chlamydia* that invades the arterial wall as a result of endothelial dysfunction contributes to the atherosclerosis process [20]. Its demonstrated presence in atheromatous plaques and smooth muscle cells, as well as in macrophage and foam cells, is the main feature that distinguishes *C. pneumoniae* from other microorganisms [21, 22].

2.1 Discovery of Chlamydia

2.1.1 Production in culture

Ramirez et al. [23] reported the first case of *C. pneumoniae* that could be isolated from a coronary artery plaque and cultured in vitro in 1996. Jackson et al [24].

demonstrated the presence of *Chlamydia* by immunohistochemical, PCR, or electron microscopy in 75% of 25 patients with carotid endarterectomy, whereas culture was positive in only one patient. A small proportion of atherosclerotic plaques with *Chlamydia* presence confirmed using other diagnostic methods have been successfully cultured [25, 26]. Karlsson et al. [27] demonstrated the presence of *C. pneumoniae* immunohistochemically in 20 of 26 abdominal aortic aneurysm tissue specimens, but were able to isolate *Chlamydia* in culture media in 10 cases. *Chlamydia* are reported to be difficult bacteria to culture because of their biphasic life cycle. It is accepted that in vitro culture has low sensitivity in demonstrating the presence of *Chlamydia* in tissue examinations [28].

2.1.2 Serological investigations

While some of the studies using serological tests showed a positive relationship between *C. pneumoniae* infection and coronary atherosclerosis, some studies reported that this relationship could not be accepted as sufficient evidence for the etiology of atherosclerosis [29–31].

Some studies revealed a relationship between *C. pneumoniae*-specific IgG and IgA positivity and atherosclerosis development, whereas other researchers did not observe this relationship [32–35]. Serological tests are based on the detection of anti-chlamydial antibodies (IgA, IgG) in blood samples. However, these antibodies are indicators of the immune response rather than active infection. They also show cross-reactivity with other *Chlamydia* species. Danesh et al. [36] conducted a meta-analysis of 14 prospective studies including a total of 3619 patients and reported that there was no relationship between *C. pneumoniae* antibodies and atherosclerotic heart disease. This is similar to the presence of antituberculosis antibodies in serological tests after tuberculosis vaccination. The presence of antibodies may not mean there is active infection. In addition, it was shown that serological tests were negative even though the presence of *Chlamydia* could be demonstrated in the atherosclerotic plaques of immunodeficient individuals [19]. In general, pathogenic processes that cause an inflammatory response (such as smoke exposure, hypertension, hyperlipidemia, malignancy, and hyperglycemia) are known to cause errors in serological tests, which reduces their specificity. As a result, it is accepted that serological studies are not useful and are insufficient in the detection of *Chlamydia*.

2.1.3 Techniques for demonstrating Chlamydia *in atheromatous plaques*

Although most studies conducted in different centers in many parts of the world were able to demonstrate the presence of *Chlamydia* in atherosclerotic lesions, they could not be detected in other studies. This was thought to be related to differences or technical incompatibilities between the imaging methods, leading to debate regarding which diagnostic methods are most appropriate. As a result, polymerase chain reaction (PCR), immunohistochemistry (microimmunofluorescence), and electron microscopy imaging are the most widely accepted techniques. These studies focus on the bacteria's DNA signature or directly demonstrate bacterial presence instead of utilizing indirect methods.

PCR is a diagnostic method for detecting chlamydial DNA or RNA and focuses on the bacteria's genetic material [37]. It is a sensitive and specific test based on the degradation of genetic material in atheromatous plaques by electrophoresis [38, 39]. Immunogold labeling is based on the direct observation of *Chlamydia* bacteria with

DOI: http://dx.doi.org/10.5772/intechopen.109745

an electron microscope. The detection of monoclonal antibodies clearly demonstrates the presence of *Chlamydia*. Immunocytochemistry (ICC) is based on the demonstration of anti-chlamydial immunoglobulins adhering to the *Chlamydia* bacteria using immunofluorescent microscopy. This method has lower specificity and sensitivity than PCR. Serologic studies are based on the measurement of the host response to chlamydial invasion. Results are obtained by demonstrating host immunoglobulins. It has low specificity and sensitivity.

In most studies using ICC, PCR, and culture methods for *C. pneumoniae*, detection rates were higher in atherosclerotic vessels than in those without atherosclerosis [40, 41].

3. Atherosclerosis

Atherosclerosis can be defined as a disease that causes progressive arterial stenosis and obstruction due to intimal plaques containing lipids, fibroblasts, macrophages, smooth muscle cells, and extracellular substances in varying proportions, leading to loss of the elasticity and antithrombotic properties of the arterial walls. Atherosclerosis is a multifactorial, morbid and mortal systemic disease that affects not only the coronary vessels but all arterial structures. The coronary arteries, internal carotid arteries, and abdominal aorta are vessels most commonly affected [42].

Atherosclerotic lesions appear as focal thickenings in the intima and subintimal space of arteries. When the content of the thickened region is examined, it is seen to contain vascular endothelial cells, smooth muscle cells, connective tissue, and lipid deposits, as well as inflammatory and immune cells from the blood. Historically, with our nascent understanding of atherosclerosis, treatment focused on cholesterol-lowering drugs and a low-cholesterol diet. However, research on therapeutic processes started to diversify after the role of inflammation in atherosclerosis came to light.

3.1 Atherosclerosis and inflammation

Atherosclerotic vascular disease is a typical environment-gene interaction. Environmental risk factors trigger a proinflammatory response in people with genetic predisposition. Epidemiological studies have demonstrated the role of risk factors such as cigarette exposure, cholesterol, hypertension, and diabetes mellitus in the development of atherosclerosis. Experimental studies have shown that these risk factors induce a general inflammatory response, causing a widespread reaction in the body. In response to risk factors, systemic acute phase reactants are activated and there is the onset of signal traffic from the endothelium. In light of this information, atherosclerosis is defined as a multifactorial disease that is associated with the inflammatory process and in which chronic inflammation plays a role in every stage, from onset to progression [43–45].

At the onset of atherosclerosis, leukocytes and macrophages attach to the endothelium and cross into the subendothelial space. This occurs because of adhesion molecules [46, 47]. The best-known adhesion molecules are endothelial leukocyte adhesion molecule 1 (ELAM-1), membrane-bound vascular cell adhesion molecule 1 (VCAM-1), and intracellular adhesion molecule 1 (ICAM-1) [48, 49].

Cytokines are also an integral factor in the inflammatory process. The best-known proinflammatory cytokines are tumor necrosis factor alpha (TNF-α), interleukin (IL)-1, and IL-6. TNF-α is released from macrophages, vascular smooth muscle cells, and endothelial cells. These cytokines trigger the production of other cytokines in the inflammatory cycle [50].

Another marker is plasma fibrinogen values, which are an indicator of both the inflammatory response and the thrombotic response. Increased fibrinogen values have been shown to significantly increase coronary event risk. In addition, elevated fibrinogen levels have been detected in healthy individuals with a family history of atherosclerosis [51, 52].

C-reactive protein (CRP) is a good indicator of inflammation because its values are stable over time [53, 54]. It does not increase due to anything other than inflammation. It can be measured with a highly sensitive and inexpensive test. Studies have shown that CRP levels have an additive effect on other risk markers. The cholesterol/high-density lipoprotein (HDL) ratio is a strong indicator of cardiovascular risk [55]. However, the risk predictivity increases when CRP values are added. The PROVE-IT study showed that highest risk group is those with both high total cholesterol/HDL ratio and high CRP levels [56].

Elevated CRP levels, increased leukocyte counts in peripheral blood counts, and high serum fibrinogen levels are strong predictors of coronary artery disease and atherosclerotic diseases [57, 58].

The normal arterial structure consists of three main layers, the intima, media, and adventitia from innermost to outermost. The intima layer is covered with a single cell layer endothelium. The intact endothelial surface is resistant to thrombus formation because it secretes nitric oxide (NO) and prostacyclin (PGI2) and is covered with heparin sulfate.

3.2 Endothelial inflammation

The endothelium is the first vascular structure affected by risk factors [59, 60]. Normally shiny, slippery, and antithrombotic, risk factors cause the endothelium to lose its slipperiness and become sticky and prothrombotic. Endothelial cells exposed to risk factors from an early age start producing adhesion molecules (VCAM-1, ICAM), growth factors (platelet-derived growth factor [PDGF], basic fibroblast growth factor [FGF], *transforming growth factor beta* [TGF-β], IL-1, TNF-α), and cytokines (macrophage colony-stimulating factor [M-CSF], granulocyte-macrophage colony stimulating factor [GM-CSF]). VCAM-1 binds both monocytes and T lymphocytes. Atherosclerosis-related leukocyte adhesion molecule, or athero-ELAM, is released from endothelial cells, triggering mononuclear cell migration [61]. This initiates the chemotactic process on monocytes, macrophages, and lymphocytes and triggers the inflammation process [62]. The result is a vicious cycle in which inflammation stimulates cytokine release and cytokines increase inflammation. These proteins, which are expressed due to the vascular inflammatory response, are the main cause of early atherosclerotic lesions [62].

On the one hand, there is an inflammatory response in the endothelium, while on the other hand, there is subclinical systemic inflammation. Proinflammatory risk factors such as oxidized low-density lipoprotein (LDL) activate IL-1 and TNF-α, which are called primary proinflammatory cytokines [53, 63]. These primary proinflammatory cytokines activate IL-6, resulting in the release of acute phase reactants. The presence of subclinical systemic inflammation can be understood by measuring some acute phase reactants such as CRP, fibrinogen, factor 7, plasminogen activator inhibitor-1 (PAI-1), tissue plasminogen activator (tPA), and lipoprotein (a) in the blood or by measuring endothelium-derived peripheral markers [53, 64, 65].

3.3 Medial inflammation

In the atherosclerosis process, smooth muscle cells migrate from the media to the intima and there is a reduction in the contractile protein content and an increase in the number of synthetic organelles. Smooth muscle cells migrating to intima change from the contractile phenotype to the synthetic phenotype and contribute to proliferation. Smooth muscle cells in the media respond to vasoconstrictors such as endothelin, catecholamine, angiotensin II, and vasodilators such as NO and PGI2, while those in the intima respond to mitogens such as PDGF. In addition, the balance shifts from vasodilation to vasoconstriction, from antithrombotic to prothrombotic, and from antiproliferative to proliferative properties. Adhesion molecules, cytokines (IL-1, TNF-α), chemokines (monocyte chemoattractant protein-1 [MCP-1], IL-8), and growth factors (PDGF, FGF) are released from dysfunctional endothelial cells. IL-8 triggers the inflammatory cascade by binding to chemokine receptor 2 on leukocytes [66]. MCP-1 mediates selective directed migration of monocytes to the subendothelial space. Transgenic experimental animals unable to express MCP-1 were found to have nearly absent subendothelial lipid accumulation [67] All these processes allow defense cells to migrate to the inflammation site, leading to the onset of volumetric thickening of the vessel wall.

3.4 Lipid deposition and atherosclerosis

Lipids are a key cell component that serves as one of the main building blocks of cell membranes and organelles, as well as having nutrient and energy functions. Fatty acids, the simplest lipid form, are divided into different classes depending on the length of their structure, the number of carbon atoms, and whether the bonds are saturated or unsaturated. Phosphoglycerides are the main class of lipids comprising cell membranes. Cholesterols are also part of a large group of fats called sterols and are another important component of cellular membranes. LDL particles in the blood are made of lipids and protein, including cholesterol esters, triglycerides, phospholipids, and apoB-100 protein.

Many studies indicate that atherosclerosis begins with endothelial damage. However, histopathological studies have revealed atherosclerotic plaque formations with an intact endothelial structure [68, 69]. This raises the question of how lipid and cell passage into the subendothelial space occurs without endothelial damage.

It has been observed that eating even a single meal of excessively fatty food disrupts endothelial function, raises CRP levels, and increases adhesion molecules [70]. Animal experiments have shown that in subjects fed a high-cholesterol diet, the endothelium becomes sticky and begins expressing adhesion molecules within a few weeks [71–73]. The first alteration in the arterial endothelium of experimental animals fed a cholesterol-rich diet was shown to be leukocyte adhesion [74].

The main damage caused by cholesterol particles occurs through LDL. LDL particles are believed to penetrate the arterial wall by passing through the endothelial cells and initiate a number of remarkable changes involving various different processes. Subintimal lipid particles have been shown to be ingested by macrophages and smooth muscle cells, where they are degraded in the intracellular lipid oxidation and peroxidation chains. In the sub intimal space, LDL particles are modified with a different phospholipid and fatty ester structure and begin to form lipid clusters [75]. These lipid clusters trigger free radicals produced by chain chemical reactions, induce the inflammatory process, and cause chemotaxis.

3.5 Fibrous plaque–fibrous cap

Although immunohistochemical studies have demonstrated a cascade mechanism that allows inflammatory cells to infiltrate the subintimal layer at this early stage of atherosclerosis, pathological studies show that the endothelium is intact at this stage and there is no physical damage to this layer on microscopic examination [68]. Light microscopy examination of very small early lesions showed that primary damage occurred in the muscle cell component of the intima.

Monocytes accumulated in the subendothelial space transform into macrophages and begin to express scavenger receptors. This enables them to phagocytose the oxidized LDL.

As cholesterol esters accumulate in the macrophages, foam cells are formed. Macrophages accumulate lipids while continuing to release inflammatory mediators. M-CSF released from activated endothelial cells increases macrophage accumulation in the region. M-CSF also stimulates the immune system. A proinflammatory cytokine called CD40 ligand is one of the inflammatory mediators that contribute to progression. T cells accumulate in the subendothelial space due to the effect of different chemokines (e.g., interferon gamma-induced protein 10 [IP-10], monokine induced by interferon gamma [MIG]). Mast cells have recently been shown to accumulate via similar mechanisms. T lymphocytes also accumulate in the intima and continue to release proinflammatory cytokines. Another interesting function of T cells is to activate macrophages to stimulate the release of collagen, matrix metalloproteinases (MMP), and cytokines. Thus, the atheromatous plaque gradually grows. Oxidized LDL and heat shock protein (HSP) increase inflammation by stimulating toll-like receptors [76, 77]. Experimental studies have shown that toll-like receptor blockade can reduce atherosclerosis. Toll-like receptors accelerate atherosclerosis by triggering cytokine release in the inflammation cascade and stimulating the immune response [78].

As the lesions progress, extracellular lipids begin to accumulate. The extracellular lipid pool is largely a result of foam cell apoptosis and the release of their stored cholesterol esters. A very small proportion comprises lipoproteins that pass from the lumen. The "fibrous plaque" that begins to form in the subintimal layer initially appears microscopically as lipid nuclei, large amounts of smooth muscle cells, macrophages, foam cells, T lymphocytes, and extracellular matrix, and macroscopically as white lesions that enlarge mostly towards the artery lumen [3].

Smooth muscle cells in the fibrous plaque continue to produce extracellular matrix, while macrophages degrade the connective tissue. This construction and destruction is mediated by numerous cytokines. Even if fibrous plaques significantly narrow the vessel lumen, they are believed not to cause significant clinical events as long as they remain intact. The structure on the luminal side of this plaque is called the "fibrous cap." A thicker fibrous cap is associated with greater plaque stability.

Plaques that are rich in lipids and inflammatory cells and have a thin fibrous cap have higher risk of rupture (vulnerable plaque). Metalloproteinases (collagenase, elastase, stromelysin) secreted by macrophages surrounding the lipid nucleus degrade the collagenous matrix of the fibrous cap. In addition, the synergistic effect of IL-1β and TNF-α released from activated macrophages and interferon gamma (IFN-γ) released by T lymphocytes results in smooth muscle cell death and reduced extracellular matrix. As a result of increased destruction and decreased construction, the fibrous cap weakens and eventually ruptures. Procoagulant substances in plaques with a disrupted fibrous cap interact with blood elements and clotting factors, triggering thrombus formation [65].

The ruptured plaque remains unstable for some time, after which the healing process begins. Smooth muscle cells capable of making extracellular matrix act as reparative cells. Smooth muscle cells produce large amounts of matrix proteins, such as glycosaminoglycan, elastin, and collagen, which are needed to repair the vessel and form the fibrous cap over the lipid-rich plaque nucleus. By synthesizing its contents, they enable the plaque capsule to stabilize the atherosclerotic lesion and separate the thrombogenic lipid-rich plaque nucleus from the platelets and coagulation cascade proteins in the blood. Thus, vascular smooth muscle cells have a critical role in ensuring plaque stability and inhibiting fatal thrombogenic outcomes. Some authors have argued that smooth muscle cells migrating into the intima play a constructive and reparative role, rather than a destructive role, in atherosclerosis [45, 79].

3.6 Atherosclerosis and immune response

It has recently become understood that both the natural and adaptive immune systems play important roles in the development of atherosclerosis [80, 81]. The natural immune system is responsible for the initial inflammatory response to a microorganism or pathogen. Immune cells, namely T cells, monocytes, macrophages and mast cells, circulating through various tissues (including the atherosclerotic artery) seeking antigen. When T cells encounter and bind to an antigen, a series of cytokines are released to launch an inflammatory response. Scavenger and toll-like receptors are the main receptors responsible for natural immunity in atherothrombosis [82]. Toll-like receptors are found on fibroblasts and macrophages in the intimal and adventitial layers of coronary atherothrombotic plaques.

The adaptive immune system is more specific than the natural immune system. This system includes an organized immune response leading to the formation of T and B cell receptors and immunoglobulins that recognize foreign antigens. Modified lipoproteins, HSPs, beta$_2$-glycoprotein I, and infectious agents can stimulate the adaptive immune system [83].

4. *Chlamydia pneumoniae* and atherosclerosis

The first findings regarding the association of *C. pneumoniae* and coronary artery disease were presented by Shor et al. [84] in 1992. Their study examined coronary artery atherosclerosis and vascular fatty streaks in seven autopsy studies and demonstrated the presence of TWAR-like *C. pneumoniae*. In a later, extended autopsy study, Kuo et al. [21] demonstrated the presence of *C. pneumoniae* in atherosclerotic lesions by PCR and culture studies.

In a 1998 study by Saiku et al. including 40 patients with acute myocardial infarction, 30 patients with coronary artery disease and 41 controls, chlamydial IgA and IgG antibodies were detected in 68% and 50% by micro immunofluorescence, respectively. Both frequencies were significantly higher than in the controls (7.17%). In 68% of patients with acute myocardial infarction, a significant seroconversion was demonstrated in enzyme immunoassay with LPS antigen; this response was absent in patients with coronary heart disease and in all but one of the controls [85].

The presence of *C. pneumoniae* organisms in atherosclerotic lesions was later demonstrated using immunohistochemistry, PCR, in situ DNA hybridizations, and electron microscopy [21, 86–88].

Chlamydia has been detected not only in plaques in the coronary arteries, but also in the aortic tissue, aortic aneurysms, and plaques in the carotid and peripheral arteries [22, 24, 89–92].

4.1 *Chlamydia pneumoniae* and the immune response

In studies demonstrating the relationship between *C. pneumoniae* and atherosclerosis, circulating cholesterol-containing immune complexes were shown to be present in 50–70% of patients with acute myocardial infarction [93, 94]. These immune complexes (comprising IgG and apolipoprotein (a)) have a proatherogenic effect [95]. Patients with immunocomplexes containing *C. pneumoniae*-specific IgG and apolipoprotein (a) were found to have a 3.8 times higher risk of developing acute myocardial infarction than the control group [96].

Several mechanisms have been proposed to explain the formation of immunocomplexes containing *C. pneumoniae*-specific IgG and apolipoprotein (a). According to one mechanism, structurally similar elements in *C. pneumoniae* and apolipoprotein (a), which is found in lipoprotein (a), causes anti-*C. pneumoniae* antibodies to form an immune complex with apolipoprotein (a) [34, 35, 97].

Another mechanism involves the formation of antibodies against apolipoprotein (a) in association with HLA tissue groups, which is facilitated by *C. pneumoniae* infection. It was reported that HLA class II DR genotypes were more common in patients with high lipoprotein (a) levels and early coronary artery disease compared to the healthy control group. This finding indicates that an immune response to apolipoprotein (a) may occur in connection with the HLA system [95, 98].

Many of the properties of the single-cell-layer endothelium that forms the innermost layer of the arteries are mediated by NO. NO is synthesized from L-arginine by NO synthetase, an endothelial enzyme. NO is a potent inhibitor of platelet aggregation on endothelial cells and a potent vasodilator that acts by reducing vascular tone. In addition, it inhibits atherosclerosis at every stage through its anti-inflammatory properties, which it exerts by preventing the expression of genes that synthesize molecules that cause inflammation, such as ICAM-1, VCAM-1, MCP-1, and P selectin. Conditions known to predispose to atherosclerosis, such as hypertension, diabetes mellitus, smoking, or increased super oxide levels, have been associated with reduced endothelial production or increased destruction of NO [99]. Chlamydial infection in the endothelial layer results in the disruption of these endothelial properties. Stimulation of the release of endothelin 1, which is an especially powerful vasoconstrictor, causes endothelial cells to revert to their proliferative form, initiating the atherosclerosis process [100]. Chlamydial infection also stimulates the release of ELAM-1, VCAM-1, and ICAM-1 from the endothelium. Studies have shown that *C. pneumoniae* is associated with damage to the endothelium, which forms the intima layer of the arteries, in the early stages of the atherosclerosis process [84].

Host monocytes infected with *C. pneumoniae* begin secreting the adhesion molecules E-selectin, ICAM-1, and VCAM-1. These molecules allow adhesion of monocytes from the endothelium to the subendothelium. There the monocytes turn into macrophages and start to increase their cytokine production. Macrophages enlarged from the phagocytosis of oxidized LDL rupture, releasing the bacteria within them into the atherosclerotic plaque to infect neighboring cells [92].

In addition, *C. pneumoniae* proliferating within monocytes and macrophages stimulates the release of IL-6, TNF-ɑ, monocyte chemoattractant protein-1 (MCP-1), and macrophage inflammatory protein 1-a (MIP1-a) [84].

Another mechanism that may explain the relationship between *C. pneumoniae* infection and atherosclerosis is based on the similarities in structure between the heat shock protein (HSP-60) produced by nearly all bacteria and the HSP produced by humans. Antibodies against the HSP-60 in bacteria may cross-react with human HSP [40]. The immune response to *C. pneumoniae* and/or human HSP in the vascular wall is thought to activate atherosclerosis. Wong et al. showed that *C. pneumoniae* and human HSPs coexisted in atherosclerotic lesions, and incubating mouse macrophages with this HSP caused an increase in matrix-degrading metalloproteinases and TNF-α activity. *Chlamydia*-infected endothelial cells trigger smooth muscle cell proliferation by stimulating the synthesis of endogenous HSP-60 and PDGF [40].

In addition, *C. pneumoniae* HSP has been shown to increase the secretion of lectin-like oxidized LDL receptor 1 (LOX-1) in hypercholesterolemic rabbit endothelial cells. Increased LOX-1 disrupts the LDL regulation system in the host and induces oxidized-LDL-mediated atherosclerosis. LOX-1 forces macrophages to phagocytose oxidized LDL, thereby turning macrophages into foam cells through the phagocytosis of high amounts of oxidized LDL, and foam cells are known to be one of the main players in the atherosclerotic process [74].

Chlamydia has been shown to stimulate the toll-like receptor system in host tissue. Toll-like receptor stimulation is considered one of the factors that initiates and promotes atherosclerosis by triggering the cytokine and inflammatory cascade. Thus, smooth muscle cell migration into the media layer is stimulated and the macrophage/foam cell diapedesis process that causes subintimal thickening progresses [101].

An experimental study by Justin et al. [102] showed that after contaminating porcine coronary arteries with *C. pneumonia* in culture medium, *Chlamydia* proliferating in the arterial wall quickly stimulated smooth muscle cell proliferation in the medial layer of the artery and caused atherosclerosis and significant narrowing in the lumen.

4.2 *Chlamydia pneumoniae* and lipid metabolism

C. pneumoniae has been shown to adversely affect the regulation of lipid metabolism in host tissue. *C. pneumoniae* continues to live in immune cells after undergoing phagocytosis and thus can survive even in chronic inflammation environments [103].

The unmodified, natural level of LDL is controlled by LDL receptors and does not normally lead to the formation of macrophage-derived foam cells. However, the oxidation of LDL due to chlamydial infection disrupts this balance. It has been shown that *C. pneumoniae*-infected macrophages incubated with LDL turn into foam cells within 22 hours [40]. This effect occurs mostly through the induction of LDL oxidation, phagocytosis of oxidated LDL, and induction of lipid accumulation within cells and in the atherosclerotic plaque. Liu et al. [104] reported that both active and inactive *Chlamydia* trigger lipid accumulation and induce foam cell formation.

A study conducted by Zhao et al. [105] showed that *C. pneumoniae* negatively affects lipid metabolism by decreasing ATP-binding cassette transporter A1 (ABCA1) level, which has an important role in cholesterol transport in macrophages. In a study conducted by Tumurkhuu et al. [106] on the same system, it was shown that *C. pneumoniae* infection affected the lipid reuptake system by stimulating extracellular IL-1β and caused intracellular cholesterol accumulation by reducing the synthesis of ABCA1 and G protein-coupled receptor 109A (GPR109a), which are involved in the niacin and ketone receptor system.

In a study on the effects of *Chlamydia* on lipid metabolism in humans, it was found that chronic inflammation associated with *C. pneumoniae* infection caused a significant increase in cardiovascular risk in individuals with familial hypercholesterolemia [104].

In experimental studies, rabbits intranasally infected with *C. pneumoniae* exhibited findings consistent with early atherosclerosis characterized by aortic inflammation when fed a high-fat diet but not in those fed a normal diet [107, 108]. The combination of hyperlipidemia and *C. pneumoniae* infection has been shown to significantly increase the development of atherosclerosis.

Blessing et al. [109, 110] demonstrated in their study that *C. pneumoniae* inoculation causes inflammation in the heart and aorta in normolipidemic C57BL/6J mice. In the same model, atherosclerosis was shown to accelerate and become widespread when the animals were fed a high-cholesterol diet.

Lantos et al. [111] showed that hyperlipidemic diet-induced atherosclerosis in ApoB100only/LDLR−/− mice accelerated threefold in the presence of *C. pneumoniae* infection.

Apolipoprotein E (apoE) is involved in chylomicron and very-low-density lipoprotein (VLDL) metabolism and has a key role in LDL and cholesterol metabolism. ApoE deficiency leads to dyslipidemia and increases susceptibility to atherosclerosis. In mice with apoE enzyme deficiency, even a single dose of *Chlamydia* inoculation significantly increased atherosclerosis compared to uninfected subjects [112].

New Zealand rabbits do not develop atherosclerosis unless they are fed a hyperlipidemic diet. However, when infected with *C. pneumoniae*, atherosclerosis was observed in these animals within 2 weeks despite being fed a normal diet [113]. These results suggest that *C. pneumoniae* also triggers atherosclerosis independently of lipid levels and acts as an independent factor in the development of atherosclerosis.

In their study on C57BL/6J mice fed a high-cholesterol diet, Zafiratos et al. [114] concluded that the coexistence of *Chlamydia* infection and hyperlipidemia significantly increased levels of TNF receptors 1 and 2 and caused inflammation when compared with hyperlipidemia or *Chlamydia* infection alone. Similarly, a study conducted on IL-17A-deficient mice showed that a hyperlipidemic diet did not result in a significant difference in inflammation or atherosclerosis compared to the control group. However, after infection with *C. pneumoniae*, the control group exhibited significant elevation in inflammation markers in the blood (IL-12p40 and IFN-γ) and increased macrophage accumulation in atherosclerotic plaques compared to the IL-17A-deficient group. This showed that IL-17A plays a role in the *Chlamydia*-induced atherosclerosis process in hyperlipidemic subjects [115].

These studies demonstrate the important role of *Chlamydia*, both independent of lipid physiology and as a cofactor of hyperlipidemia, in the different stages of initiating and advancing atherosclerosis.

5. Treatment strategies

5.1 Antibiotic studies

The multitude of studies indicating that *C. pneumoniae* plays a role in the pathogenesis of atherosclerosis led to the investigation of whether this pathogenesis can be treated with antibiotic therapy. Some experimental studies showed that antichlamydial antibiotherapy slowed atherosclerosis to some extent [116].

The ACADEMIC study included 302 coronary artery patients with positive *Chlamydia* IgG tests. Of these, 152 patients received a placebo and 150 patients received azithromycin for 6 months. At the end of the study, there were significant decreases in CRP, IL-1, IL-6, and TNF levels in the azithromycin group, but the expected significant change in serological tests was not observed. In addition, there was no difference in terms of rates of clinical events related to coronary artery disease [117]. This supports the theory that inflammation can be reduced with antichlamydial antibiotherapy.

However, in a multi-center antichlamydial antibiotic study including more than 15,000 people in total, although there were significant changes in laboratory parameters, it unfortunately did not yield the expected results in terms of reducing rates of clinical symptoms and events [118–120].

The failure of antibiotic therapy to provide secondary protection against atherosclerosis complications in individuals infected with *C. pneumoniae* has been attributed to the treatment being too late. It is believed that the atherosclerosis process is already triggered in people infected with *C. pneumoniae* and that antichlamydial treatment does not protect against infection. Experimental studies have indicated that antibiotic treatment initiated immediately after chlamydial infection may protect against atherosclerosis [121, 122]. Research on this subject is ongoing.

5.2 Vaccine studies

Could the failure to obtain expected results in antibiotic studies be due to late treatment? Taking measures before inflammatory and immune responses are induced might facilitate the management of the process. Antichlamydial vaccine studies are the focus in this regard.

Due to the different strains and pathogenetic mechanisms in the *Chlamydia* family, vaccines against all chlamydial species have long been a research topic of interest. *C. trachomatis* is the most common sexually transmitted disease in the world and causes health problems of concern to all of humanity in both men and women, from urinary tract infection to infertility, from pneumonia to blindness. Thus, antichlamydial vaccine development started about 100 years ago with *C. trachomatis*. Using the inactivated EB form for immunization provided results, but the short duration of immunity was disappointing [123].

Chlamydia contain two main bacteria-specific antigens: HSP-60 and major outer membrane protein (MOMP). MOMP activates both cellular and humoral immunity. Most current antichlamydial vaccine studies are focused on MOMP. HSP-60 is a receptor that can be found in many bacterial species and human cells, and no significant progress has been made to date in vaccine studies targeting this antigen [124].

Li et al. [125] demonstrated that administering a recombinant chlamydial protease-like activity factor (rCPAF) and IL-2 vaccine slowed the atherosclerosis process in their study on mice in which atherosclerosis was induced by a hyperlipidemic diet.

Recombinant protein vaccine studies have also yielded promising results in terms of reducing the immune response occurring after chlamydial contamination [126].

There have been nearly 200 antichlamydial vaccine studies to date, and an average of 10–12 new studies are conducted each year. However, although antichlamydial vaccine studies have investigated numerous specific antigenic targets and achieved partial success in mice, the results from whole-cell vaccine targets have not yet reached the clinical implementation stage [123].

5.3 Treatments targeting inflammation triggers (risk factors)

There is ample evidence regarding the anti-inflammatory effect of lifestyle modification. Regular exercise have been shown to both directly improve endothelial function and reduce inflammatory mediators, as well as mitigate risk factors [54, 55 83]. Adipose tissue is an important source of IL-6, which is known to be elevated and linked to inflammation in people with obesity. Lipid-lowering diet and treatments are effective in reducing inflammation. Statins not only have a strong lipid-lowering effect, but anti-inflammatory activity is known to be one of their pleiotropic effects. Statins reduce the release of adhesion molecules and inflammatory cytokines. In addition, they correct endothelial function, reduce oxidative stress, inhibit platelet aggregation, prevent clustering of T cell antigen receptors due to immune activation, and generally stabilize vulnerable plaques. The anti-inflammatory effects of statins have been demonstrated in patients with rheumatoid arthritis. In clinical studies, statins have been shown to reduce CRP values independently of LDL levels. In the CARE study, subgroup analyses revealed that the patient group with high CRP levels benefited more from statin treatment, which was more effective in reducing coronary events in this group [127, 128]. In the PROVE-IT study, the greatest benefit was seen in the group with aggressively reduced LDL and decreased CRP, which demonstrated that patients with the most inflammation benefited most and supported the use of statins in acute coronary syndromes [129]. In the JUPITER study, statin therapy resulted in significant reduction of cardiovascular events in individuals with high CRP but without high LDL, offering further evidence of the importance of reducing inflammation [130]. That study included 17,802 healthy individuals with normal LDL-cholesterol level and CRP above 2 mg/l who were randomized to receive rosuvastatin 20 mg or a placebo, and was terminated after only 1.9 years because of the significant reduction in cardiovascular events in the rosuvastatin arm. This rapid benefit was thought to be a result of the anti-inflammatory effect of rosuvastatin rather than its lipid-lowering effect [131].

There are studies on treatment methods that target risk factors, as well as treatments that directly target inflammation [73]. Some evidence has indicated that acetyl salicylic acid also has an important anti-inflammatory effect in addition to its inhibition of platelet aggregation [73].

An emerging treatment method that is still mostly in the animal testing phase is cytokine blockade. The newly identified CD40 pathway has been shown to play an important role in inflammation, the increase in adhesion molecules, and thrombosis. Blockade of this pathway with monoclonal antibodies has allowed a reduction in the development of atherosclerotic lesions in animal experiments [132].

Another treatment method based on cytokine blockade is polyclonal IgG injection. With polyclonal IgG injections, it is possible to block receptors in phagocytic cells and inhibit antibody synthesis and cytokine production. In mouse studies, intravenous IgG injection prevented the development of fatty streaks at several sites and reduced the area of atheromatous plaques [133]. The latest method of cytokine blockade are treatments to shrink atheromatous plaques with IL-10 injection, but these are still in the animal trial stage [134].

Anti-atherosclerosis vaccine development studies have intensified in recent years. The basic principle here is to modulate the immune response and protect against the development of atherosclerosis. For example, developing antibodies against oxidized LDL and creating antibodies by activating B lymphocytes have been shown to have a protective effect against atherosclerosis. In brief, inflammation is a fundamental mechanism that is present at every stage of atherosclerosis and must be suppressed. The anti-inflammatory effects of lifestyle modification, statin therapy, and some other treatments have been demonstrated, while the search for new anti-inflammatory therapies continues.

6. Conclusions

The presence of *C. pneumoniae* in human atherosclerotic plaques is now a generally accepted fact. Numerous studies in various centers have repeatedly confirmed this with many different diagnostic methods, laboratory tests, and imaging techniques.

The association between *C. pneumoniae* and the atherosclerosis process leads to new questions. Is *Chlamydia* a cause of atherosclerosis, or is it a risk factor that participates in the process and predisposes to its complications?

The active pathogenic mechanism of the bacteria, which involves the ability to live within the cytoplasm, persist long-term and even multiple within vacuoles, cause cell necrosis and lysis, and infect the surrounding cells, and its detection even in the fatty streaking stage, which is the initial stage of atherosclerosis, can be regarded as evidence of its role as a triggering factor. However, its ability to survive in macrophages and lymphocytes, cause cell necrosis and fibrosis, and exist and reproduce in plaque inclusion bodies can be regarded as evidence that it is a co-factor associated with and contributing to the atherosclerotic process.

As a result, the pathophysiological mechanisms of Chlamydial infection shown to play a role in atherosclerosis can be summarized under the main headings as follows:

- Arterial wall infection resulting from *Chlamydia* entering the bloodstream via the respiratory system and invading the arterial wall (initiation of atherosclerosis),
- Systemic inflammation induced by inflammatory mediators released into the circulation in response to infection,
- Chronic infection and a chronic inflammation process due to the biphasic life cycle of *Chlamydia*,
- Triggering of adhesion and inflammation in the arteries,
- Bacterial infection and consequent accumulation of inflammatory cells in the sub-intimal area,
- *Chlamydia*-associated lipoprotein deposition and fibro-fatty plaque induction (advancement of atherosclerosis)
- Autoimmunity caused by the host immune response to *Chlamydia*-specific components,
- Proatherogenic effects of specific bacterial toxins produced by *Chlamydia*.

Considerable research continues on atherosclerosis and related cardiovascular diseases, which are leading causes of mortality and morbidity worldwide. Vascular interventional techniques and bypass surgeries are performed as palliative interventions. However, atherosclerosis is a major disease that has no definitive treatment and is still awaiting a solution.

Studies on the role of *C. pneumoniae* in the pathogenesis of atherosclerosis, vaccine studies, and advances in immune response regulation remain scientists' focus of attention for the treatment of atherosclerosis.

Abbreviations

ABCA-1	ATP-binding cassette transporter A1
apoE	apolipoprotein E
EB	elementary body
ELAM-1	endothelial leukocyte adhesion molecule 1
HSP	heat shock protein
FGF	fibroblast growth factor
ICAM-1	intracellular adhesion molecule 1
ICC	immunohistochemistry
IFN-γ	interferon gamma
IL	interleukin
LOX-1	lectin-like oxidized LDL receptor 1
LPS	lipopolysaccharide
MCP-1	monocyte chemoattractant protein-1
M-CSF	macrophage colony stimulating factor
MIP1-a	macrophage inflammatory protein 1-a
MMP	matrix metalloproteinase
NO	nitric oxide
PAI-1	plasminogen activator inhibitor-1
PCR	polymerase chain Rreaction
PDGF	platelet derived growth factor
PGI2	prostocyclin
TNF-ɑ	tumor necrosis factor alpha
tPA	tissue plasminogen activator
RB	reticulate body
VCAM-1	vascular cell adhesion molecule 1

Author details

Mehmet Besir Akpinar
Faculty of Medicine, Cardio-Vascular Surgery Department, Istinye University, Istanbul, Turkey

*Address all correspondence to: besirakpinar@gmail.com

References

[1] Tanaka K, Masuda J, Imamura T, Sueishi K, Nakashima T, Sakurai I, et al. A nation-wide study of atherosclerosis in infants, children and young adults in Japan. Atherosclerosis. 1988;**72**(2-3):143-156

[2] Berenson GS, Srinivasan SR, Bao W, Newman WP, Tracy RE, Wattigney WA. Association between multiple cardiovascular risk factors and atherosclerosis in children and young adults. The New England Journal of Medicine. 1998;**338**(23):1650-1656

[3] Allan Shor. Chlamydia atherosclerosis lesion discovery, diagnosis and treatment [Internet]. London; 2007 [cited 2022 Nov 21]. Available from: https://primo.qatar-weill.cornell.edu/discovery/fulldisplay?vid=974WCMCIQ_INST:VU1&tab=Everything&docid=alma991000118139706691&lang=en&context=L&adaptor=Local%20Search%20Engine&query=sub,exact,%20stents%20,AND&mode=advanced

[4] Sarier M, Sepin N, Keles Y, Imir L, Emek M, Demir M, et al. Is there any association between urothelial carcinoma of the bladder and human papillomavirus? A Case-Control Study. Urologia Internationalis. 2020;**104**(1-2):81-86

[5] Rosenfeld M, Ann Campbell L. Pathogens and atherosclerosis: update on the potential contribution of multiple infectious organisms to the pathogenesis of atherosclerosis. Thrombosis and Haemostasis. 2011;**106**(11):858-867

[6] Lawson JS. Multiple infectious agents and the origins of atherosclerotic coronary artery disease. Front Cardiovasc Med. 2016;**3**:30

[7] Sarier M. Prevalence of polymicrobial infection in urethritis. Journal of Urological Surgery. 2019;**6**(3):180-183

[8] Kern JM, Maass V, Maass M. Molecular pathogenesis of chronic Chlamydia pneumoniae infection: a brief overview. Clinical Microbiology and Infection. 2009;**15**(1):36-41

[9] Grayston JT, Kuo CC, Wang SP, et al. A new Chlamydia psittaci strain, TWAR, isolated in acute respiratory tract infections. The New England Journal of Medicine. 1986;**315**(3):161-168

[10] Porritt RA, Crother TR. Chlamydia pneumoniae ınfection and ınflammatory diseases. For Immunopathol Dis Therap. 2016;**7**(3-4):237-254

[11] Choroszy-Król I, Frej-Mądrzak M, Hober M, Sarowska J, Jama-Kmiecik A. Infections caused by Chlamydophila pneumoniae. Advances in Clinical and Experimental Medicine. 2014;**23**(1):123-126

[12] von Hertzen LC. Role of persistent infection in the control and severity of asthma: focus on Chlamydia pneumoniae. The European Respiratory Journal. 2002;**19**(3):546-556

[13] Contini C, Grilli A, Badia L, Guardigni V, Govoni M, Seraceni S. Detection of Chlamydophila pneumoniae in patients with arthritis: significance and diagnostic value. Rheumatology International. 2011;**31**(10):1307-1313

[14] Sriram S, Stratton CW, Yao S, Tharp A, Ding L, Bannan JD, et al. Chlamydia pneumoniae infection of the central nervous system in multiple sclerosis. Annals of Neurology. 1999;**46**(1):6-14

[15] Balin BJ, Gérard HC, Arking EJ, Appelt DM, Branigan PJ, Abrams JT, et al. Identification and localization

of Chlamydia pneumoniae in the Alzheimer's brain. Medical Microbiology and Immunology. 1998;**187**(1):23-42

[16] McClarty G. Chlamydiae and the biochemistry of intracellular parasitism. Trends in Microbiology. 1994;**2**(5):157-164

[17] AbdelRahman YM, Belland RJ. The chlamydial developmental cycle. FEMS Microbiology Reviews. 2005;**29**(5):949-959

[18] di Pietro M, Filardo S, Romano S, Sessa R. Chlamydia trachomatis and Chlamydia pneumoniae Interaction with the host: latest advances and future prospective. Microorganisms. 2019;**7**(5):140

[19] Saikku P. Seroepidemiology in Chlamydia pneumoniae — atherosclerosis association. European Heart Journal. 2002;**23**(4):263-264

[20] Evani SJ, Ramasubramanian AK. Biophysical regulation of Chlamydia pneumoniae-infected monocyte recruitment to atherosclerotic foci. Scientific Reports. 2016;**6**(1):19058

[21] Kuo C, c., Shor A, Campbell LA, Fukushi H, Patton DL, Grayston JT. Demonstration of Chlamydia pneumoniae in atherosclerotic lesions of coronary arteries. Journal of Infectious Diseases. 1993;**167**(4):841-849

[22] Kuo CC, Gown AM, Benditt EP, Grayston JT. Detection of Chlamydia pneumoniae in aortic lesions of atherosclerosis by immunocytochemical stain. Arteriosclerosis and Thrombosis. 1993;**13**(10):1501-1504

[23] Ramirez JA. Isolation of Chlamydia pneumoniae from the coronary artery of a patient with coronary atherosclerosis. Annals of Internal Medicine. 1996;**125**(12):979

[24] Jackson LA, Campbell LA, Kuo C, Rodriguez DI, Lee A, Grayston JT. Isolation of Chlamydia pneumoniae from a carotid endarterectomy specimen. The Journal of Infectious Diseases. 1997;**176**(1):292-295

[25] Maass M, Bartels C, Engel PM, Mamat U, Sievers HH. Endovascular presence of viable Chlamydia pneumoniaeIs a common phenomenon in coronary artery disease. Journal of the American College of Cardiology. 1998 Mar;**31**(4):827-832

[26] Apfalter P, Loidl M, Nadrchal R, Makristathis A, Rotter M, Bergmann M, et al. Isolation and continuous growth of Chlamydia pneumoniae from arterectomy specimens. European Journal of Clinical Microbiology & Infectious Diseases. 2000;**19**(4):305-308

[27] Karlsson L, Gnarpe J, Nääs J, Olsson G, Lindholm J, Steen B, et al. Detection of viable Chlamydia pneumoniae in abdominal aortic aneurysms. European Journal of Vascular and Endovascular Surgery. 2000;**19**(6):630-635

[28] Lewis ME, Belland RJ, AbdelRahman YM, Beatty WL, Aiyar AA, Zea AH, et al. Morphologic and molecular evaluation of Chlamydia trachomatis growth in human endocervix reveals distinct growth patterns. Frontiers in Cellular and Infection Microbiology. 2014;**4**:71

[29] Jm O, Ejm F, De Vries A, Ce V, Kromhout D. Chlamydia pneumoniae is a risk factor for coronary heart disease in symptom-free elderly men, but Helicobacter pylori and cytomegalovirus are not. Epidemiology and Infection. 1998;**120**(1):93-99

[30] Kark J, Leinonen M, Paltiel O, Saikku P. Chlamydia pneumoniae and

acute myocardial infarction in Jerusalem. International Journal of Epidemiology. 1997;**26**(4):730-738

[31] Altman R, Rouvier J, Scazziota A, Gonzalez C, Absi RS. Lack of association between prior infection with chlamydia pneumoniaeand acute or chronic coronary artery disease. Clinical Cardiology. 1999;**22**(2):85-90

[32] Saikku P. Chronic Chlamydia pneumoniae infection as a risk factor for coronary heart disease in the Helsinki Heart Study. Annals of Internal Medicine. 1992;**116**(4):273

[33] Miettinen H, Lehto S, Saikku P, Haffner SM, Ronnemaa T, Pyorala K, et al. Epidemiology and prevention: association of Chlamydia pneumoniae and acute coronary heart disease events in non-insulin dependent diabetic and non-diabetic subjects in Finland. European Heart Journal. 1996;**17**(5):682-688

[34] Leinonen M, Linnanmäki E, Mattila K, Nieminen MS, Valtonen V, Leirisalo-Repo M, et al. Circulating immune complexes containing chlamydial lipopolysaccharide in acute myocardial infarction. Microbial Pathogenesis. 1990;**9**(1):67-73

[35] Ieven MM, Hoymans VY. Involvement of Chlamydia pneumoniae in atherosclerosis: more evidence for lack of evidence. Journal of Clinical Microbiology. 2005;**43**(1):19-24

[36] Danesh J. Chlamydia pneumoniae IgG titres and coronary heart disease: prospective study and meta-analysis commentary: adjustment for potential confounders may have been taken too far. BMJ. 2000;**321**(7255):208-213

[37] Sarier M, Sepin N, Emek M, Germen AT, Hoscan MB, Konuk E, et al. Evaluating the utility of the A.F. Genital System test for pathogen diagnosis in acute male urethritis. Andrologia. 2022;**54**(4)

[38] Diaz MH, Winchell JM. Detection of Mycoplasma pneumoniae and Chlamydophila pneumoniae directly from respiratory clinical specimens using a rapid real-time polymerase chain reaction assay. Diagnostic Microbiology and Infectious Disease. 2012;**73**(3):278-280

[39] Sarıer M, Duman İ, Göktaş Ş, Demirorcid.org M, Kukul E. Results of multiplex polymerase chain reaction assay to identify urethritis pathogens. Journal of Urological Surgery. 2017;**4**(1):18-22

[40] Wong YK, Gallagher PJ, Ward ME. Chlamydia pneumoniae and atherosclerosis. Heart. 1999;**81**(3):232-238

[41] Boman J, Hammerschlag MR. Chlamydiapneumoniaeandatherosclerosis: critical assessment of diagnostic methods and relevance to treatment studies. Clinical Microbiology Reviews. 2002;**15**(1):1-20

[42] Gimbrone MA. Vascular endothelium, hemodynamic forces, and atherogenesis. The American Journal of Pathology. 1999;**155**(1):1-5

[43] Mallika V, Goswami B, Rajappa M. Atherosclerosis pathophysiology and the role of novel risk factors: a clinicobiochemical perspective. Angiology. 2007;**58**(5):513-522

[44] Falk E, Shah PK, Fuster V. Coronary plaque disruption. Circulation. 1995;**92**(3):657-671

[45] Libby P. Molecular bases of the acute coronary syndromes. Circulation. 1995;**91**(11):2844-2850

[46] Munro JM, Cotran RS. The pathogenesis of atherosclerosis:

atherogenesis and inflammation. Laboratory Investigation. 1988;**58**(3):249-261

[47] Albelda SM, Smith CW, Ward PA. Adhesion molecules and inflammatory injury. The FASEB Journal. 1994;**8**(8):504-512

[48] Blankenberg S, Barbaux S, Tiret L. Adhesion molecules and atherosclerosis. Atherosclerosis. 2003;**170**(2):191-203

[49] Libby P, Li H. Vascular cell adhesion molecule-1 and smooth muscle cell activation during atherogenesis. Journal of Clinical Investigation. 1993;**92**(2):538-539

[50] van Snick J. Interleukin-6: an overview. Annual Review of Immunology. 1990;**8**(1):253-278

[51] Stefanadis C, Diamantopoulos L, Dernellis J, Economou E, Tsiamis E, Toutouzas K, et al. Heat production of atherosclerotic plaques and ınflammation assessed by the acute phase proteins in acute coronary syndromes. Journal of Molecular and Cellular Cardiology. 2000;**32**(1):43-52

[52] Ma J, Hennekens CH, Ridker PM, Stampfer MJ. A prospective study of fibrinogen and risk of myocardial infarction in the physicians' health study. Journal of the American College of Cardiology. 1999;**33**(5):1347-1352

[53] Alizadeh Dehnavi R, de Roos A, Rabelink TJ, van Pelt J, Wensink MJ, Romijn JA, et al. Elevated CRP levels are associated with increased carotid atherosclerosis independent of visceral obesity. Atherosclerosis. 2008;**200**(2):417-423

[54] Ridker PM, Silvertown JD. Inflammation, C-reactive protein, and atherothrombosis. Journal of Periodontology. 2008;**79**(8s):1544-1551

[55] Ridker PM, Cushman M, Stampfer MJ, Tracy RP, Hennekens CH. Inflammation, aspirin, and the risk of cardiovascular disease in apparently healthy men. The New England Journal of Medicine. 1997;**336**(14):973-979

[56] Cannon CP, Braunwald E, McCabe CH, Rader DJ, Rouleau JL, Belder R, et al. Intensive versus moderate lipid lowering with statins after acute coronary syndromes. The New England Journal of Medicine. 2004;**350**(15):1495-1504

[57] Ridker PM, Hennekens CH, Buring JE, Rifai N. C-reactive protein and other markers of ınflammation in the prediction of cardiovascular disease in women. The New England Journal of Medicine. 2000;**342**(12):836-843

[58] Gram J, Bladbjerg EM, Moller L, Sjol A, Jespersen J. Tissue-type plasminogen activator and C-reactive protein in acute coronary heart disease. A nested case-control study. Journal of Internal Medicine. 2000;**247**(2):205-212

[59] Sima Av, Stancu CS, Simionescu M. Vascular endothelium in atherosclerosis. Cell and Tissue Research. 2009;**335**(1):191-203

[60] Virani SS, Polsani VR, Nambi V. Novel markers of inflammation in atherosclerosis. Current Atherosclerosis Reports. 2008;**10**(2):164-170

[61] Cybulsky MI, Gimbrone MA. Endothelial expression of a mononuclear leukocyte adhesion molecule during atherogenesis. Science 1991. 1979;**251**(4995):788-791

[62] Libby P. Inflammatory mechanisms: the molecular basis of ınflammation and disease. Nutrition Reviews. 2008;**65**:S140-S146

[63] Abbas MA, Guenther A, Galantucci S, Fawi G, Comi G, Kwan J, et al. Microbial

risk factors of cardiovascular and cerebrovascular diseases: potential therapeutical options. Open Neuroimaging Journal. 2008;**2**(1):20-24

[64] Rizzo M, Corrado E, Coppola G, Muratori I, Novo G, Novo S. Markers of inflammation are strong predictors of subclinical and clinical atherosclerosis in women with hypertension. Coronary Artery Disease. 2009;**20**(1):15-20

[65] Halvorsen B, Otterdal K, Dahl TB, Skjelland M, Gullestad L, Øie E, et al. Atherosclerotic plaque stability—what determines the fate of a plaque? Progress in Cardiovascular Diseases. 2008;**51**(3):183-194

[66] Singh RB, Mengi SA, Xu YJ, Arneja AS, Dhalla NS. Pathogenesis of atherosclerosis: a multifactorial process. Experimental and Clinical Cardiology. 2002;**7**(1):40-53

[67] Smith JD, Trogan E, Ginsberg M, Grigaux C, Tian J, Miyata M. Decreased atherosclerosis in mice deficient in both macrophage colony-stimulating factor (op) and apolipoprotein E. Proceedings of the National Academy of Sciences of the United States of America. 1995;**92**(18):8264-8268

[68] Cahill PA, Redmond EM. Vascular endothelium – gatekeeper of vessel health. Atherosclerosis. 2016;**248**:97-109

[69] von Eckardstein A, Rohrer L. Transendothelial lipoprotein transport and regulation of endothelial permeability and integrity by lipoproteins. Current Opinion in Lipidology. 2009;**20**(3):197-205

[70] O'Keefe JH, Gheewala NM, O'Keefe JO. Dietary strategies for improving post-prandial glucose, lipids, inflammation, and cardiovascular health. Journal of the American College of Cardiology. 2008;**51**(3):249-255

[71] Montecucco F, Mach F. Common inflammatory mediators orchestrate pathophysiological processes in rheumatoid arthritis and atherosclerosis. Rheumatology. 2008;**48**(1):11-22

[72] Zhang C. The role of inflammatory cytokines in endothelial dysfunction. Basic Research in Cardiology. 2008;**103**(5):398-406

[73] Athyros VG, Kakafika AI, Karagiannis A, Mikhailidis DP. Do we need to consider inflammatory markers when we treat atherosclerotic disease? Atherosclerosis. 2008;**200**(1):1-12

[74] Lin FY, Lin YW, Huang CY, Chang YJ, Tsao NW, Chang NC, et al. GroEL1, a heat shock protein 60 of Chlamydia pneumoniae, induces lectin-like oxidized low-density lipoprotein receptor 1 expression in endothelial cells and enhances atherogenesis in hypercholesterolemic rabbits. Journal of Immunology. 2011;**186**(7):4405-4414

[75] Oörni K, Pentikäinen MO, Ala-Korpela M, Kovanen PT. Aggregation, fusion, and vesicle formation of modified low density lipoprotein particles: molecular mechanisms and effects on matrix interactions. Journal of Lipid Research. 2000;**41**(11):1703-1714

[76] Inia JA, O'Brien ER. Role of heat shock protein 27 in modulating atherosclerotic inflammation. Journal of Cardiovascular Translational Research. 2021;**14**(1):3-12

[77] Cook DN, Pisetsky DS, Schwartz DA. Toll-like receptors in the pathogenesis of human disease. Nature Immunology. 2004;**5**(10):975-979

[78] Lee GL, Yeh CC, Wu JY, Lin HC, Wang YF, Kuo YY, et al. TLR2 promotes vascular smooth muscle cell chondrogenic differentiation and

consequent calcification via the concerted actions of osteoprotegerin suppression and IL-6–mediated RANKL induction. Arteriosclerosis, Thrombosis, and Vascular Biology. 2019;**39**(3):432-445

[79] Stary HC, Chandler AB, Dinsmore RE, Fuster V, Glagov S, Insull W, et al. A Definition of advanced types of atherosclerotic lesions and a histological classification of atherosclerosis. Circulation. 1995;**92**(5):1355-1374

[80] Hansson GK, Libby P, Schönbeck U, Yan ZQ. Innate and adaptive ımmunity in the pathogenesis of atherosclerosis. Circulation Research. 2002;**91**(4):281-291

[81] Bodi V, Sanchis J, Nunez J, Mainar L, Minana G, Benet I, et al. Uncontrolled immune response in acute myocardial infarction. American Heart Journal. 2008;**156**(6):1065-1073

[82] Gordon S. Pattern recognition receptors. Cell. 2002;**111**(7):927-930

[83] Matsuura E, Kobayashi K, Lopez LR. Atherosclerosis in autoimmune diseases. Current Rheumatology Reports. 2009;**11**(1):61-69

[84] Shor A, Kuo CC, Patton DL. Detection of Chlamydia pneumoniae in coronary arterial fatty streaks and atheromatous plaques. South African Medical Journal. 1992;**82**(3):158-161

[85] Saikku P, Mattila K, Nieminen MS, Huttunen JK, Leinonen M, Ekman MR, et al. Serological evidence of an association of a novel chlamydia, twar, with chronic coronary heart disease and acute myocardial infarction. The Lancet. 1988;**332**(8618):983-986

[86] Campbell LA, Kuo C, cho. Chlamydia pneumoniae — an infectious risk factor for atherosclerosis? Nature Reviews. Microbiology. 2004;**2**(1):23-32

[87] Watson C, Alp NJ. Role of Chlamydia pneumoniae in atherosclerosis. Clinical Science. 2008;**114**(8):509-531

[88] Izadi M, Fazel M, Akrami M, Saadat SH, Pishgoo B, Nasseri MH, et al. Chlamydia pneumoniae in the atherosclerotic plaques of coronary artery disease patients. Acta Medica Iranica. 2013;**51**(12):864-870

[89] Kuo CC, Coulson AS, Campbell LA, Cappuccio AL, Lawrence RD, Wang SP, et al. Detection of Chlamydia pneumoniae in atherosclerotic plaques in the walls of arteries of lower extremities from patients undergoing bypass operation for arterial obstruction. Journal of Vascular Surgery. 1997;**26**(1):29-31

[90] Vikatmaa P, Lajunen T, Ikonen TS, Pussinen PJ, Lepäntalo M, Leinonen M, et al. Chlamydial lipopolysaccharide (cLPS) is present in atherosclerotic and aneurysmal arterial wall—cLPS levels depend on disease manifestation. Cardiovascular Pathology. 2010;**19**(1):48-54

[91] Otani T, Nishihira K, Azuma Y, Yamashita A, Shibata Y, Asada Y, et al. Chlamydia pneumoniae is prevalent in symptomatic coronary atherosclerotic plaque samples obtained from directional coronary atherectomy, but its quantity is not associated with plaque ınstability: an ımmunohistochemical and molecular study. Clinical. Pathology. 2022;**15**:2632010X2211251

[92] Assar O, Nejatizadeh A, Dehghan F, Kargar M, Zolghadri N. Association of Chlamydia pneumoniae ınfection with atherosclerotic plaque formation. Global Journal of Health Science. 2015;**8**(4):260

[93] Farrell C, bloth B, Nielsen H, Daugharty H, Lundman T, Svehag Se. A survey for circulating ımmune complexes in patients with acute myocardial

infarction. Scandinavian Journal of Immunology. 2008;**6**(12):1233-1240

[94] Mfl L-V, Kj H, Agarwal R, Nl B, Virella G, Investigators V. Pro-apoptotic and inflammatory markers enhance the ability of MDA-LDL in circulating immune complex to predict acute myocardial infarction in the VADT Study. Diabetes. 2018:67(Supplement_1):430-P

[95] Glader C. The proatherogenic properties of lipoprotein(a) may be enhanced through the formation of circulating immune complexes containing Chlamydia pneumoniae-specific IgG antibodies. European Heart Journal. 2000;**21**(8):639-646

[96] Tertov VV, Orekhov AN, Sayadyan KS, Serebrennikov SG, Kacharava AG, Lyakishev AA, et al. Correlation between cholesterol content in circulating immune complexes and atherogenic properties of CHD patients' serum manifested in cell culture. Atherosclerosis. 1990;**81**(3):183-189

[97] Dahlén GH. Indications of an autoimmune component in LP(a) associated disorders. European Journal of Immunogenetics. 1994;**21**(5):301-312

[98] Dahlén GH, Boman J, Birgander LS, Lindblom B. Lp(a) lipoprotein, IgG, IgA and IgM antibodies to Chlamydia pneumoniae and HLA class II genotype in early coronary artery disease. Atherosclerosis. 1995;**114**(2):165-174

[99] Li H, Förstermann U. Nitric oxide in the pathogenesis of vascular disease. The Journal of Pathology. 2000;**190**(3):244-254

[100] Kern J, Maass V, Rupp J, Maass M. Proliferative stimulation of the vascular endothelin-1 axis in vitro and ex vivo by infection with Chlamydia pneumoniae. Thrombosis and Haemostasis. 2009;**102**(10):743-753

[101] Wang B, Zhang L, Zhang T, Wang H, Zhang J, Wei J, et al. Chlamydia pneumoniae infection promotes vascular smooth muscle cell migration through a toll-like receptor 2-related signaling pathway. Infection and Immunity. 2013;**81**(12):4583-4591

[102] Deniset JF, Cheung PKM, Dibrov E, Lee K, Steigerwald S, Pierce GN. Chlamydophila pneumoniae infection leads to smooth muscle cell proliferation and thickening in the coronary artery without contributions from a host immune response. The American Journal of Pathology. 2010;**176**(2):1028-1037

[103] Flego D, Bianco M, Quattrini A, Mancini F, Carollo M, Schiavoni I, et al. Chlamydia pneumoniae modulates human monocyte-derived dendritic cells functions driving the induction of a Type 1/Type 17 inflammatory response. Microbes and Infection. 2013;**15**(2):105-114

[104] Liu W, He P, Cheng B, Mei CL, Wang YF, Wan JJ. Chlamydia pneumoniae disturbs cholesterol homeostasis in human THP-1 macrophages via JNK-PPARγ dependent signal transduction pathways. Microbes and Infection. 2010;**12**(14-15):1226-1235

[105] Zhao GJ, Mo ZC, Tang SL, Ouyang XP, He PP, Lv YC, et al. Chlamydia pneumoniae negatively regulates ABCA1 expression via TLR2-Nuclear factor-kappa B and miR-33 pathways in THP-1 macrophage-derived foam cells. Atherosclerosis. 2014;**235**(2):519-525

[106] Tumurkhuu G, Dagvadorj J, Porritt RA, Crother TR, Shimada K, Tarling EJ, et al. Chlamydia pneumoniae hijacks a host autoregulatory IL-1β loop to drive foam cell formation and accelerate atherosclerosis. Cell Metabolism. 2018;**28**(3):432-448.e4

[107] Laitinen K, Laurila A, Pyhälä L, Leinonen M, Saikku P. Chlamydia pneumoniae infection induces inflammatory changes in the aortas of rabbits. Infection and Immunity. 1997;**65**(11):4832-4835

[108] Moazed TC, Kuo C, Patton DL, Grayston JT, Campbell LA. Experimental rabbit models of Chlamydia pneumoniae infection. The American Journal of Pathology. 1996;**148**(2):667-676

[109] Blessing E, Lin TM, Campbell LA, Rosenfeld ME, Lloyd D, Kuo CC. Chlamydia pneumoniae induces inflammatory changes in the heart and aorta of normocholesterolemic C57BL/6J mice. Infection and Immunity. 2000;**68**(8):4765-4768

[110] Blessing E, Campbell LA, Rosenfeld ME, Kuo CC. Chlamydia pneumoniae and hyperlipidemia are co-risk factors for atherosclerosis: infection prior to induction of hyperlipidemia does not accelerate development of atherosclerotic lesions in C57BL/6J mice. Infection and Immunity. 2002;**70**(9):5332-5334

[111] Lantos I, Endrész V, Virok DP, Szabó A, Lu X, Mosolygó T, et al. Chlamydia pneumoniae infection exacerbates atherosclerosis in ApoB100 only/LDLR −/− mouse strain. BioMed Research International. 2018;**2018**:1-12

[112] Sorrentino R, Yilmaz A, Schubert K, Crother TR, Pinto A, Shimada K, et al. A single infection with Chlamydia pneumoniae is sufficient to exacerbate atherosclerosis in ApoE deficient mice. Cellular Immunology. 2015;**294**(1):25-32

[113] Fong IW, Chiu B, Viira E, Fong MW, Jang D, Mahony J. Rabbit model for Chlamydia pneumoniae infection. Journal of Clinical Microbiology. 1997;**35**(1):48-52

[114] Zafiratos MT, Cottrell JT, Manam S, Henderson KK, Ramsey KH, Murthy AK. Tumor necrosis factor receptor superfamily members 1a and 1b contribute to exacerbation of atherosclerosis by Chlamydia pneumoniae in mice. Microbes and Infection. 2019;**21**(2):104-108

[115] Chen S, Shimada K, Zhang W, Huang G, Crother TR, Arditi M. IL-17A is proatherogenic in high-fat diet-induced and chlamydia pneumoniae infection-accelerated atherosclerosis in mice. Journal of Immunology. 2010;**185**(9):5619-5627

[116] Muhlestein JB, Anderson JL, Hammond EH, Zhao L, Trehan S, Schwobe EP, et al. Infection with Chlamydia pneumoniae accelerates the development of atherosclerosis and treatment with azithromycin prevents it in a rabbit model. Circulation. 1998;**97**(7):633-636

[117] Anderson JL, Muhlestein JB. The ACADEMIC study in perspective (azithromycin in coronary artery disease: elimination of myocardial infection with Chlamydia). The Journal of Infectious Diseases. 2000;**181**(s3):S569-S571

[118] O'Connor CM, Dunne MW, Pfeffer MA, Muhlestein JB, Yao L, Gupta S, et al. Azithromycin for the secondary prevention of coronary heart disease events. Journal of the American Medical Association. 2003;**290**(11):1459

[119] Grayston JT, Kronmal RA, Jackson LA, Parisi AF, Muhlestein JB, Cohen JD, et al. Azithromycin for the secondary prevention of coronary events. The New England Journal of Medicine. 2005;**352**(16):1637-1645

[120] Cannon CP, Braunwald E, McCabe CH, Grayston JT, Muhlestein B, Giugliano RP, et al. Antibiotic treatment of chlamydia pneumoniae after acute coronary syndrome. The New England Journal of Medicine. 2005;**352**(16):1646-1654

[121] Fong IW, Chiu B, Viira E, Jang D, Fong MW, Peeling R, et al. Can an antibiotic (macrolide) prevent chlamydia pneumoniae -induced atherosclerosis in a rabbit model? Clinical and Diagnostic Laboratory Immunology. 1999;**6**(6):891-894

[122] Rothstein NM, Quinn TC, Madico G, Gaydos CA, Lowenstein CJ. Effect of azithromycin on murine arteriosclerosis exacerbated by Chlamydia pneumoniae. The Journal of Infectious Diseases. 2001;**183**(2):232-237

[123] Phillips S, Quigley BL, Timms P. Seventy years of chlamydia vaccine research – limitations of the past and directions for the future. Frontiers in Microbiology. 2019;**10**:70

[124] Birkelund S, Christiansen G. Chlamydia trachomatis and chlamydia pneumoniae vaccines. In: Ellis & Brodeur, editor, New Bacterial Vaccines. Landes bioscience/Kluwer Academic/Plenum Publishers. 2003. p. 91-109

[125] Li W, Gudipaty P, Li C, Henderson KK, Ramsey KH, Murthy AK. Intranasalimmunizationwithrecombinant chlamydial protease-like activity factor attenuates atherosclerotic pathology following Chlamydia pneumoniae infection in mice. Immunology and Cell Biology. 2019;**97**(1):85-91

[126] Lu X, Xia M, Endresz V, Faludi I, Szabo A, Gonczol E, et al. Impact of multiple antigenic epitopes from ApoB100, hHSP60 and Chlamydophila pneumoniae on atherosclerotic lesion development in Apobtm2SgyLdlrtm1Her J mice. Atherosclerosis. 2012;**225**(1):56-68

[127] Sacks FM, Pfeffer MA, Moye LA, Rouleau JL, Rutherford JD, Cole TG, et al. The effect of pravastatin on coronary events after myocardial infarction in patients with average cholesterol levels. The New England Journal of Medicine. 1996;**335**(14):1001-1009

[128] Ridker PM, Rifai N, Pfeffer MA, Sacks F, Braunwald E. Long-term effects of pravastatin on plasma concentration of C-reactive protein. Circulation. 1999;**100**(3):230-235

[129] Khush KK, Waters D. Lessons from the PROVE-IT trial. Higher dose of potent statin better for high-risk patients. Cleveland Clinic Journal of Medicine. 2004;**71**(8):609-616

[130] Ridker PM, Danielson E, Fonseca FAH, Genest J, Gotto AM, Kastelein JJP, et al. Rosuvastatin to prevent vascular events in men and women with elevated C-reactive protein. The New England Journal of Medicine. 2008;**359**(21):2195-2207

[131] Albert MA, Danielson E, Rifai N, Ridker PM, for the PRINCE Investigators. Effect of Statin Therapy on C-Reactive Protein Levels. Journal of the American Medical Association. 2001;**286**(1):64

[132] Poznyak AV, Bharadwaj D, Prasad G, Grechko AV, Sazonova MA, Orekhov AN. Anti-inflammatory therapy for atherosclerosis: focusing on cytokines. International Journal of Molecular Sciences. 2021;**22**(13):7061

[133] Nardulli M, Durlach V, Pepe G, Anglés-Cano E. Mechanism for the homocysteine-enhanced antifibrinolytic potential of lipoprotein(a) in human plasma. Thrombosis and Haemostasis. 2005;**94**(07):75-81

[134] Almer G, Frascione D, Pali-Schöll I, Vonach C, Lukschal A, Stremnitzer C, et al. Interleukin-10: an anti-inflammatory marker to target atherosclerotic lesions via PEGylated liposomes. Molecular Pharmaceutics. 2013;**10**(1):175-186

Chapter 12

Chlamydia Infection's Role in Neurological Diseases

Nurgül Uzun

Abstract

Chlamydia infections are common infections that are transmitted through sexual *C. pneumonia* is a pathogen that causes different acute and chronic infections. Due to the increase in biological knowledge and the use of more sensitive and specific techniques in the detection of the pathogen in recent years, it is thought that *C. pneumonia* has a role in various cardiovascular and central nervous system (CNS) diseases. There is increasing evidence that *C. pneumonia* may have a role in various chronic neurologic diseases, especially Alzheimer's disease (AD) and multiple sclerosis (MS). *C. pneumonia* crosses the blood-brain barrier via monocytes and triggers neuroinflammation in the central nervous system. Various diagnostic methods (molecular, histopathologic, and culture) have shown the presence of *C. pneumonia* in patients with late-onset AD dementia. It is thought that *C. pneumonia* may be a cofactor in the development of MS disease by causing chronic permanent brain infection in MS patients. There are also reports of *C. pneumonia* causing other CNS diseases such as Guillaine Barre syndrome, encephalitis/meningoencephalitis, and cerebellar ataxia. In this section, the relationship between Chlamydia infections and neurological diseases will be discussed based on scientific research.

Keywords: Chlamydia, neuroinflamation, stroke, neurologic disease, chlamydia infection

1. Introduction

Chlamydiae have been identified as viruses because they have a life cycle within the host cell and are smaller than bacteria. However, they were later classified as bacteria because they can also live outside the cell. With these conditions, they were named as "obligate intracellular bacteria" [1].

There are four species in the genus Chlamydia: *C. pecorum*, *C. psittaci*, *C. trachomatis* and *C. pneumoniae*. These species are classified according to their disease, antigenic structures, and intracellular inclusions. *C. pecorum* does not cause disease in humans. Others may cause disease in humans.

C. trachomatis is the most frequently sexually transmitted bacterium today [2]. It most commonly causes urethritis in men and cervicitis most commonly in women. If left untreated, it can progress to pelvic inflammatory disease in women. *C. trachomatis* is the most common cause of nongonococcal urethritis [3]. As a significant proportion of patients are asymptomatic, they continue to be contagious and act as vector [4].

IntechOpen

This complicates the management of the disease and results in a serious socioeconomic burden, even in developed countries [5]. The three main clinical manifestations of urethritis—urethral discharge, itching, and dysuria—are mild or absent in some cases [6]. Therefore, diagnosing *C. trachomatis* infection is important. Although conventional diagnostic methods have low efficiency, PCR tests have high sensitivity and specificity and are currently the gold standard in the diagnosis of *C. trachomatis* infection. *C. trachomatis* can also cause ocular trachoma, lymphogranuloma venerum, and neonatal infections [7].

Chlamydia Psittaci; it causes a systemic disease that often progresses with pneumonia, being more common in occupational groups that come into contact with birds.

C. pneumoniae; it causes respiratory tract (such as pneumonia, bronchitis, sinusitis, and pharyngitis) infections and is also associated with atherosclerosis and cardiovascular diseases [8].

Chlamydia pneumonia is transmitted from person to person by direct respiratory route. The infection spreads slowly [9, 10]. It has a longer incubation period than many pathogens that cause respiratory tract disease, and this period is about a few weeks [11]. If it is within the family, the infection spreads in a shorter time [12].

Chlamydiae are obligate intracellular parasites and have a biphasic life cycle. They can grow and multiply using the host cell's ATP. Chlamydia are in the bacteria class because they are sensitive to antibiotics, reproduce by division, contain both DNA and RNA, and have cell membranes similar to gram-negative bacteria [13, 14].

Chlamydia reproduces by forming inclusion bodies in the cytoplasm of host cells. Chlamydia pneumonia has two forms called "Elementary body" (EB) and "Reticulate body" (RB). These two forms are functionally and morphologically different from each other and undergo regular change. The EB form is the metabolically inactive, extracellular form and causes contamination. It attaches to the mucosal surfaces of the respiratory tract by inhalation and enters the host cell by endocytosis, where it transforms into the RB form.

The RB form is metabolically active and utilizes the host cell's metabolism. It multiplies in the host cell, breaks up this cell, spreads around as newly formed elementary body bodies and continues to be transmitted. In its RB form, it is protected from the host cell's endocytic lysosomal digestive tract, where it can be stored for years. In this way, it causes a chronic inflammatory process in the body [15, 16].

Being located intracellularly provides the ability of this bacterium to transform into a resistant form [8, 17].

C. pneumonia lives in the host cell as a non-degradable inclusion separate from the cytoplasm of the cell. For this reason, it is protected from the host cell's defense systems by arranging the signal pathways used by the host cell for defense. In this way, *C. pneumoniae* cannot be eliminated because the host defense mechanisms are insufficient and may lead to persistent infection [18–20]. While *C. pneumoniae* lives in mononuclear cells, it multiplies from time to time and creates a chronic infection. In this chronic infection, heat shock protein ((HsP) and proinflammatory cytokine production takes place, and this process can initiate an autoimmunity process over time. As a result of chronic infection, *C. pneumonia* increases the expression of its own HsP60 proteins. The immune response of the host to microbial HsP60 is over time to human HsP60. This may contribute to the development of chronic diseases such as asthma, atherosclerosis, and coronary artery disease [11, 21, 22].

In recent years, there has been a great deal of information about the physiological effects of chlamydia infection on the host cell [23]. Although it is not known exactly how *C. pneumonia* may cause chronic infection in the central nervous system by affecting apoptotic pathways [24, 25].

In recent years, it has been determined that *C. pneumonia* may have a role in other chronic diseases in addition to respiratory tract diseases, as more powerful tests have been developed to show the presence of *C. pneumonia* [26].

It has also been shown to cause progressive diseases with chronic inflammation processes such as lung cancer, Alzheimer's disease, multiple sclerosis, arthritis, and atherosclerosis [18, 27–31].

The demonstration that various human cells (smooth muscle, monocytes, lymphocytes, macrophages, endothelium, and epithelium) are infected by *C. pneumonia* after a respiratory infection supports the systemic spread after respiratory tract infection [32]. Thus, *C. pneumonia* spreads everywhere through the circulatory system. Chlamydia, which invades the arterial wall as a result of endothelial damage, participates in the atherosclerosis process [33].

Chlamydia that invades the arterial wall as a result of endothelial dysfunction contributes to the atherosclerosis process [33]. However, *C. pneumoniae* infection has also been shown to promote monocytic migration via human brain endothelial cells, which is thought to be a mechanism by which the organism is able to enter the CNS. This mechanism may explain how the organism enters the CNS and causes chronic damage [34].

This chapter examines the potential role of chlamydial infections in different neurological diseases and the underlying mechanisms in light of the literature.

2. Chlamydial infection and cerebrovascular disease

At present, cerebrovascular diseases constitute an important public health problem because of the associated mortality and functional losses in the acute and chronic period. According to studies conducted in the USA, 500,000 new or recurrent stroke cases are observed every year [35]. Approximately 80–85% of these are cases of ischemic stroke [36, 37].

Although studies have identified many etiological factors for stroke, none of these factors can be identified in approximately 40% of cases. The number of patients with no detectable risk factors is increasing, especially in the patient population under 45 years of age [38]. The research, identification, and (if possible) treatment of potential risk factors have become a priority in order to reduce the incidence and consequences of the disease [35, 39, 40].

Many researchers have suggested that viruses play a role in the development of atherosclerosis and have shown that these pathogens are closely linked to the rapidly progressive CAD that develops in heart transplant recipients [41–45].

The main infectious agents implicated are *C. pneumoniae*, cytomegalovirus, *Helicobacter pylori*, *Streptococcus mutans*, *Porphyromonas gingivalis*, *Actinobacillus*, and *Prevotella intermedia*. Although there are a few publications in the literature on the role of *C. pneumoniae* in ischemic cerebrovascular diseases, the number of studies on this subject is steadily increasing [46–57].

Çalık et al. investigated the presence of *C. pneumoniae* antibodies in patients and healthy controls and did not detect IgM positivity, an indicator of acute *C. pneumoniae* infection, in either group. Both IgA and IgG antibodies were more common in the patient group, with IgG antibodies detected in 37 (74%) of patients and 28 (56%) of controls, and IgA antibodies detected in 31 (62%) of patients and 16 (32%) of controls. However, the difference was statistically significant only for IgA antibodies ($P < 0.01$). Chronic persistent *C. pneumoniae* infection was not present in any of the controls but was detected in eight patients (16%). Findings of atherosclerosis in the carotid and vertebral arteries were statistically more frequent in the patient group. When they compared patients with and without atherosclerosis on Doppler ultrasound, those with atherosclerosis showed higher rates of *C. pneumoniae* IgG and IgA positivity, higher mean titers of these antibodies, and more frequent chronic persistent infection. However, the differences were not statistically significant [41].

Studies have generally shown that IgA antibodies are associated with ischemic cerebrovascular disease while IgG antibodies are not [49, 50, 53].

In a study by Cook et al., acute *C. pneumoniae* infection or reinfection was found to be associated with ischemic cerebrovascular disease [55].

IgG positivity is an indicator of a previous infection and can remain positive for years [11]. However, IgA antibodies have a very short half-life of 5–6 days on average. Therefore, IgA antibodies are useful in determining persistent and active carrier status. Based on observations, anti-*Chlamydia* IgA antibodies become positive (titer of 1/16 or higher) early in primary chlamydial infections, and the titer increases 2–4 times within 20–40 days, even if the patient is treated. This elevated titer rapidly decreases to former values after treatment [58]. However, infection status can be ascertained by simultaneously determining IgG and IgM antibody status. The presence of IgM antibodies is a definitive indicator of acute infection. In chronic or re-infection, IgM antibodies do not rise at all or are positive at very low titers. Thus, IgM negativity and IgA positivity ($\geq$1/32) accompanied by IgG positivity ($\geq$1/128) indicate chronic or re-infection [11, 53, 56, 59].

Acute *C. pneumoniae* infection was not detected in any of the patients included in the study by Çalık et al. [41]. Similarly, Elkind et al. reported not detecting IgM antibodies in any of the patients in their ischemic stroke study [53].

Although criteria have been established for the diagnosis of chronic persistent infection, a positive IgA titer is an indirect indicator that the causative pathogen is present in the body [60].

Studies have emphasized the relationship between *C. pneumoniae* infections and atherosclerosis, focusing mostly on the coronary and carotid arteries [17, 46, 51, 61].

Schmidt et al. reported that *C. pneumoniae* seropositivity was associated with an increase in intima media thickness in the main carotid arteries [51]. Grayston et al. demonstrated the presence of *C. pneumoniae* in endarterectomy specimens by PCR and immunocytochemistry and concluded that *C. pneumoniae* infections may cause atherosclerosis or play a role in its pathogenesis [62]. The findings support that *C. pneumoniae* infections may be a strong risk factor for atherosclerosis and related vascular diseases [41]. However, the mechanism underlying this relationship has not been elucidated. Different mechanisms have been described in relation to the contribution of infections in the formation or emergence of atherosclerotic diseases. Infections have both direct and indirect effects on the vasculature. The main direct effects are endothelial cell destruction or dysfunction, smooth muscle cell proliferation, and local inflammation. Indirect effects include chronic systemic inflammation, cross-immunoreactivity of antibodies against the pathogen with host tissues, and the impact of the host response to the pathogen on known atherosclerotic risk factors.

C. pneumoniae can infect various types of cells. Among the cells it infects are endothelial cells, vascular smooth muscle cells, and macrophages, all of which have important roles in the pathogenesis of atherosclerosis. Changes in the function and structure of these cells are an expected result of direct invasion by the pathogen [41]. Indeed, many studies have demonstrated the presence of *C. pneumoniae* in vascular endothelium affected by atherosclerosis [62, 63]. In addition to local vessel wall invasion and destruction, *C. pneumoniae* induces a procoagulant state by causing tumor necrosis factor (TNF) and interleukin (IL)-2 release and affecting lipoprotein levels and tissue factors because of its lipopolysaccharide cell wall components [50, 62]. Hsp60, one of the antigens in the protein structure of *C. pneumoniae*, can trigger atherogenesis indirectly through certain immunological mechanisms [64]. The effects of chronic *C. pneumoniae* infection on blood clotting factors have also been demonstrated. Toss et al. determined that chronic persistent *C. pneumoniae* infection was associated with increased serum fibrinogen levels but were unable to explain the mechanism behind this increase [65].

C. pneumoniae infections were also reported to have a number of effects on the blood lipid profile, which has an important role in the development of atherosclerosis [64]. In their study including 1053 patients, Laurila et al. showed that individuals with *C. pneumoniae* IgG antibody titer values of 1/128 and above had higher serum triglyceride levels and lower HDL/total cholesterol ratio compared to individuals with lower antibody titers [66]. The host response to the lipopolysaccharides in the structure of *C. pneumoniae* found in the atherosclerotic region alters the synthesis of certain cytokines. These cytokines cause a complex set of changes in the serum lipid profile [64].

In summary, evidence pointing to the relationship between *C. pneumoniae* and atherosclerosis is as follows: (a) sero-epidemiological studies have demonstrated its association with atherosclerotic diseases (CAD, ischemic cardiovascular disease, and carotid atherosclerosis); (b) the pathogen has been demonstrated in atherosclerotic lesions; and (c) several small clinical studies have shown the benefits of using anti-inflammatory antibiotics in the secondary prevention in patients with CAD [52]. If the possible relationship between infections and vascular occlusive diseases such as ischemic cardiovascular disease and CAD is confirmed, adding antibiotics to treatment protocols for stroke and coronary events may help prevent ischemic events [50].

3. *C. pneumoniae* and neurodegenerative and demyelinating diseases

Information regarding the role of *C. pneumoniae* in chronic neurological diseases has been increasing recently. This was supported by the detection of *C. pneumoniae* genomic material in the cerebrospinal fluid of MS and AD patients [11, 18–20, 34].

3.1 *C. pneumoniae* and multiple sclerosis

MS is a chronic autoimmune and demyelinating disease that affects the CNS, usually in young adults [67]. MS was first described in 1838. During the six decades following its identification, German and French physicians determined the clinical and pathological features of the disease. Previously documented only as cases, MS became one of the most common diseases in neurology at the turn of the twentieth century. The disease is characterized by damage to the myelin sheaths, oligodendrocytes, and to a lesser extent, axons and neurons. There are currently 2.5 million people with MS worldwide, and their treatment and care cost billions of dollars [68]. MS is a highly heterogeneous disease and can present with widely variable clinical signs and symptoms including motor, sensory, autonomic, and cognitive disorders, depending on the part of the CNS affected [69].

MS develops in genetically predisposed individuals as a result of a combination of environmental factors, viral or bacterial pathogens, cytokines secreted in inflammatory and autoimmune response, and other yet unidentified etiological agents. Various lesions can be seen in patients with MS, such as CNS inflammatory infiltrates, astrogliosis, demyelination, and early axonal damage [70–72].

In MS, CD4+ T helper (Th)-1 and Th17 cells perceive myelin sheath components as foreign antigens and develop an autoreaction against myelin [67].

3.1.1 Axonal and neuronal damage in MS

Inflammatory CNS damage in MS has frequently been associated with axonal damage. Although MS is classically defined as a condition primarily characterized by axonal myelin loss, axonal damage has also been described in the early pathological findings of MS lesions. Modern techniques have yielded definitive findings showing axonal damage. Antibodies to amyloid precursor proteins (APP) reveal damaged axons in the active areas of MS lesions [72].

The distinctive pathological feature of MS is demyelinating plaques, which represent areas of demyelination and gliosis around blood vessels [73]. Acute lesions show macrophage infiltration and phagocytosis of myelin membranes, as well as perivascular lymphocytes and plasma cells. The continuous destruction and regeneration of myelin has been demonstrated within progressive MS plaques [74]. Toll-like receptors (TLR) are strongly associated with many neurodegenerative and demyelinating disorders, including MS, with a significant increase in TLR expression in MS lesions. PCR studies have shown that TLR1–8 s are expressed in microglial cells obtained from MS patients [75]. In addition, healthy white matter from MS patients does not contain TLR, whereas active lesions are associated with increased TLR3 and TLR4 expression by microglia and astrocytes. Late active lesions also contain astrocytes with surface expression of TLR3 and TLR4 [75]. This indicates that early lesions are characterized by microglial infiltration, while astrocytes are also active in late active lesions. However, the exact role of TLR3 and TLR4 activation in these lesions remains unclear. TLRs have been shown to recognize highly conserved sites (pathogen-associated molecular patterns) in various microorganisms, including *C. pneumoniae*, thereby stimulating a strong inflammatory response that contributes to pathogen clearance [76]. In one study, overexpression of TLR-2 and TLR-4 messenger RNA (mRNA) was detected in the peripheral blood, but not in the CSF of MS patients with the relapsing-remitting form, and the combined activation of these TLR has been reported to play a significant role in activating and modulating cellular immune response during chronic *C. pneumoniae* infection [77].

Based on epidemiological observations, it has been suggested that along with genetic predisposition, exposure to an environmental factor such as an infectious agent may play a role in the pathogenesis of MS [78].

The risk of MS is increased by the presence of specific genes in the human MHC, or human leukocyte antigen (HLA) complex, on chromosome 6. In particular, HLA-DR and HLA-DQ genes, which are involved in antigen presentation, are strongly associated with the development of disease. However, although the risk of disease is higher in monozygotic than in dizygotic twins (approximately 30% and 5%, respectively), the low concurrence rate among identical twins suggests that nongenetic factors may contribute to the etiology of MS. In this regard, the etiopathogenesis of MS is complex and remains a subject of debate.

To date, about 20 microorganisms, including viruses, have been associated with MS [79]. The screening techniques used in these studies varied from serology to PCR, and the quality and number of controls examined varied greatly. The most recent pathogen associated with MS is *C. pneumoniae* [26].

Sriram et al. reported the first evidence pointing to the potential role of *C. pneumoniae* in the pathogenesis of MS [80]. A year later, a larger study from the same group strongly confirmed that the frequency of *C. pneumoniae* in the CSF of individuals with MS was significantly higher than in control patients with other neurological diseases (OND) [18]. Specifically, *C. pneumoniae* was isolated in culture in 24/37 (65%) of MS patients and 3/27 (11%) of OND patients; CSF PCR for major outer membrane protein (MOMP) was positive in 36/37 (97%) of MS patients and 5/27 positive (18%) of OND patients, and CSF anti-*C. pneumoniae* IgG test by enzyme-linked immunosorbent assay (ELISA) was positive in 32/37 (86%) of MS patients and none of the OND patients. After this groundbreaking report, a number of studies suggested that *C. pneumoniae* infection may be associated with MS, while no association could be established in others [81, 82].

In recent years, the possible role of *C. pneumoniae* in the development of MS has been supported by sero-epidemiological, cultural, molecular, immunological, and therapeutic studies. However, the fact is that there are not many studies supporting the role of the organism in MS. Firstly, some reports have shown that *C. pneumoniae* seropositivity is associated with the risk of developing progressive forms of MS but only moderately associated with the developing MS [83], while others found no association between serum anti-*Chlamydia* antibody titers and MS risk [84]. Secondly, the microorganism was detected in the throat with increasing serological titers during MS relapses [85]. Thirdly, MS relapses have long been known to follow respiratory tract infections, including sore throats or pneumonia, a typical clinical pattern of respiratory tract infection caused by *C. pneumoniae*. However, studies to isolate the pathogen in cultures of CSF and brain tissue have repeatedly failed in MS patients or shown culture positivity in only a small proportion of MS patients [86–90].

Dong-Si et al. reported gene transcription of *C. pneumoniae* mRNA in the CSF of MS patients, a finding that supports active infection with this pathogen [91].

In another study, active transcription of DNA of the organism indicating in a persistent and metabolically active state was detected in cultured CSF and PBMCs from MS patients but not controls [92]. Other investigators were able to culture *C. pneumoniae* in buffy coat samples from a healthy blood donor population and demonstrated 24.6% carriage of *Chlamydia* in the circulating white blood cells. Because of the difficulties of isolating *C. pneumoniae* in culture, PCR-based nucleic acid amplification methods have become the preferred method for the detection of this microorganism. However, PCR procedures also often differ in several aspects that may affect their sensitivity, reproducibility, and specificity [26]. In this context, collaborative studies involving different laboratories examining the presence of *C. pneumoniae* in blinded CSF samples further highlighted the lack of an accepted standardized PCR protocol [93, 94]. A series of PCR studies failed to provide evidence of *C. pneumoniae* DNA in the CSF of MS patients. Most of these studies were conducted using single or nested PCR targeting the MOMP or 16 s ribosomal (rRNA) chlamydial genes [26].

In contrast, a substantial number of studies from around the world have provided clear evidence that *C. pneumoniae* has a role in MS. In this setting, most studies found positive PCR results, with rates of DNA or mRNA positivity ranging from 2.9–69% [26]. Some reports also showed that *C. pneumoniae* DNA was more common in the CSF of MS patients with gadolinium-enhancing lesions on MRI [95, 96]. Furthermore, detection of 16 s rRNA and Hsp60 mRNA by reverse transcriptase (RT)-PCR of CSF was more frequent in MS patients than controls, indicating the presence of high gene transcription and thus a more active *C. pneumoniae* metabolism in MS [91]. In 2004, a new amplification program for the MOMP gene was developed by analyzing CSF samples from patients with MS, other inflammatory neurological disorders (OIND), and non-inflammatory neurological disorders (NIND), and using three gene targets in parallel (MOMP, 16 s rRNA, and Hsp70) to achieve high sensitivity and specificity [97]. PCR positivity for MOMP and 16 s rRNA in CSF was present in a small proportion of MS patients (37%), OIND (28%), and NIND (37%), and there was no difference between MS and controls. Also, PCR positivity for MOMP and 16 s rRNA in CSF was more frequent in relapsing-remitting MS than in its progressive forms, as well as clinically and MRI stable MS compared to clinically and MRI active MS. In contrast, CSF PCR positivity for HsP70 was observed in only three patients with active relapsing-remitting MS. Therefore, the presence of *C. pneumoniae*, especially in a specific subgroup of active relapsing-remitting MS patients, cannot be disregarded. Early in the disease course, activated infected blood-derived monocytes cross the blood-brain barrier via transendothelial migration, resulting in inflammatory immune activation in the CNS. Alternatively, the presence of *C. pneumoniae* DNA in the CSF at high rates in this subset of MS patients may reflect selective infiltration of monocytes to the brain only after activation, thus suggesting that *C. pneumoniae* plays a role only as a silent passenger. In a PCR study targeting multiple genes in both CSF and PBMCs, 64% of active relapsing-remitting MS patients were positive for *C. pneumoniae* DNA and mRNA, while only three control patients were found to be positive for *Chlamydia*, showing that *C. pneumoniae* may exist in a persistent and metabolically active state at both the peripheral and intrathecal levels in MS patients but not in controls [92]. *C. pneumoniae* DNA was found in PBMCs, which can cross the blood-brain barrier into the intrathecal area and induce a chronic persistent brain infection that may be a cofactor in the development of the disease. Recently, they found that intrathecal synthesis of anti-*C. pneumoniae* IgG evaluated by antibody specific index was more common in MS (16.9%) and OND (21.6%) than in NIND (1.9%) patients, as well as in progressive forms of MS than in relapsing-remitting MS [98]. In addition, in patients with intrathecally produced anti-*C. pneumoniae* IgG, it was shown that CSF *C. pneumoniae*-specific high affinity antibodies are more common in the subgroup of patients with progressive forms of MS than in patients with OND and were not found at all in patients with remitting-relapsing MS and NIND. To further examine a possible relationship between *C. pneumoniae* infection and MS, Sriram et al. published a study examining autopsy samples of brain tissue and CSF using immunohistochemical staining with anti-*C. pneumoniae* monoclonal antibodies in addition to molecular and ultrastructural methods [99]. These techniques provided evidence for the presence of *C. pneumoniae,* which was more common in MS patients (90, 62, and 55%, respectively) than in control patients. The authors first demonstrated the presence of chlamydial EBs on the ependymal surfaces and periventricular regions by electron microscopy in 40% of patients with MS but not in the control group. Collectively, MS patients are more likely to have detectable levels of *C. pneumoniae* compared with patients with OND. However, a review of 26 studies including 1332 MS patients and 1464 controls reported that the findings were insufficient to establish an etiological relationship between *C. pneumoniae* and MS after controlling for the confounding effects of gender differences [88].

Treatment targeting the inflammatory process is only partly effective on the course of MS. In relapsing-remitting MS, this type of therapy slows the progression of disability, while the same therapy has been shown to have little or no effect on the progression of disability in primary progressive MS. Reports regarding antimicrobial therapy in MS have also yielded conflicting results. In one trial, the antibiotic minocycline resulted in a reduction in the number of gadolinium-enhancing lesions detected by MRI [100]. Another study showed that anti-chlamydial therapy reduced brain atrophy, but showed no beneficial effect on the number of gadolinium-enhancing lesions on MRI [101].

From the data presented, there is evidence that *Chlamydia* does not have a causal role in MS disease. Therefore, the findings on this topic are still confusing. While some studies have stated that the presence of *Chlamydia* is merely an epiphenomenon of ongoing inflammation in MS, others have reported that it plays a role as a cofactor in the development and progression of the disease by enhancing a pre-existing immune response in a subgroup of MS patients, as supported by recent immunological and molecular findings [81, 92].

There are also studies showing a possible association between MS and *Parachlamydia*-like organisms, which are thought to act alone or in conjunction with *C. pneumoniae* as a cofactor in the development and progression of MS [102].

Finally, we cannot rule out the possibility that other pathogens could be involved in the development of MS. Viruses are often considered potential candidates because they are known to cause demyelinating disease in experimental animals and humans and are generally known to cause diseases that have prolonged latent periods and manifest clinically with relapsing and remitting symptoms [103]. However, research conducted to date has not identified any single virus that plays an important role in MS. Among the viruses proposed as MS cofactors are ubiquitous members of the Herpesviridae family, human herpesvirus 6, and Epstein-Barr virus [26]. The MS-related human retrovirus of the endogenous retrovirus family has also been identified as a potential pathogen in MS [104].

3.2 C. *pneumoniae* and Alzheimer's disease

AD is among the most severe dementias and is increasing as the population ages. AD is associated with neuronal atrophy/death in certain areas of the brain and occurs in two main forms: an early-onset form that is primarily genetically determined, and late-onset AD, which is a non-familial, progressive neurodegenerative disease that is currently the most common and severe form of dementia in older adults. The descriptive neuropathology of both familial and sporadic AD includes neuritic senile plaques (NSPs), consisting mainly of amyloid-β protein, and neurofibrillary tangles (NFTs), the major component of which is modified *tau* protein, which affect nerve synapses and nerve-nerve cell communication. Genetic, biochemical, and immunological analyses have provided relatively detailed information about these entities [31]. The disease usually initially presents as a gradual loss in short-term memory and later progresses to major cognitive dysfunction. Later it can manifest with various behavioral disorders, disorientation, language difficulties, and impairment in activities of daily living [105]. Estimates of the gross incidence of AD range from 7.03 to 23.8 per 1000 person-years [106, 107]. The incidence of AD increases with age in both sexes. Women have approximately 33% higher incidence and prevalence than men [105–109]. Although AD was discovered by Alois Alzheimer in 1907, the cause of this pathology and neurodegeneration is unknown. CNS infections have been shown to stimulate inflammatory responses that may result in neurodegeneration [110]. Several groups have investigated the relationship between various infectious agents and AD, but none of these pathogens were confirmed as etiological factors of disease development or worsening of neuropathology. Interesting insights came from a study that identified herpes simplex virus 1 infection as a risk factor for AD development in subjects expressing the apolipoprotein-E (APOE)-4 allele [110, 111].

Viruses such as the measles virus, adenovirus, lentiviruses, and others were initially evaluated but later ruled out [112, 113]. Bacterial pathogens, including *C. trachomatis*, *Coxiella burnetii*, *Mycoplasma* species, and spirochetes, have also been investigated for involvement in the neuropathogenesis of AD and were rejected [114, 115].

Prions were also considered but later excluded [116].

The first article reporting an association between *C. pneumoniae* infection and late-onset AD was published by Balin et al. [31]. In this study, highly sensitive and specific PCR tests for *C. pneumoniae* were performed on different brain regions (hippocampus, cerebellum, temporal cortex, and prefrontal cortex) showing varying degrees of AD pathology and were positive in 90% of the brains [117]. Electron microscope studies revealed *C. pneumoniae*-like particles containing EBs and RBs in brain tissue, and immunohistochemical analysis showed strong labeling in the parts of the brain most affected by AD, while no labeling was observed in controls. Furthermore, *C. pneumoniae* were detected and visualized in some CNS cells associated with plaques and tangles, RNA transcripts of *C. pneumoniae* showing metabolically active organisms were demonstrated by RT-PCR of frozen tissue samples, and the organisms were subsequently isolated and grown in cell culture. As demonstrated in reactive arthritis, Balin et al. reported a strong correlation between the APOE-4 genotype and *C. pneumoniae* infection in 58% (11/19) of patients with AD, suggesting that the APOE-4 gene may support some aspects of *C. pneumoniae* pathobiology in AD [31]. This report attracted great interest from the public and science, and attempts to replicate their findings were made at reputable laboratories worldwide. Two independent research teams (Ossewaarde et al., 2000 and Mahony et al., 2000, unpublished data) found *C. pneumoniae* in the brains of patients with AD using PCR and immunohistochemistry, confirming the results of Balin et al. However, subsequent studies conducted by different authors using the same procedures but different protocols in paraffin-embedded brain tissues yielded conflicting results [26]. The contradictory results obtained in these studies may be related to differences in diagnostic criteria or demographic differences such as the patients' geographic location, season of death, and history.

AD patients included in the Balin study may have recently been exposed to *C. pneumoniae* and therefore may have been at high risk of systemic dissemination from the respiratory tract to sites within the CNS where advanced AD pathology was already present [118]. As an extension of these findings, 2 years later Gerard demonstrated the presence of *C. pneumoniae* in 80% of AD specimens and 11.1% of controls using a technique targeting two *Chlamydia* genes [1046, 0695] genes. Although the AD patients (mean age: 79.3 years) and controls (65.9 years) were as well matched for age and sex as possible, the controls were younger and only 22.7% were male [119]. Cultures of brain specimens showed that the organism was viable in the AD brain, and further reverse-transcriptase PCR analyses identified primary rRNA gene transcripts from *C. pneumoniae,* demonstrating metabolic activity of the organism in these tissues. Interestingly, immunohistochemical analyses have also shown that astrocytes, microglia, and neurons all serve as host cells for *C. pneumoniae*. These infected cells were found in the AD brain close to both NSPs and NFTs.

Recent studies in cultured astrocytes and microglia have shown that *C. pneumoniae* exhibits an active rather than persistent growth phenotype, indicating possible simultaneous destruction with the rupture of some host cell components at the end of this cycle [120].

In the years immediately following Balin et al.'s study, some experimental discoveries provided insight into the pathogenetic mechanisms of AD. First, there is a relationship between carriage of the APOE-4 allele and the pathobiology of *C. pneumoniae*, and the *C. pneumoniae* load in the AD brain varies by ApoE genotype [121, 122]. Second, infection of human microvascular endothelial cells cultured with *C. pneumoniae* results in an increase in the expression of proteins involved in the organism's CNS access, including N-cadherin and b-catenin [123]. Third, the expression of occluding, a protein associated with tight connections was attenuated in *C. pneumoniae*-infected cells. Fourth, infection with *C. pneumoniae* via the olfactory pathways in nontransgenic young female BALB/c mice, which generally do not develop AD, was shown to promote the production of extracellular amyloid-like plaques [124]. Because *C. pneumoniae* resides in the respiratory tract and has a tendency to infect epithelial cells, the olfactory epithelium in the nasal passages is a possible target of infection. After entry into these epithelia, potential damage and/or cell death may occur in the main olfactory bulb and olfactory cortex, opening the way for further retrograde neuronal damage [117, 125].

In a recent study by Chacko et al., it was shown that *C. pneumoniae* rapidly infects both the olfactory and trigeminal nerves that nasal epithelial injury exacerbated peripheral nerve infection but reduced brain infection and that *C. pneumoniae* inclusions in the olfactory nerve and bulb were associated with amyloid-β deposits. It was also reported that *C. pneumoniae* replication occurred in the glial cells of the olfactory/trigeminal nerves and the brain and that *C. pneumoniae* infection may lead to differential regulation of the genes associated with AD. Thus, *C. pneumoniae* can spread very quickly from the periphery to the CNS via the nerves connecting the nasal cavity and the brain, without infecting the bloodstream. This study demonstrated in vivo that there is a rapid accumulation of amyloid-β in response to *C. pneumoniae* infection of the primary olfactory nervous system. *C. pneumoniae* inclusions were detected in the olfactory bulb and nerve fiber layer/glomerular layer. The detection of inclusion bodies in the olfactory piriform cortex as well suggested that *C. pneumoniae* progressed deeper into the olfactory bulb, as previously reported.

The ability to infect glia is considered the key to invading the CNS via cranial neural pathways. The study by Chacko et al. demonstrated that *C. pneumoniae* could infect, survive, and replicate (form inclusions) within the glia of the peripheral nervous system (olfactory ensheathing cells and trigeminal Schwann cells) and the CNS (astrocytes and microglia). *C. pneumoniae* antigens have been detected in both astrocytes and microglia in human brains post-mortem. Olfactory ensheathing cells, Schwann cells, and astrocytes are all innate immune cells that can respond to and phagocytose bacteria, and microglia (macrophages of the CNS) are well-characterized professional phagocytes. The ability of *C. pneumoniae* to form inclusions in these cells suggests that the bacteria may overcome phagocytic destruction, at least to some extent, which may be an important mechanism that allows this bacterium to invade and establish long-term infection of the CNS.

In addition, their study also revealed localized amyloid-β accumulation adjacent to *C. pneumoniae* inclusion bodies and in the olfactory bulb 7 days and 28 days after inoculation. Diffuse/scattered amyloid-β immunoreactivity was also present in these tissues in control mice, but the common localization of amyloid-β deposits and *C. pneumoniae* inclusions in vaccinated mice was clear and pronounced. Their findings and those of previous studies suggest that amyloid-β secretion occurs in response to infection. One reason for this may be that amyloid-β is secreted as an antimicrobial agent, but alternatively, it may be secreted in response to infection due to pathway activation for subsequent processing of APP into secreted amyloid-β. Future studies may clarify the secretion and role of amyloid-β in this context.

Thus, the secretion of amyloid-β may be a normal immune response to any microbe that might invade the nervous system, and if the infection is cleared, the accumulated amyloid-β can be cleared by phagocytic glia. However, if the bacteria are not cleared and instead become persistent or latent in neural cells, continuous amyloid-β deposition may occur, which contributes to late-onset dementia and/or accelerates amyloid-β accumulation in familial AD. In the case of *C. pneumoniae*, one study in wild-type mice showed that amyloid-β deposits from infection were subsequently cleared, while another study showed that deposits did not disappear for several months [125].

C. pneumoniae infection also leads to the upregulation of key pathways involved in the pathogenesis of AD. The pathological features of AD, such as the production of activated microglia, inflammatory mediators, and reactive oxygen species, were highly regulated in infected brain tissue after inoculation. These neuroinflammatory responses are considered an important driving factor in patients with neurodegeneration and AD pathology, which begins in the early stages of the disease, before the formation of amyloid-β plaques in the brain. After infection, activated microglia and astrocytes (which were shown to be hosts for *Chlamydia*) have been shown to secrete pro-inflammatory cytokines including IL-1β, TNFα, and IL-6. These cytokines are neurotoxic and can directly increase amyloid-β production through activation of β-secretase, which cleaves APP and initiates the amyloid cascade. Microglial activation reduces amyloid-β accumulation in the brain by increasing phagocytosis, clearance, and degradation. However, neuroinflammation associated with AD may be a double-edged sword, as persistent microglia activation stimulated by microglia binding to amyloid-β may increase the production of inflammatory mediators and reactive oxygen species, further strengthening the neuroinflammatory response [125].

In addition to considering key pathways, it is also useful to consider changes in individual gene expression. Long-term *C. pneumoniae* infection triggered downregulation of many other key genes involved in the pathogenesis of AD. Most importantly, the downregulation of the protective Hsp (*Hspa1b or Hsp70–2*), which was associated with increased oxidative stress and the onset of AD pathology, and of Bag2, a B-cell lymphoma-2-associated co-chaperone gene that controls Hsp70 functionality, which led to further failure of the system to protect cells from oxidative damage. Persistent infection was also reported to be associated with AD by leading to mitochondrial dysfunction, gene modulations, increased unfolded protein response, and oxidative stress. In fact, long-term infection has also been associated with low expression of CD2-associated protein, which was previously associated with AD pathology exacerbated by increased amyloid-β deposition and *tau*-induced neurotoxicity. In this study, it was concluded that nerves extending between the nasal cavity and brain constitute invasion pathways by which *C. pneumoniae* was able to rapidly invade the CNS, triggering genetic and molecular changes in the longer term and contributing to the initiation of AD pathogenesis [125].

Because chlamydial chronic infections are characterized by a "chlamydial persistent state" inaccessible to traditional antichlamydial agents, there have been several clinical studies determining the efficacy of antibiotic therapy against *C. pneumoniae* in AD. In a first randomized, placebo-controlled, multicenter clinical trial to determine whether a 3-month course of doxycycline and rifampin reduced the decline in cognitive function in AD patients, the antibiotic group exhibited significantly less cognitive decline at 6 months and less dysfunctional behavior at 3 months compared to controls [126]. Although these observations did not show a causal relationship between *C. pneumoniae* and CNS infection, they paved the way for further research on the eradication of chronic *C. pneumoniae* infection and AD neuropathogenesis. In this context, animal modeling will be required to describe in detail how chlamydial infection can lead to AD-related pathological changes in CNS and to provide a better understanding of infection parameters. In vitro and mouse model studies have shown that metal protein attenuating compounds support the dissolution and clearing of extracellular senile plaques composed of amyloid-β. The antiprotozoal metal chelator clioquinol, which has been reported to reduce amyloid-β plaques, possibly through chelation associated with copper and zinc, is currently in clinical trials as a potential treatment for AD [127, 128].

Scientific knowledge about AD and *C. pneumoniae* infection is still growing. Standardization of diagnostic techniques will certainly allow for better comparability of studies. However, other systemic infections should also be considered as potential contributors to AD pathogenesis.

3.3 *C. pneumoniae* and AIDS dementia

Many authors have investigated the possibility that *C. pneumoniae* is involved in neurodegenerative disorders other than AD. However, the available data are few and not significant. One study investigated the possible link between AIDS-dementia complex and *C. pneumoniae* [129]. AIDS-dementia complex is an HIV-induced neuropathological disease characterized by infection of macrophages and microglial cells and release of proinflammatory cytokines into the parenchyma [130]. In this report, *C. pneumoniae* was identified in the CNS by PCR. Four (17.4%) of 23 HIV-infected patients with stage 3 AIDS-dementia complex diagnosed according to the AIDS-dementia complex scheme and confirmed by autopsy were found to have *C. pneumoniae* in their CNS by PCR for *C. pneumoniae* MOMP and 16 s rRNA gene. Sequence analysis revealed important homologies with *C. pneumoniae* when compared with *C. trachomatis* and *C. psittaci*. In addition, ELISA demonstrated high mean levels of CSF specific anti-*C. pneumoniae* antibodies and significantly elevated *C. pneumoniae* antibody-specific index values in these patients. These findings suggest that although the low rate of isolation does not represent the incidence of *C. pneumoniae*, an increase in the "trafficking" of monocytes containing *C. pneumoniae* to the brain in the late stages of HIV infection may carry this organism to regions that are major reservoirs of productive HIV replication and contribute to neuronal damage in HIV-infected patients [129]. Furthermore, the possibility cannot be ruled out that in a subset of patients this organism exists is not an "innocent bystander," as in atherosclerosis and other chlamydial diseases, but is able to survive and reproduce in CNS macrophages [26].

4. *C. pneumoniae* and other neurological complications

A number of reports have focused on the involvement of C. pneumoniae in other CNS disorders, particularly encephalitis or meningoencephalitis. Reported cases have not been not very frequent [26]. Most patients were young patients presenting with different neurological symptoms and/or neuro-radiological changes on computed tomography or MRI. In most cases, there were also accompanying well-defined respiratory symptoms, although in some cases these occurred prior to the onset of neurological records. Three patients had cerebellar ataxia, acute demyelinating encephalitis, and Guillain-Barrè syndrome. *Chlamydia* was almost always detected serologically using microimmunofluorescence test (four-fold increase in IgG titer) and ELISA techniques based on the detection of specific anti-*C. pneumoniae* antibodies. One study found the presence of IgA-type antibodies, suggesting re-infection [131]. One note reported the use of PCR in a tracheal swab and increased *Chlamydia* IgM antibody titers [132]. These cases and a review of the literature have shown that *C. pneumoniae* infection, in addition to other *Chlamydia* species, can present with significant neurological symptoms. Therefore, the differential diagnosis of respiratory tract infections with neurological presentation should include chlamydial infections as well as *Mycoplasma* and *Legionella* infections.

5. Conclusions

Thanks to the deep knowledge of *Chlamydia* biology of and the use of more advanced techniques than those traditionally used, the presence of *C. pneumoniae* genomic material has been demonstrated in a large number of people suffering from different acute and chronic diseases. Over the past 10 years, an increasing number of reports have indicated a possible link between *C. pneumoniae* and atherosclerosis and CNS diseases including various neurobehavioral disorders, MS, and AD. The main obstacle to determining the exact role of *C. pneumoniae* in chronic diseases is the lack of any method to safely and reliably diagnose chronic infection. The causal role of *C. pneumoniae* infection in cardiovascular disease has not been definitively established. Despite molecular and genetic studies of the role of *C. pneumoniae* in the progression of atherosclerosis, some important questions urgently need answers, such as whether *C. pneumoniae* is an innocent passenger or whether it is actively involved in the onset or progression of atherosclerotic disease. In particular, *C. pneumoniae* Hsp60 should be further investigated as a potential culprit and therapeutic target [86]. Efforts should be made to find a truly effective treatment targeting chronic *C. pneumoniae*. At the same time, the development of an effective vaccine should continue [133].

Although astrocytes, microglia, and neurons have been shown to be host cells for *C. pneumoniae* in the brain of patients with AD, and infected cells can be found near both NSPs and NFTs, most studies have been conducted with different diagnostic methods, none of which have yet been standardized. This has led to wide variation in interlaboratory test performance even when using the same test and the same criteria. Therefore, the actual involvement of *C. pneumoniae* in AD remains a subject of debate and requires further understanding through standardized cultural and molecular protocols.

Recent molecular, ultrastructural, and cultural developments have provided evidence that *C. pneumoniae* is viable and metabolically active in different biological compartments such as CSF and PBMCs in MS patients compared to controls, suggesting a relationship between this pathogen and the disease. The role of *Chlamydia* has been demonstrated in a subgroup of relapsing-remitting MS patients with clinical and MRI disease activity who experience the early inflammatory phase representing the development of the disease [81, 82, 92, 96]. However, growing evidence suggests that *C. pneumoniae* is not just an innocent bystander epiphenomenon due to ongoing MS inflammation, but is a cofactor in the development and progression of the disease by strengthening a pre-existing autoimmune response in a subset of MS patients [81, 92, 134].

For both AD and MS, there is an urgent need for further well-designed studies to determine the importance of C. pneumoniae involvement in the disease and the usefulness of antibiotic treatment.

Abbreviations

C	*Chlamydia*
CNS	Central nervous system
MS	Multiple sclerosis
AD	Alzheimer's disease
TWAR	*Chlamydia pneumoniae*
USA	United States of America
EB	Elementary body
RB	Reticulate body
Hsp	Heat shock protein
PCR	Polymerase chain reaction
CAD	Coronary artery disease
TNF	Tumor necrosis factor
IL	Interleukin
CSF	Cerebrospinal fluid
APC	Antigen-presenting cell
FLAIR	Fluid-attenuated inversion recovery
MHC	Major histocompatibility complex
APP	Amyloid precursor protein
TLR	Toll-like receptor
mRNA	Messenger RNA
HLA	Human leukocyte antigen
OND	Other neurologic diseases
MOMP	Major outer membrane protein
ELISA	Enzyme-linked immunosorbent assay
PBMC	Peripheral blood mononuclear cell
rRNA	Ribosomal RNA
OIND	Other inflammatory neurological disease
NIND	Non-inflammatory neurological disease
NSP	*Neuritic senile plaques*
NFT	Neurofibrillary tangles
APOE	Apolipoprotein-E

Author details

Nurgül Uzun
Department of Neurology, Medical Park Hospital, Antalya, Turkey

*Address all correspondence to: uzunnurgul2@gmail.com

References

[1] Shor A. Chlamydia Atherosclerosis Lesion Discovery, Diagnosis and Treatment. London: Springer Science & Business Media; 2007

[2] Sarier M, Kukul E. Classification of non-gonococcal urethritis: A review. International Urology and Nephrology. 2019;**51**(6):901-907

[3] Sarier M, Sepin N, Emek M, Germen AT, Hoscan MB, Konuk E, et al. Evaluating the utility of the a.F. genital system test for pathogen diagnosis in acute male urethritis. Andrologia. 2022;**54**(4):e14377. DOI: 10.1111/and.14377. Epub 2022 Jan 22

[4] Sarier M, Demir M, Turgut H, Hizel A, Emek M, Kukul E, et al. New approach to microscopy of gram-stained urethral smear: The kissing slide method. Sexually Transmitted Diseases. 2020;**47**(10):712-715

[5] Sarıer M. Prevalence of Polymicrobial infection in urethritis. Journal of Urological Surgery. 2019;**6**(3):180-183

[6] Sarier M, Sepin N, Duman I, Demir M, Hizel A, Göktaş Ş, et al. Microscopy of gram-stained urethral smear in the diagnosis of urethritis: Which threshold value should be selected? Andrologia. 2018;**50**(10):e13143. DOI: 10.1111/and.13143. Epub 2018 Sep 20. PMID: 30238498

[7] Sarıer M, Duman İ, Göktaş Ş, Kukul E. Results of multiplex polymerase chain reaction assay to identify urethritis pathogens. Journal of urological. Surgery. 2017;**4**(1):18-22

[8] Kern JM, Maass V, Maass M. Molecular pathogenesis of chronic chlamydia pneumoniae infection: A brief overview. Clinical Microbiology and Infection. 2009;**15**(1):36-41

[9] Saikku P, Mattila K, Nieminen MS, Huttunen JK, Leinonen M, Ekman MR, et al. Serological evidence of an association of a novel chlamydia, TWAR, with chronic coronary heart disease and acute myocardial infarction. The Lancet. 1988;**332**(8618):983-986

[10] Kleemola M, Saikku P, Visakorpi R, Wang SP, Grayston JT, Kleemola M. Epidemics of pneumonia caused by twar, a new chlamydia organism, in military trainees in Finland. Journal of Infectious Diseases. 1988;**157**(2):230-236

[11] Chou KC, Jackson LA, Ann Campbell L, Thomas Grayston J. Chlamydia pneumoniae (TWAR). Clinical Microbiology Reviews. 1995;**8**:451-461

[12] Mordhorst CH, Wang SP, Grayston JT. Outbreak of chlamydia pneumoniae infection in four farm families. European Journal of Clinical Microbiology & Infectious Diseases. 1992;**11**(7):617-620

[13] McClarty G. Chlamydiae and the biochemistry of intracellular parasitism. Trends in Microbiology. 1994;**2**(5):157-164

[14] Everett KDE. Chlamydia and Chlamydiales: More than meets the eye. Veterinary Microbiology. 2000;**75**(2):109-126

[15] AbdelRahman YM, Belland RJ. The chlamydial developmental cycle. FEMS Microbiology Reviews. 2005;**29**(5):949-959

[16] di Pietro M, Filardo S, Romano S, Sessa R. Chlamydia trachomatis and chlamydia pneumoniae interaction with the host: Latest advances and

future prospective. Microorganisms. 2019;7(5):140

[17] Saikku P. Seroepidemiology in chlamydia pneumoniae — Atherosclerosis association. European Heart Journal. 2002;**23**(4):263-264

[18] Yucesan C, Sriram S. Chlamydia pneumoniae infection of the central nervous system. Curr Opin Neurol. 2001;**14**(3):355-359

[19] Stratton CW, Mitchell WM. The immunopathology of chlamydial infections. Antimicrobics and Infectious Diseases Newsletter. 1997;**16**(12):89-94

[20] Stratton CW, Sriram S. Association of Chlamydia pneumoniae with central nervous system disease. Microbes and Infection. 2003;**5**(13):1249-1253

[21] Palikhe A, Lokki ML, Saikku P, Leinonen M, Paldanius M, Seppänen M, etal.AssociationofChlamydiapneumoniae infection with HLA-B*35 in patients with coronary artery disease. Clinical and Vaccine Immunology. 2008;**15**(1):55-59

[22] Ciervo A, Visca P, Petrucca A, Biasucci LM, Maseri A, Cassone A. Antibodies to 60-kilodalton heat shock protein and outer membrane protein 2 of chlamydia pneumoniae in patients with coronary heart disease. Clinical and Diagnostic Laboratory Immunology. 2002;**9**(1):66-74

[23] Byrne GI. Chlamydia uncloaked. Proceedings of the National Academy of Sciences of the United States of America. 2003;**100**(14):8040-8042

[24] Byrne GI, Ojcius DM. Chlamydia and apoptosis: Life and death decisions of an intracellular pathogen. Nature Reviews Microbiology. 2004;**2**(10):802-808

[25] Byrne GI. Chlamydia uncloaked. Proceedings of the National Academy of Sciences of the United States of America. 2003;**100**(14):8040-8042

[26] Contini C, Seraceni S, Cultrera R, Castellazzi M, Granieri E, Fainardi E. Chlamydophila pneumoniae infection and its role in neurological disorders. Interdisciplinary Perspectives on Infectious Diseases. 2010;**2010**:273573

[27] Porritt RA, Crother TR. Chlamydia pneumoniae infection and inflammatory diseases. For Immunopathol Dis Therap. 2016;**7**(3-4):237-254

[28] Choroszy-Król I, Frej-Mądrzak M, Hober M, Sarowska J, Jama-Kmiecik A. Infections caused by Chlamydophila pneumoniae. Advances in Clinical and Experimental Medicine. 2014;**23**(1):123-126

[29] von Hertzen LC. Role of persistent infection in the control and severity of asthma: Focus on chlamydia pneumoniae. European Respiratory Journal. 2002;**19**(3):546-556

[30] Contini C, Grilli A, Badia L, Guardigni V, Govoni M, Seraceni S. Detection of Chlamydophila pneumoniae in patients with arthritis: Significance and diagnostic value. Rheumatology International. 2011;**31**(10):1307-1313

[31] Balin BJ, Gérard HC, Arking EJ, Appelt DM, Branigan PJ, Abrams JT, et al. Identification and localization of chlamydia pneumoniae in the Alzheimer's brain. Medical Microbiology and Immunology. 1998;**187**(1):23-42

[32] Boman J, Söderberg S, Forsberg J, Slunga Birgander L, Allard A, Persson K. et al, High prevalence of chlamydia pneumoniae DNA in peripheral blood mononuclear cells in patients with cardiovascular disease and in middle-aged blood donors. J Infect Dis. 1998;**178**(1):274-277

[33] Evani SJ, Ramasubramanian AK. Biophysical regulation of chlamydia pneumoniae-infected monocyte recruitment to atherosclerotic foci. Scientific Reports. 2016;**6**(1):19058

[34] MacIntyre A, Abramov R, Hammond CJ, Hudson AP, Arking EJ, Little CS, et al. Chlamydia pneumoniae infection promotes the transmigration of monocytes through human brain endothelial cells. Journal of Neuroscience Research. 2003;**71**(5):740-750

[35] Eslie L, Ronner LB, Anter ASK, Nn JOA, Anson EM. Medical progress review articles primary prevention of stroke. 1995.

[36] Demirci, Şahin A, Üstü Y, Işık D. Serebrovasküler Hastalıklarda Önlenebilen Risk Faktörlerinin Yönetimi. Ankara Medical Journal. 2015;**15**(2)

[37] Akpinar MB, Sahin V, Sahin N, Abacilar AF, Kiris I, Uyar IS, et al. Previous chronic cerebral infarction is predictive for new cerebral ischemia after carotid endarterectomy. Journal of Cardiothoracic Surgery. 2015;**10**(1):141

[38] Jose B, Duracher A. Ischemic cerebrovascular disease. In: Jose B, editor. Practical Neurology. Washington: Lipincott-Raven Publishers; 1997. pp. 379-391

[39] Bova IY, Bornstein NM, Korczyn. Acute infection as a risk factor for ischemic stroke. Stroke. 1996;**27**(12):2204-2206

[40] Uyar IS, Sahin V, Akpinar MB, Abacilar F, Okur FF, Ozdemir U, et al. Does oral hygiene trigger carotid artery intima-media thickness? Heart Surgery Forum. 2013;**16**(4):E232-E236. DOI: 10.1532/HSF98.20121137. PMID: 23958538

[41] Calik M, Uyar Y, Onar MK, Gunaydin M. Investigation of the relation between ischemic cerebrovascular disease and chlamydia pneumoniae infections. Turkish journal of. Cerebrovascular Diseases. 2013;**19**(2):56-63

[42] Zhou YF, Leon MB, Waclawiw MA, Popma JJ, Yu ZX, Finkel T, et al. Association between prior cytomegalovirus infection and the risk of restenosis after coronary Atherectomy. New England Journal of Medicine. 1996;**335**(9):624-630

[43] Speir E, Modali R, Huang ES, Leon MB, Shawl F, Finkel T, et al. Potential role of human cytomegalovirus and p53 interaction in coronary restenosis. Science (1979). 1994;**265**(5170):391-394

[44] Epstein SE, Speir E, Zhou YF, Guetta E, Leon M, Finkel T. The role of infection in restenosis and atherosclerosis: Focus on cytomegalovirus. Lancet. 1996;**348**(Suppl.1):s13-s17

[45] Adam E, Probtsfield JL, Burek J, Mccollum CH, Melnick JL, Petrie BL, et al. High levels of cytomegalovirus antibody in patients requiring vascular surgery for atherosclerosis. The Lancet. 1987;**330**(8554):291-293. 2886763

[46] Bandaru VCSS, Boddu DB, Laxmi V, Neeraja M, Kaul S. Seroprevalence of chlamydia pneumoniae antibodies in stroke in young. Canadian Journal of Neurological Sciences. 2009;**36**(6):725-730

[47] Atik B, Johnston SC, Dean D. Association of Carotid Plaque Lp-PLA2 with macrophages and chlamydia pneumoniae infection among patients at risk for stroke. PLoS One. 2010;**5**(6):e11026. DOI: 10.1371/journal.pone.0011026. PMID: 20543948; PMCID: PMC2882946

[48] Elkind MSV, Tondella MLC, Feikin DR, Fields BS, Homma S, di Tullio MR.

Seropositivity to chlamydia pneumoniae is associated with risk of first ischemic stroke. Stroke. 2006;**37**(3):790-795

[49] Rai NK, Choudhary R, Bhatia R, Singh MB, Tripathi M, Prasad K, et al. Chlamydia pneumoniae seropositivity in adults with acute ischemic stroke: A case-control study. Annals of Indian Academy of Neurology. 2011;**14**(2):93-97

[50] Wimmer MLJ, Sandmann-Strupp R, Saikku P, Haberl RL. Association of chlamydial infection with cerebrovascular disease. Stroke. 1996;**27**(12):2207-2210

[51] Schmidt C, Hulthe J, Wikstrand J, Gnarpe H, Gnarpe J, Agewall S, et al. Chlamydia pneumoniae seropositivity is associated with carotid artery intima-media thickness. Stroke. 2000;**31**(7):1526-1531

[52] Muhlestein JB. Chronic infection and coronary artery disease. Cardiol Clin. 2000;**84**(1):333-362

[53] Elkind MSV, Lin IF, Grayston JT, Sacco RL. Chlamydia pneumoniae and the risk of first ischemic stroke: The northern Manhattan stroke study. Stroke. 2000;**31**(7):1521-1525

[54] Elkind MS, Lin IF, Grayston JT, Sacco RL. Chlamydia pneumoniae and the risk of first ischemic stroke. Stroke. 2000;**31**(7):1521-1525

[55] Cook PJ, Honeybourne D, Lip GYH, Beevers DG, Wise R, Davies P. Chlamydia pneumoniae antibody titers are significantly associated with acute stroke and transient cerebral ischemia: The West Birmingham stroke project. Stroke. 1998;**29**(2):404-410

[56] Ameriso SF, Fridman EA, Leiguarda RC, Sevlever GE. Detection of helicobacter pylori in human carotid atherosclerotic plaques. Stroke. 2001;**32**(2):385-391

[57] Elkind MS, Sacco RL. Stroke risk factors and stroke prevention. Seminars in Neurology. 1998;**18**:429-440

[58] Demir S. In: Demir S, editor. Virus Riketsiya ve Klamidya Hastalıkları. Vol. 1. Istanbul: Nobel Tip Kitabevi; 1996. pp. 94-115

[59] Birnie DH, Holme ER, McKay IC, Hood S, McColl KEL, Hillis WS. Association between antibodies to heat shock protein 65 and coronary atherosclerosis. Possible mechanism of action of helicobacter pylori and other bacterial infections in increasing cardiovascular risk. European Heart Journal. 1998;**19**(3):387-394

[60] Linnanmaki E, Leinonen M, Mattila K, Nieminen MS, Valtonen V, Saikku P. Chlamydia pneumoniae-specific circulating immune complexes in patients with chronic coronary heart disease. Circulation. 1993;**87**(4):1130-1134

[61] Yamashita K, Ouchi K, Shirai M, Gondo T, Nakazawa T, Ito H. Distribution of chlamydia pneumoniae infection in the atherosclerotic carotid artery. Stroke. 1998;**29**(4):773-778

[62] Grayston JT, Kuo CC, Coulson AS, Campbell LA, Lawrence RD, Lee MJ, et al. Chlamydia pneumoniae (TWAR) in atherosclerosis of the carotid artery. Circulation. 1995;**92**(12):3397-3400

[63] Campbell LA, O'brien ER, Cappuccio AL, Kuo CC, Wang SP, Stewart D, et al. Detection of chlamydia pneumoniae TWAR in human coronary atherectomy tissues. Journal of Infectious Diseases. 1995;**172**(2):585-588

[64] Leinonen M. Pathogenetic mechanisms and epidemiology of chlamydia pneumoniae. European Heart Journal. 1993;**14**(Suppl K):57-61

[65] Toss H, Gnarpe J, Gnarpe H, Siegbahn A, Lindahl B, Wallentin L. Increased fibrinogen levels are associated with persistent chlamydia pneumoniae infection in unstable coronary artery disease. European Heart Journal. 1998;**19**(4):570-577

[66] Laurila A, Bloigu A, Näyhä S, Hassi J, Leinonen M, Saikku P. Chlamydia pneumoniae antibodies and serum lipids in Finnish men: Cross sectional study. BMJ. 1997;**314**(7092):1456-1457

[67] Hafler DA, Slavik JM, Anderson DE, O'Connor KC, de Jager P, Baecher-Allan C. Multiple sclerosis. Immunological Reviews. 2005;**204**(1):208-231

[68] Alastair C, Christian C, Hans L, McDonald Ian R, David M, John N. In: Alastair C, editor. The Story of Multiple Sclerosis. Philadelphia: Churchill Livingstone Elsevier; 2006 3 p

[69] Noseworthy JH, Lucchinetti C, Rodriguez M, Weinshenker BG. Multiple Sclerosis. New England Journal of Medicine. 2000;**343**(13):938-952

[70] Lucchinetti C, Bruck W, Parisi J, Scheithauer B, Rodriguez M, Lassmann H. Heterogeneity of multiple sclerosis lesions: Implications for the pathogenesis of demyelination. Annals of Neurology. 2000;**47**(6):707-717

[71] Compston A, Coles A. Multiple sclerosis. Lancet. 2002;**359**:1221-1231

[72] Serra Ö, Güneş A, Ferah K, Muzaffer S. Multiple Sclerosis. Akd Med J. 2017;**3**:137-147

[73] Barnett MH, Sutton I. The pathology of multiple sclerosis: A paradigm shift. Current Opinion in Neurology. 2006;**19**(3):242-247

[74] Prineas JW, Kwon EE, Cho E-S, Sharer LR. Continual breakdown and regeneration of myelin in progressive multiple sclerosis plaques. Annals of the New York Academy of Sciences. 1984;**436**(1):11-32

[75] Bsibsi M, Ravid R, Gveric D, van Noort JM. Broad expression of toll-like receptors in the human central nervous system. Journal of Neuropathology and Experimental Neurology. 2002;**61**(11):1013-1021

[76] Yang X, Joyee A. Role of toll-like receptors in immune responses to chlamydial infections. Current Pharmaceutical Design. 2008;**14**(6):593-600

[77] Miranda-Hernandez S, Baxter AG. Role of toll-like receptors in multiple sclerosis. Am J Clin Exp Immunol. 2013;**2**(1):75-93

[78] Gilden DH. Infectious causes of multiple sclerosis. Lancet Neurology. 2005;**4**:195-202

[79] Steiner I, Nisipianu P, Wirguin I. Infection and the etiology and pathogenesis of multiple sclerosis. Current Neurology and Neuroscience Reports. 2001;**1**(3):271-276

[80] Sriram S, Mitchell W, Stratton C. Multiple sclerosis associated with chlamydia pneumoniae infection of the CNS. Neurology. 1998;**50**(2):571-572

[81] Fainardi E, Castellazzi M, Seraceni S, Granieri E, Contini C. Under the microscope: Focus on chlamydia pneumoniae infection and multiple sclerosis. Current Neurovascular Research. 2008;**5**(1):60-70

[82] Stratton CW, Wheldon DB. Multiple sclerosis: An infectious syndrome involving Chlamydophila pneumoniae. Trends in Microbiology. 2006;**14**(11):474-479

[83] Munger KL, Peeling RW, Hernán MA, Chasan-Taber L, Olek MJ, Hankinson SE, et al. Infection with chlamydia pneumoniae and risk of multiple sclerosis. Epidemiology. 2003;**14**(2):141-147

[84] Munger KL, DeLorenze GN, Levin LI, Rubertone M, Vogelman JH, Peck CA, et al. A prospective study of chlamydia pneumoniae infection and risk of MS in two US cohorts. Neurology. 2004;**62**(10):1799-1803

[85] Buljevac D, Verkooyen RP, Jacobs BC, Hop W, van der Zwaan LA, van Doorn PA, et al. Chlamydia pneumoniae and the risk for exacerbation in multiple sclerosis patients. Annals of Neurology. 2003;**54**(6):828-831

[86] Leinonen M, Saikku P. Evidence for infectious agents in cardiovascular disease and atherosclerosis. Lancet Infectious Diseases. 2002;**2**:11-17

[87] Layh-Schmitt G, Bendl C, Hildt U, Dong-Si T, Jüttler E, Schnitzler P, et al. Evidence for infection with chlamydia pneumoniae in a subgroup of patients with multiple sclerosis. Annals of Neurology. 2000;**47**(5):652-655

[88] Bagos PG, Nikolopoulos G, Ioannidis A. Chlamydia pneumoniae infection and the risk of multiple sclerosis: A meta-analysis. Multiple Sclerosis. 2006;**12**(4):397-411

[89] Boman J, Roblin PM, Sundström P, Sandström M, Hammerschlag MR. Failure to detect chlamydia pneumoniae in the central nervous system of patients with MS. Neurology. 2000;**54**(1):265

[90] Hammerschlag MR, Ke Z, Lu F, Roblin P, Boman J, Kalman B. Is chlamydia pneumoniae present in brain lesions of patients with multiple sclerosis? Journal of Clinical Microbiology. 2000;**38**(11):4274-4276

[91] Dong-Si T, Weber J, Liu YB, Buhmann C, Bauer H, Bendl C, et al. Increased prevalence of and gene transcription by chlamydia pneumoniae in cerebrospinal fluid of patients with relapsing-remitting multiple sclerosis. Journal of Neurology. 2004;**251**(5):542-547

[92] Contini C, Seraceni S, Castellazzi M, Granieri E, Fainardi E. Chlamydophila pneumoniae DNA and mRNA transcript levels in peripheral blood mononuclear cells and cerebrospinal fluid of patients with multiple sclerosis. Neuroscience Research. 2008;**62**(1):58-61

[93] Kaufman M, Gaydos CA, Sriram S, Boman J, Tondella ML, Norton HJ. Is chlamydia pneumoniae found in spinal fluid samples from multiple sclerosis patients? Conflicting results. Multiple Sclerosis. 2002;**8**(4):289-294

[94] Sriram S, Yi YS, Stratton C, Calabresi P, Mitchell W, Ikejima H, et al. Comparative study of the presence of chlamydia pneumoniae in cerebrospinal fluid of patients with clinically definite and monosymptomatic multiple sclerosis. Clinical and Diagnostic Laboratory Immunology. 2002;**9**(6):1332-1337

[95] Hao Q, Miyashita N, Matsui M, Wang HY, Matsushima T, Saida T. Chlamydia pneumoniae infection associated with enhanced MRI spinal lesions in multiple sclerosis. Multiple Sclerosis. 2002;**8**(5):436-440

[96] Grimaldi LME, Pincherle A, Martinelli-Boneschi F, Filippi M, Patti F, Reggio A, et al. An MRI study of chlamydia pneumoniae infection in Italian multiple sclerosis patients. Multiple Sclerosis. 2003;**9**(5):467-471

[97] Contini C, Cultrera R, Seraceni S, Castellazzi M, Granieri E, Fainardi E. Cerebrospinal fluid molecular demonstration of chlamydia pneumoniae

DNA is associated to clinical and brain magnetic resonance imaging activity in a subset of patients with relapsing-remitting multiple sclerosis. Multiple Sclerosis. 2004;**10**(4):360-369

[98] Fainardi E, Castellazzi M, Casetta I, Cultrera R, Vaghi L, Granieri E, et al. Intrathecal production of chlamydia pneumoniae-specific high-affinity antibodies is significantly associated to a subset of multiple sclerosis patients with progressive forms. Journal of the Neurological Sciences. 2004;**217**(2):181-188

[99] Sriram S, Ljunggren-Rose A, Yao SY, Whetsell WO. Detection of chlamydial bodies and antigens in the central nervous system of patients with multiple sclerosis. Journal of Infectious Diseases. 2005;**192**(7):1219-1228

[100] Metz LM, Zhang Y, Yeung M, Patry DG, Bell RB, Stoian CA, et al. Minocycline reduces gadolinium-enhancing magnetic resonance imaging lesions in multiple sclerosis. Annals of Neurology. 2004;**55**:756

[101] Sriram S, Yao SY, Stratton C, Moses H, Narayana PA, Wolinsky JS. Pilot study to examine the effect of antibiotic therapy on MRI outcomes in RRMS. Journal of the Neurological Sciences. 2005;**234**(1-2):87-91

[102] Contini C, Seraceni S, Cultrera R, Castellazzi M, Granieri E, Fainardi E. Molecular detection of Parachlamydia-like organisms in cerebrospinal fluid of patients with multiple sclerosis. Multiple Sclerosis. 2008;**14**(4):564-566

[103] Gilden DH, Devlin ME, Burgoon MP, Owens GP. The search for virus in multiple sclerosis brain. Multiple Sclerosis. Vol. 2. Houndmills, Basingstoke, England; 1996;**2**(4):179-183

[104] Dolei A. MSRV/HERV-W/syncytin and its linkage to multiple sclerosis: The usability and the hazard of a human endogenous retrovirus. Journal of Neurovirology. 2005;**11**(2):232-235

[105] Keefover RW. The clinical epidemiology of Alzheimer's disease. Neurologic Clinics. 1996;**14**(2):337-351

[106] Kawas C, Gray S, Brookmeyer R, Fozard J, Zonderman A. Age-specific incidence rates of Alzheimer's disease: The Baltimore longitudinal study of aging. Neurology. 2000;**54**(11):2072-2077

[107] di Carlo A, Baldereschi M, Amaducci L, Lepore V, Bracco L, Maggi S, et al. Incidence of dementia, Alzheimer's disease, and vascular dementia in Italy. The ILSA study. Journal of the American Geriatrics Society. 2002;**50**(1):41-48

[108] Ravaglia G, Forti P, Maioli F, Martelli M, Servadei L, Brunetti N, et al. Incidence and etiology of dementia in a large elderly Italian population. Neurology. 2005;**64**(9):1525-1530

[109] Brookmeyer R, Gray S, Kawas C. Projections of Alzheimer's disease in the United States and the public health impact of delaying disease onset. American Journal of Public Health. 1998;**88**(9):1337-1342

[110] Lue LF, Brachova L, Civin WH, Rogers J. Inflammation, Aβ deposition, and neurofibrillary tangle formation as correlates of Alzheimer's disease neurodegeneration. Journal of Neuropathology and Experimental Neurology. 1996;**55**(10):1083-1088

[111] Itzhaki RF, Lin WR, Shang D, Wilcock GK, Faragher B, Jamieson GA. Herpes simplex virus type 1 in brain and risk of Alzheimer's disease. Lancet. 1997;**349**(9047):241-244

[112] Itzhaki RF, Dobson CB, Lin WR, Wozniak MA. Association of HSV1 and

apolipoprotein E-ε4 in Alzheimer's disease. Journal of NeuroVirology. 2001;7:570-571

[113] Pogo BGT. A study of viral genomes and antigens in brains of patients with alzheimer's disease. Brain. 1987;**110**(4):907-915

[114] Friedland RP, May C, Dahlberg J. The viral hypothesis of Alzheimer's disease: Absence of antibodies to lentiviruses. Archives of Neurology. 1990;**47**(2):177-178

[115] Renvoize EB, Awad LO, Hambling MH. A sero-epidemiological study of conventional infectious agents in alzheimer's disease. Age and Ageing. 1987;**16**(5):311-314

[116] Miklossy J. Alzheimer's disease--a spirochetosis? Neuroreport. 1993;**4**:841-848

[117] Balin BJ, Appelt DM. Role of infection in Alzheimer's disease. Journal of the American Osteopathic Association. 2001;**101**(12 Suppl Pt 1):1-6

[118] Robinson SR, Dobson C, Lyons J. Challenges and directions for the pathogen hypothesis of Alzheimer's disease. Neurobiology of Aging. 2004;**25**(5):629-637

[119] Gérard HC, Dreses-Werringloer U, Wildt KS, Deka S, Oszust C, Balin BJ, et al. Chlamydophila (chlamydia) pneumoniae in the Alzheimer's brain. FEMS Immunology and Medical Microbiology. 2006;**48**(3):355-366

[120] Dreses-Werringloer U, Bhuiyan M, Zhao Y, Gérard HC, Whittum-Hudson JA, Hudson AP. Initial characterization of Chlamydophila (chlamydia) pneumoniae cultured from the late-onset Alzheimer brain. International Journal of Medical Microbiology. 2009;**299**(3):187-201

[121] Gérard HC, Wang GF, Balin BJ, Schumacher HR, Hudson AP. Frequency of apolipoprotein E (APOE) allele types in patients with chlamydia-associated arthritis and other arthritides. Microbial Pathogenesis. 1999;**26**(1):35-43

[122] Gérard HC, Wildt KL, Whittum-Hudson JA, Lai Z, Ager J, Hudson AP. The load of chlamydia pneumoniae in the Alzheimer's brain varies with APOE genotype. Microbial Pathogenesis. 2005;**39**(1-2):19-26

[123] Little CS, Hammond CJ, MacIntyre A, Balin BJ, Appelt DM. Chlamydia pneumoniae induces Alzheimer-like amyloid plaques in brains of BALB/c mice. Neurobiology of Aging. 2004;**25**(4):419-429

[124] Apfalter P, Assadian O, Blasi F, Boman J, Gaydos CA, Kundi M, et al. Reliability of nested PCR for detection of chlamydia pneumoniae DNA in atheromas: Results from a multicenter study applying standardized protocols. Journal of Clinical Microbiology. 2002;**40**(12):4428-4434

[125] Chacko A, Delbaz A, Walkden H, Basu S, Armitage CW, Eindorf T, et al. Chlamydia pneumoniae can infect the central nervous system via the olfactory and trigeminal nerves and contributes to Alzheimer's disease risk. Scientific Reports. 2022;**12**(1):2759

[126] Loeb MB, Molloy DW, Smieja M, Standish T, Goldsmith CH, Mahony J, et al. A randomized, controlled trial of doxycycline and rifampin for patients with Alzheimer's disease. Journal of the American Geriatrics Society. 2004;**52**(3):381-387

[127] Finefrock AE, Bush AI, Doraiswamy PM. Current status of metals as therapeutic targets in Alzheimer's disease. Journal of the American Geriatrics Society. 2003;**51**:1143-1148

[128] Cahoon L. The curious case of clioquinol. Nature Medicine. 2009;**15**(4):356-359

[129] Contini C, Fainardi E, Seraceni S, Granieri E, Castellazzi M, Cultrera R. Molecular identification and antibody testing of Chlamydophila pneumoniae in a subgroup of patients with HIV-associated dementia complex. Preliminary results. Journal of Neuroimmunology. 2003;**136**(1-2)

[130] Gartner S. HIV infection and dementia. Science. 2000;**287**

[131] Airas L, Kotilainen P, Vainionpää R, Marttila RJ. Encephalitis associated with chlamydia pneumoniae. Neurology. 2001;**56**:12

[132] Heick A, Skriver E. Chlamydia pneumoniae-associated ADEM. European Journal of Neurology. 2000;**7**:4

[133] Contini C. International conference on chlamydial and mycoplasma human infections. Future Microbiology. 2007;7

[134] Tang YW, Sriram S, Li H, Yao SY, Meng S, Mitchell WM, et al. Qualitative and quantitative detection of Chlamydophila pneumoniae DNA in cerebrospinal fluid from multiple sclerosis patients and controls. PLoS One. 2009;**4**(4)

Chapter 13

The Probable Role of *Chlamydia pneumoniae* Infection in Acute Stroke

Atakan Yanikoglu

Abstract

Cardiovascular diseases are the most leading cause of worldwide mortality. According to USA statistics, about 1 of 6 cardiovascular deaths is due to stroke. Stroke is the second most common cause of death and a chief cause of disability due to EU data. Treatment, care providing, rehabilitation costs and with the labor loss, the overall cost in EU due to stroke was estimated about €45 billion in year 2017. Acute stroke due to infectious diseases *via* several possible mechanisms with various clinical presentations were previously reported in the literature. *Chlamydia pneumoniae* is an obligate intracellular bacteria and extremely common in adult individuals. Besides it being a major cause of pneumonia in adults, association between atherosclerosis and vascular diseases was demonstrated by several sero-epidemiological studies and by direct detection of organism in atherosclerotic lesions by electron microscopy, immunohistochemistry, polymerase chain reaction. Also, several sero-epidemiological studies have demonstrated a link between *Chlamydia pneumoniae* infection and acute stroke. In this chapter, we will summarize the data in literature regarding the association between *Chlamydia pneumoniae* infection and acute stroke and we will try to explain the possible mechanisms that could be responsible in pathophysiology of stroke in these patients.

Keywords: Chlamydia pneumonia, stroke, atherosclerosis, cerebral infarction, acute stroke

1. Introduction

Several previous studies have demonstrated a possible association between the infection by *Chlamydia pneumoniae* and atherosclerosis and stroke. The demonstration of the presence of the pathogen in the atherosclerotic parts of the infarct-related arteries and the increased Chlamydia pneumonia antibody titers in stroke patients raises suspicions about the role of Chlamydia pneumonia infections in development of stroke. Besides these, several animal and *in vitro* studies support the hypothesis that Chlamydia pneumonia has role in atherosclerosis development, and its complications resulting in the stroke. In this chapter, we will summarize the epidemiology, pathophysiology, and its associations with the infections and the possible pathophysiological mechanisms of the Chlamydia pneumonia in the

 IntechOpen

development of atherosclerosis and atherosclerosis-related complications resulting in the cerebral infarcts.

2. Acute stroke

2.1 Definition and epidemiology

Abrupt disturbance of cerebral circulation due to thrombosis or embolism which results in focal neurologic deficit that persist for at least 24 hours is termed as stroke. Cerebral ischemia due to arterial occlusion results in an irreversibly damaged core area with a surrounding reversibly dysfunctional area, which is called penumbra. Cerebral ischemia owing to occluded arterial supply produces focal symptoms and signs that correlate with the influenced cerebral territory. Diagnosis is made by history and detailed neurological examination and confirmed by imaging studies (computerized tomography and magnetic resonance imaging). Further investigations are carried out in order to determine a specific cause responsible for the cerebral ischemia [1]. Yearly more than 13.7 million people have stroke, and 5.8 million people die as a result of stroke in the world [2]. Ischemic stroke comprises about 70% of stroke cases, and this proportion is estimated at about 85–87% in USA [3]. Stroke is the second most common cause of death and adult disability and it affects about 1.1 million people every year in European Union (EU) countries. According to EU cardiovascular disease statistics, treatment and care costs and costs due to labor loss because of stroke were estimated about €45 billion in year 2017 [4, 5].

2.2 Pathology, etiology, and pathophysiology

Oxygen and glucose insufficiency due to ischemia result in depletion of energy stores of neural cells to maintain membrane potentials and transmembrane ion gradients. Leak of potassium and increased calcium entry due to depolarization initiate series of events resulting in activation of calcium-dependent enzymes. This enhanced enzymatic activity of catabolic enzymes and their metabolic products with the oxygen-free radicals result in cell death. Prolonged ischemia leads to irreversible injury results with infarctions and persistent neurologic sequella [1, 6]. Pathological examinations defines two types of cerebral infarctions: First, the infarctions in a major cerebral artery distribution; both the gray and white matter are influenced and acute ischemic changes in neurons, destruction of glial cells, disruption of axons and myelins, and interstitial edema are visible changes in pathology. The second is the lacunar infarctions that are usually seen in chronic hypertensive people; small infarction cavities in size from 0.5 to 1.5 diameter due to occlusion of small cerebral arterioles are the characteristic of pathological finding [1].

The thrombosis comprises about two thirds of ischemic stroke cases. Thrombotic strokes are produced by occlusion of large cerebral arteries. Embolic strokes are produced from thrombi from heart, aortic arch, and large cerebral arteries. The distinction between them is very difficult and the establishment of the source necessitates detailed clinical examination [1].

Vascular disorders as a result of atherosclerosis of the large extracranial arteries in the neck and at the base of the brain are responsible for the cerebral ischemia in the great majority of cases. Atherosclerosis affects large and medium-sized elastic and muscular arteries of cerebral circulation. This complex chronic inflammation initiates in endothelial injury, and followed by the migration of monocytes with T-lymphocytes, transforming of these monocytes into lipid-laden macrophages and in continuation with the vascular smooth muscle cell proliferation; finally, the lesion proceeds into atheroma. The process of atherosclerosis is prevalent in patients with hypertension, diabetes mellitus, hypercholesterolemia/ hypertriglyceridemia, homocystinuria, and cigarette smokers. The enlargement and/or ulcerations of the atheroma would result in cerebral circulation disturbances. The severity of the circulatory problem and the localization of the threatened cerebral territory present with various clinical/neurologic scenarios. The detailed explanation of the arise and evolution of the atherosclerotic lesions and the probable role of Chlamydia pneumonia (CP) will be discussed in detail in this chapter [1, 7].

Inflammatory disorders other than atherosclerosis with arterial involvement can also result in cerebral ischemic syndromes: Giant cell arteritis, systemic lupus erythematous, polyarteritis nodosa, granulomatous angiitis, syphilitic arteritis are some examples of these diseases with central nervous system involvement due to vasculitis of arteries/arterioles. Fibromuscular dysplasia, carotid or vertebral artery dissection, lacunar infarctions in hypertensive individuals, vasculitis and vasopasms in drug abusers (cocaine, amphetamines, etc.), and multiple progressive intracranial arterial occlusions (Moyamoya disease) are other vascular causes of cerebral strokes [8–10].

Cardiac diseases comprises about one quarter of ischemic strokes [11]. Mural thrombus formation especially after first weeks of myocardial infarction is a well-documented source of cardiac embolism. Atrial fibrillation is a very common and preventable cause of cardiac embolism especially in patients with risk factors for hypercoagulable state. Infective and marantic endocarditis, atrial myxoma, and paradoxical embolus from venous system through a patent foramen ovale (PFO) are other rare causes of cardiac embolism [12].

Chronic myeloproliferative disorders such as thrombocytosis and polycythemia vera, sickle cell anemia, hypercoagulable states due to paraproteinemias, hereditary thrombophilia syndromes are the mostly recognized hematological disorders that cause cerebral strokes chiefly due to increased blood viscosity and thrombophilia [1].

2.3 Acute stroke and infectious diseases

Various infections may cause cerebrovascular complications, mainly due to involvement of the CNS vasculature by the pathogen itself usually with an inflammatory reaction of the immune system. The activation of pro-thrombotic mechanisms as a result of infection, and cardiac embolization in case of an infective endocarditis are other pathogenic mechanisms in the development of stroke [13]. Cerebral infarctions can be seen in viral infections such as HIV and VZV. The underlying mechanism in HIV infection was thought to be direct vasculopathy and hypercoagulable state [14, 15]. Syphilitic arteritis and inflammatory vasculopathy in Lyme's disease, which is caused by *Borrelia burgdorferi*, are good examples for spirochetal infections that cause cerebral infarctions [16, 17]. *Hemophilus influenzae, Neisseria meningitidis*, and *Streptococcus pneumoniae*—the pathogens causing pyogenic meningitis may lead to cerebral infarctions as a result of disturbance of larger arteries at the skull base by a purulent exudate, and arterial spasm in response to inflammation [18]. Infective endocarditis is a well-documented cause of strokes due to occlusion of intracranial arteries by an embolic material derived from vegetations [19].

3. *Chlamydia pneumoniae* (CP) and atherosclerosis

3.1 Is CP just a respiratory tract infection agent?

Chlamydia species are gram-negative obligate intracellular bacteria [20]. They can cause infections in both humans and animals. The Chlamydia pneumonia (CP) and the *Chlamydia trachomatis* (CT) are the most common species responsible for the human infections. Particularly, the CT has a serious socioeconomical burden due to its infections are sexually transmitted [21]. The CT is the most important cause of nongonococcic urethritis in males and also, it is an important cause of cervicitis in females [22]. The control of the CT infection is challenging because the half of the infected patients are asymptomatic [23].

CP commonly causes respiratory disease such as pneumonia, bronchitis, sinusitis, and pharyngitis. According to literature data, it is estimated about the CP is the cause of 10% of community acquired pneumonia. Most of the population were infected during childhood period, and the vast majority of the adult people have serologic evidences of past infection [24]. Biological evidences of CP in atheromatous plaques, and even in influenced areas of Alzheimer's disease patients brain, cogitate about that agent could not be a just respiratory tract infection agent [25, 26].

The infectious form of CP, the elementary body (EB) which is metabolically inactive, enters the body with inhalation and attaches to mucosal surface. After receptor mediated endocytosis enters into the cells and differentiates into metabolic active form, which is called the reticulate body (RB). The RB is the replicating form of CP and it is capable of modifying host cell pathways. The final EBs are released by cell lysis after 48 to 72 hours to infect other cells. The CP can infect respiratory epithelium, vascular endothelial cells, smooth muscle cells, monocytes, and macrophages. The CP can remain persistent in the host cell by escaping cellular lysosomal pathways. Resistance of CP to the host defense mechanisms determines the chronic infectious state [27, 28]. Intracellular survival of CP in cells of pulmonary alveolar membrane may be a reservoir for the persistent infectious state [29]. CP persistence is described as long-term survival of these metabolic inactive forms in the host cells. These patients are culture negative and the infection is antibiotic resistant due to reduced ribosomal activities [30].

CP can able to spread systemically *via* bacteremia during severe pulmonary infection and could be carried from recirculating monocytes/macrophages derived from alveolar membrane [31].

3.2 The *Chlamydia pneumoniae* (CP); virulence factors, the host cells of CP, and cytokine responses and target cell activation mechanisms triggered by the CP infection

3.2.1 Virulence factors of CP

I. CP interacts with the cellular secretory pathway *via* putative receptor-mediated specific signaling and enters into cell by endocytosis. However, the exact structures of the chlamydial surface (proteins, glycolipids) which initiate and mediate contact to target cells still are not well known [32].

II. CP creates itself an adjusted intracellular environment by releasing specific proteins into cellular cytoplasm. The type III secretion apparatus is a specific

CP protein, which translocates some proteins that modulate cellular response [33]. The reactive oxygen species production in CP-infected macrophages are limited by upregulating of antioxidant enzyme systems such as superoxide dismutase (SOD) and γ-glutamylcysteine synthase (γ-GCS) thereby limits the bacteria killing ability of macrophages [34].

III. CP inhibits host cell apoptosis *via* signaling specific cascades in monocytes; pro-apoptotic proteins that stimulate apoptosis can be degraded by CP and release of apoptotic trigger cytochrome-c can be inhibited by CP and the caspase-3 activity is reduced [33, 35, 36]

All of these virulence factors of CP create an appropriate environment for replication and survival [32].

3.2.2 Host for CP is not only the respiratory epithelial cells

CP can invade various cell types other than respiratory epithelium (vascular endothelial cells, smooth muscle cells, monocytes, granulocytes, even neural glial cells) and lead to enhanced expression of numerous chemokines [37].

Infection of all these cells leads to an enhanced cytokine expression, which results in a series of events resulting with proinflammatory and proproliferating environment. The ICAM-1 (intracellular adhesion molecule), VCAM-1 (vascular cell adhesion molecule), IL-6, IL-8 cytokine and protein expressions from the endothelial cells, the IL-6, MCP-1 (monocyte chemoattractant protein) from the vascular smooth muscle cells, IL-1ß, IL-6, IL-8, MCP-1, TNFα (tumor necrosis factor α), and MMPs (matrix metalloproteinases) from monocytes are some examples for the increase expression of cytokines and proteins in CP infection. Aggravation of inflammation and vascular cell proliferation induction by these cytokines may have an effect on atherosclerosis development [32, 38–42].

3.2.3 Target cell stimulation by CP and activation of signal transduction

Several receptor systems and signaling pathways are thought to be involved in activation of host cells by CP infection. Stimulation by IL-8, ICAM-1, causes phosphorylation of various kinases, which in turn causes a proinflammatory phenotype in vascular cells [43]. The transcription factor NF-κB that mediates the pro-inflammatory cascades in cells can be activated by CP [44].

Two systems are known to be involved to activation of target cells by CP: Toll-like receptors are the extracellular receptors and Nod proteins are the intracellular receptors.

Toll-like receptor (TLR) 2 and 4 were found to be the essential mediators of CP host cell activation. TLRs are receptors of the immune system, which are responsible for recognition of pathogens. Secretion of cytokines and translocation of NF-κB in dendritic cells are dependent on TLR stimulation. Nod protein system is the intracellular part of the immune system that could be responsible for the cytokine production in chronic infections. Through several kinases finally the NF-κB is activated and immune response is mediated. Various protein kinase systems are activated after contact of CP with the endothelial cells. Mitogen-activated protein kinase family (MAPK) members that are the key elements of proinflammatory, prothrombotic and pro-proliferative responses are the most activated kinases after CP contact. The final activation of NF-κB is followed by expression of pro-inflammatory mediators: ICAM, VCAM, IL-8, MCP-1, RANTES [30].

These all responses coincide shortly after acute contact by CP. The primary infection of monocytes and the vascular smooth muscle cells resemble persistent infection rather than active infection. The less is known about the changes in the persistent CP infection in which the pro-atherosclerotic signaling cascades supervene [45, 46].

3.3 Atherosclerosis and *Chlamydia pneumoniae*

3.3.1 Endothelial dysfunction to atherosclerosis

The atherosclerosis is characterized by deposition of lipids in the artery wall and infiltration of immune cells such as macrophages, T-cell, and mast cells with a surrounding fibrous cap consisting of mainly collagen, which is formed by the vascular smooth muscle cells.

Rudolph Virchow was the first scientist who recognized the inflammatory nature of the atherosclerotic lesions in history; however, his concept of atherosclerosis consisting of the inflammatory process was complicated to comprehend at that century. Eventually, the atherosclerosis was remained to be a concept of a just an arterial cholesterol and thrombotic debris deposition disease in the last century. Thereafter with the discovery of the smooth muscle cell proliferation with the inflammatory cells in the atherosclerotic plaque in 1960s and 1970s, the inflammation was begun to be considered to be a cause of the atherogenesis [47].

Earliest change of atherosclerosis is the dysfunction of the endothelial lining of the lesion-prone areas in the vascular system. The focal permeation, entrapment, and the modification of the circulating lipoprotein particles in the subendothelial space trigger a series of immune reaction including recruitment of circulating monocytes from the circulation. The monocytes differentiate into macrophages and they become foam cells as they resume to phagocyte the modified lipoproteins. These foam cells are the hallmark of early fatty streak lesions. Initiating event in the atherogenic process was assumed to be an injury to the endothelial lining by noxious substance such as oxidized LDL, cigarette smoking contents, hyperhomocysteinemia, altered hemodynamic forces generated in hypertension. However, this type of endothelial injury was failed to be demonstrated in the animal models of natural atherosclerosis. The uncertainty of the evidences of the direct endothelial cell injury in animal studies of natural atherosclerosis and the recent findings that demonstrate the functions and phenotypic modulation of the endothelial cells raised the term endothelial dysfunction in the development of atherosclerosis [48].

The term "proinflammatory endothelial phenotype" confers to enhanced expression of various effector proteins and cytokines that are responsible for acute and chronic inflammatory responses and disease processes in endothelial cells. In the lesion-prone regions of the arterial vascular tree as a result of endothelial cell activation by the actions of pro-inflammatory cytokines and noxious stimuli, genetic regulation modifications supervene in the endothelial cells primarily driven by the transcription factor NfκB. These include enhanced expression of adhesion molecules such as VCAM-1, ICAM, increased secretion of chemokines, and prothrombotic mediators. The circulating monocytes and T-cells respond to these signals and they migrate into subendothelial space. As a result, the paracrine milieu of cytokines, growth hormones, and reactive oxygen species, which were created by the actions of all activated endothelial cells, smooth muscle cells, monocytes and T-cells all together, eventuate as a vicious cycle of chronic inflammation. This chronic inflammation establishes the pathophysiological basis of the atherosclerosis [48, 49].

Lesion-prone areas for atherosclerosis are the sites which have and disturbed laminar flow patterns. The sites with low oscillatory endothelial shear stress located near branch point of arteries are most susceptible. The abdominal aorta, coronary arteries, iliofemoral arteries, and the carotid bifurcations are the most affected sites. These predilection sites are characterized by the presence of subendothelial macrophages. Modifications of gene expression in endothelial cells are present in these sites [50].

The most of the lesion-prone areas are the bifurcation sites and the other regions with altered hemodynamics. The absence of an disrupted endothelial lining at these branch points in the detailed morphological studies undermines the arterial injury hypothesis to explain this phenomenon. Similar to the changes in lesion-prone areas *in vivo*, the enhanced endothelial cell turnover, oxidative stress, and the alterations in endothelial cell shape, and changes in cytoskeletal and junctional proteins were demonstrated *in vitro* studies. These findings suggest the hemodynamic forces might have an effect on endothelial cell dysfunction in atherogenesis [48, 51]. The association between hemodynamic forces and the various genes that are important in development of atherogenesis such as hemostasis, thrombosis, growth regulation, and proinflammatory activation was demonstrated in previous studies [52, 53]. These results suggest a presence of a system of biomechanical endothelial gene regulation [48].

3.3.2 Progression of atherosclerosis

American Heart Association (AHA) defined six lesion types according to atherosclerosis progression.

Type I lesion: initial lesions. Intimal thickening and fatty streak lesions are frequent in infants and children. The earliest vascular change is intimal thickening consisting of layers of smooth muscle cells and extracellular matrix with small isolated groups of macrophage foam cells.

Type II lesions: include fatty streaks, which are visible as yellow-colored streaks on the intimal surface of arteries. Macrophage foam cells are abundant scattered in smooth muscle cells and proteoglycan-rich intima. T cells are identified in these lesions but they are less numerous than macrophages. Foam cells, easily recognizable by light microscopy, are signs of lipoprotein-driven inflammation occurring in the vascular wall. Xanthomas are harmless and reversible in case of disappearance of the factor that caused their formation. Probably due to maternal risk factors, they are visible in some fetal aortas and infants in the first 6 months of life, but their number decreases in following years. They reappear in lesion-prone areas in adolescence period.

Type III lesions: Pathologic intimal thickening. The earliest progressive lesions are primarily composed of layers of smooth muscle cells in a proteoglycan-collagen matrix with an underlying acellular lipid pool rich in hyaluronan and proteoglycans. There is a variable accumulation of macrophages outside the lipid pool. These lesions are found in young adults.

Type IV lesions: Atheroma. The lipid core is evident with foam cells.

Type V lesions: Fibroatheroma. The lipid core is covered by a fibrous capsule. Necrotic core is present that is made up of cellular debris and this core is covered by a thick fibrous cap consisting of smooth muscle cells in a proteoglycan and collagen matrix. The fibrous cap is critical for the maintenance of the lesion.

Type VI lesions: Complicated lesions; intraplaque hemorrhage, fissures, erosions, or thrombosis.

Update to these lesions: type VII lesions, if calcification predominates; type VIII lesions if fibrosis predominates. The type IV lesions (atheroma) can evolve to any of the further stages. The progression does not need to be in a sequential manner [54]. The fate of plaque is determined by the following mechanisms: lipid retention rate, macrophage phenotype, inflammation, apoptosis and necrosis, smooth muscle cell proliferation, arterial remodeling, and stability of fibrous cap. Most of the plaques remain asymptomatic, and some become obstructive, while some of them due to complications of the plaque may elicit acute thrombosis, which present as acute coronary syndromes and stroke [55].

The higher LDL levels induce more progressive disease due to increased amount of lipid retention in the plaque. The modified and oxidized LDL exerts chronic stimulation of the immune system [56].

The phenotype of the recruited macrophages is important for the plaque progression. Macrophages with the M1-like phenotype, possibly *via* binding of modified LDL to the Toll-like receptors, secrete proinflammatory cytokines such as interleukin-1β and tumor necrosis factor-α and enzymes and reactive oxygen products, which promote further modification of LDLs. This type of proinflammatory phenotype also secretes the mediators that were demonstrated to have a role in atherosclerosis. In contrast, the macrophages with M2 phenotype secrete factors such as transforming growth factor and proresolving lipids, which cease the severity of inflammation [55, 57].

Apoptosis and secondary necrosis of foam cells and smooth muscle cells and impaired removal of the apoptotic remnants cause the formation of necrotic core in the atheroma. The enlargement of the necrotic core induces further plaque inflammation [55, 58].

New vessels can develop in the atherosclerotic lesion mainly originating from adventitial vasa vasorum. They provide an alternative entry way for the immunocytes. Intraplaque hemorrhages from these fragile vessels promote inflammation and lead to expansion of the necrotic core [59].

Smooth muscle cells of the plaque are characterized by presence of abundant secretory organelles. The contractile smooth muscle cells of the tunica media can migrate to intima and phenotypic modifications supervene in these cells. These synthetic phenotypes of smooth muscle cells increase in number with the lesion progression. The collagen, elastin, and proteoglycans of the plaque matrix are produced by these cells. Collagen-rich tissue becomes a dominant component of the plaque as the plaque expands [55].

The involved arterial segment tends to remodel in a way that does not allow the compromisation of the luminal area until plaque volume enlarges. This type of expansive remodeling is seen in fibroatheromas, and the extent of the enlargement is correlated with the plaque inflammation and necrotic core. Continued plaque growth with the shrinkage of the local vessel segment results in the stenosis of the vessel segment. This type of contrictive remodeled arterial segments contains lesions rich in fibrous tissue [55, 60].

3.3.3 Acute clinical presentations of atherosclerosis: The vulnerable plaque

Acute coronary syndromes and the vast majority of strokes are cases caused by luminal thrombi due to plaque rupture or a sudden plaque hemorrhage with or without vasopasms [61, 62]. The atherosclerotic plaque rupture occurs from the site where the cap is thinnest and most infiltrated by the foam cells. Plaque rupture is the most frequent cause of luminal thrombosis [61].

Ruptured plaques contain fewer smooth muscles cells and less collagen when compared with the intact plaques. And these lesions are demonstrated to be heavily infiltrated with macrophages rich in proteolytic activity suggesting the enhanced degradation of extracellular matrix elements. These two concurrent mechanisms leading to loss of supporting elements of the plaque are thought to explain the plaque rupture [63, 64].

Another mechanism leading to the intraluminal thrombus formation is the plaque erosion. The endothelial coating in these lesions is absent; however unlike the ruptured plaque the internal and external elastic lamina and contractile smooth muscle cells are present. The vasospasm of the involved arterial segment was suggested to be as a cause of endothelial damage and resulting thrombosis [65].

These two mechanisms whether the plaque rupture or the plaque erosion result in intraluminal thrombosis are comprised in a concept of a dynamic-active plaque that results in an acute clinical presentation: the vulnerable plaque. This term is used for the plaques to describe a group of histological features that are associated with plaque rupture and subsequent intraluminal thrombosis. The typical rupture-prone vulnerable plaque is the plaque with a thin fibrous cap containing a large necrotic core and infiltrated with abundant macrophages in the cap. Other features of this plaque include neovascularization, plaque hemorrhage, and adventitial inflammation [55, 66].

3.3.4 Infections and atherosclerosis

The traditional risk factors merely are not adequate to explain the development of atherosclerosis in all patients. Additional risk factors that predispose to atherosclerosis development are yet undetected. The triggers of the arterial injury, which result as an atherosclerotic plaque, have not been clearly identified. The oxidized LDL and heat shock proteins are identified factors, which elicit an inflammatory response through a complex autoimmune response [67–69].

The demonstration of the infectious agents in the atherosclerotic lesions by polymerase chain reaction (PCR) and immunohistochemistry (IHC), and the seroepidemiological studies suggests a presence of an inflammatory trigger pathway initiating with an infection, which results in atherosclerosis and even possibly with its complications [21, 70–72].

Infectious agents can promote atherosclerosis through direct effect of the agents on cellular components of the vessel. The Chlamydia pneumonia and cytomegalovirus infections are the mostly concerned infectious agents demonstrated to have these effects. These mechanisms include smooth muscle cell proliferation and inhibition of their apoptosis, enhancement of smooth muscle cell migration, enhanced foamy cell formation, and increased expression of cytokines and cellular adhesion molecules, which lead to endothelial cell dysfunction. Autoimmune reaction through molecular mimicry of the heat shock proteins could be other possible mechanism [69].

3.3.5 Chlamydia pneumoniae in the atherosclerotic plaque

Many of previous studies including immunohistochemistry, polymerase chain reaction, and cultures demonstrated the presence of CP in various stages of human atheromatous plaques [21, 73, 74]. The existence of these bacteria in the atherosclerotic plaque can be explained by either direct infection of the vessel and/or transportation *via* circulating infected monocytes [69].

Although the exact mechanism with the atherosclerosis development is unclear, previous *in vitro* and animal studies have demonstrated the atherosclerosis relevant alterations triggered by the CP infections; the upregulation of the atherosclerosis-related gene expression products in cultured cells such as the heat shock proteins 60 (HSP60), macrophage scavenger receptor, cytochrome p450, and VEGF165R; smooth muscle cell proliferation enhancement (mediated through platelet-derived growth factor); increased macrophage foam cell formation are some demonstrated examples of these modifications [71, 75–77].

3.3.6 The vulnerable atherosclerotic plaque, plaque complications, and Chlamydia pneumoniae

As we mentioned previously, the plaque vulnerability depends on plaque volume, both the collagen content and the macrophage population of the fibrous cap, and the cap fatigue caused by mechanical stresses on the plaque (flexion, shear, pressure alterations, etc.). The role of CP in atherosclerosis development through macrophages was demonstrated in previous studies. Cytokines produced by CP-infected macrophages (such as TNF-α, IL-1β, and IL-6) may aggravate inflammatory response resulting with fibrous cap degradation and increase necrotic core volume and thereby increase the plaque size. The activated T lymphocytes by the infected vascular cells (endothelial cells, smooth muscle cells, and macrophages) can aggravate inflammatory activation *via* the NF-κB pathway, resulting in enhanced VEGF-1 (vascular cell adhesion molecule−1) and the additional inflammatory cell recruitment. Also, these cytokines can promote thrombin generation resulting in a thrombophilic intravascular milieu [78]. All these alterations might be responsible mechanisms for the plaque vulnerability and resulting in acute events. The data are scarce regarding the association of the CP infection and the plaque vulnerability and acute events. In one study, the intimal presence of Chlamydial heat shock proteins (HSP) was demonstrated to be associated with major adverse cardiac events in 6 months following coronary intervention. Also in this study, the C reactive protein (CRP) levels as an indirect measure of the inflammation severity was demonstrated to be correlated with the major cardiac adverse events [79].

Serological studies in patients with acute coronary events demonstrated a possible association with CP infections and acute vascular events. However, this serological finding could be an indirect association and does not establish an exact causality. Moreover, this serological response may also be just a part of a nonspecific humoral response to inflammation. Further studies with using direct detection tools in the vulnerable lesions—if possible—might provide further information [80–82].

Protective effects of statins on acute cardiac events, stroke, and mortality were demonstrated in previous studies. Beyond cholesterol lowering, their effect on the modulation of the immune response was revealed by clinical studies. The reduction of the CRP (C-reactive protein) levels with statin treatment indicates their immunomodulatory actions. Either the future cardiovascular events or CRP levels—in other words the inflammation—decrease with the statin treatment. Moreover in a recent study, the reduction in major adverse cardiac events with rosuvastatin treatment and especially its efficacy in patients with increased high sensitive CRP (hs-CRP) levels were demonstrated. This study demonstrated that with statin treatment, the lower primary endpoint rate was achieved (acute coronary syndrome, stroke, confirmed cardiac death, etc.) in patients with high hs-CRP despite their low cholesterol levels. These all findings shifted the idea of preventing future vulnerable plaque-mediated events by reducing the cholesterol with statins, to the idea of prevention of these events by reducing the inflammation with statin treatment [83–86].

Statins inhibit cholesterol production by inhibition of mevalonate pathway. This inhibition also decreases the production of other downstream metabolites such as isoprenoids. Prenylation of certain proteins by certain isoprenoid compounds is essential for their function, such as post-translational modification of membrane GTPases—the members of Ras, Rho, and Rab families. These GTPases are important in various cell signaling pathways, which regulate cell growth, proliferation, and inflammation. Disturbance of these prenylation pathways by statins exert the immune modulatory effect especially through the function of macrophages. Inflammatory responses of M1 macrophages are diminished by modulation of TLR (Toll-like receptors) signaling pathways *via* inhibition of NF-κB, and modulation of the IFN-γ receptor signaling system. Inhibition of M1 response results in decreased level of cytokine expression such as IL-1ß, IL-6, IL-12, TNFα [87–89].

In vitro studies demonstrated the modification of immune response by statins in CP-infected human macrophages and endothelial cells. The increased NF-κB expression in CP-infected cells was demonstrated to be inhibited with statins. Also, it was demonstrated that in the vascular smooth muscle cells infected with CP, the reactive oxygen species production, the activity of RhoA and Rac1, and the expression of NF-κB, MCP-1, and RANTES were reduced with cerivastatin [90, 91]. The interruption of the CP-activated signal transduction cascade by statins inhibits the inflammation response in the infected vascular cells. Thereby, inhibition of the inflammation by statins in the possibly CP infected atherosclerotic plaque results in plaque stability. Despite the absence of an direct evidence, these all findings could support the hypothesis that CP infection may have a role in atherosclerosis development and plaque vulnerability *via* aggravating the immune responses in the plaque.

4. *Chlamydia pneumoniae* and stroke

Despite the presence of serologic and biologic evidences, and the information from *in vitro* and animal studies which demonstrated the possible mechanism of the CP role in atherosclerosis development, definite human atherosclerosis evidences are not present yet. Solely, from the human atherosclerosis studies we have the information of serological traces and the PCR and IHC evidences of CP. Despite their biological evidences in human atherosclerotic plaques, the definitive role in the human atherosclerotic disease is not clear. We derive the information in which the possible role of CP in atherosclerosis development from animal and *in vitro* studies. Moreover, the in-human trials with the antibiotic treatment were failed to demonstrate any atherosclerosis protective result [92, 93].

Serologic traces and PCR/IHC evidences of CP are demonstrated in stroke patients. Many studies demonstrated the increased IgG and IgA antibody titers in stroke patients. In one meta-analysis of these studies demonstrated, CP infection was significantly associated with increased risk of cerebral infarctions and the immunoglobulin A was more effective to predict the risk of stroke. However, the value of these serological studies is limited due to uncertainty in the titers of CP antibodies to diagnose acute, chronic, and chronic active infection. There are also discrepancies between the serological tests and the PCR tests, and also the inconsistency among the PCR studies [94–97].

The detection of circulating CP DNA from peripheral blood monocytes is more reliable tool to diagnose an active infection; however, this method should be performed cautiously to prevent false-positive and false-negative results. One study demonstrated the higher prevalence of CP DNA in peripheral blood monocytes in symptomatic patients with carotid artery disease. Despite controversy between similar studies, one meta-analysis demonstrated an increased risk for cerebrovascular disease. These finding of evidences of an active infection might lead a speculation of the CP inflammation-associated atherosclerotic plaque vulnerability and resulting stroke [98–100].

Controversy exits between the PCR studies from atheromatous plaques in patients with carotid artery disease. There can be problems with sensitivity and specify due to PCR testing resulting with discrepant results [101, 102].

Previous studies mainly focused on the large artery atherosclerosis etiology comprising for the stroke. In all these studies, the exact etiological evaluation is not clearly defined. Cardioembolic stroke especially due to atrial fibrillation could also be a possible cause of the stroke in these patients. Animal studies demonstrated the involvement of cardiac muscle involvement by the CP infection. Either by direct atrial tissue involvement and/or *via* the increased cytokine levels atrial fibrillation could be triggered by the CP infection. The thrombophilic milieu propensity *via* the increased cytokine levels due to infection could be another potential contributory factor for the development of stroke. Moreover, most of the patients with atrial fibrillation have also coincident widespread atherosclerosis development, which could mean the possible high burden of chronic CP infection. Further well-designed studies with a clear definition of stroke etiology might answer this question [103, 104].

There are two problems arising with the studies, which investigate the possible role of CP infection in stroke patients: First, there is not any clear diagnostic criteria in the serological evaluation of a CP infection and there are controversies between PCR tests and serology; second problem is the etiologic diagnosis of the stroke; the etiology is a vulnerable plaque complication result or a cardioembolism, should be clearly defined [102, 104].

The studies that investigate the CP role in stroke that clearly defined the clinical presentation and etiology (symptomatic carotid artery stenosis and/or stroke) have conflicting results. The PCR studies could not demonstrate the CP presence in the carotid plaques of symptomatic patients. However in a study that used the IHC method, it is demonstrated that the CP in carotid plaques is significantly associated with the cerebrovascular events [102, 105, 106].

Another interesting common finding of these studies is that of similar to finding by Elkind et al., the high serum anti chlamydial Ig-A presence in symptomatic patients. This finding could indicate the possible role of the acute and/or chronic infections of CP anywhere in the body could play a role in atherosclerotic plaque activation and plaque vulnerability [98, 102, 106].

However, it is unclear whether the possible pathophysiologic chain of the events ongoing with increased cytokine levels result in the plaque vulnerability and stroke is unique to CP infection. The epidemiological studies demonstrated the increased risk of stroke after certain infections. The pathophysiological scenario ongoing with increased cytokine levels which ends with the plaque vulnerability related events may not unique to infection by CP. Increased risk of stroke was also demonstrated after certain upper respiratory tract infections. Also, the etiology could also be an atrial fibrillation-related cardioembolism, which also shares similar pathophysiological basis due to increased cytokines. However, there is necessity for large-scale epidemiological studies in which the etiology of stroke is well defined [107–109].

The levels of proinflammatory cytokines, and the inflammatory markers such as the CRP and ESR (erythrocyte sedimentation rate) are found to be increased in symptomatic carotid stenosis patients. The cerebral ischemia/infarct, and/or the inflammation of the plaque itself could be either an explanation for the increased cytokine levels and inflammatory markers. Also, the possible aggravating etiologies which triggered this chain of events might have a role in this finding [110, 111].

5. Conclusions

The CP infection may be the relevant cause of cerebral strokes as an agent that causes and/or exacerbates atherosclerosis, or it could be a just one of the complicating agents of atherosclerosis through mechanisms of exacerbating the atherosclerotic plaque inflammation.

Further large-scale and prospective studies could find answers to this puzzle, on the condition that the exact diagnosis of recent or ongoing CP diagnosis could be established.

Author details

Atakan Yanikoglu
Cardiology Department, Medicalpark Hospital, Antalya, Turkey

*Address all correspondence to: dratakany@yahoo.com

References

[1] Greenberg DA, Simon RP, Aminoff MJ. Clinical Neurology. New York: McGraw-Hill Education; 2021

[2] Homepage [Internet]. World Stroke Organization. 2023. Available from: https://www.world-stroke.org/ [Accessed: December 9, 2022]

[3] Tsao CW, Aday AW, Almarzooq ZI, Alonso A, Beaton AZ, Bittencourt MS, et al. Heart disease and stroke statistics—2022 update: A report from the American Heart Association. Circulation. 2022;**145**(8):e153–e639. DOI: 10.1161/cir.0000000000001052

[4] Wilkins E, Wilson L, Wickramasinghe K, Bhatnagar P, Leal J, Luengo-Fernandez R, et al. European Cardiovascular Disease Statistics 2017 [Internet]. The University of Bath's Research Portal. European Heart Network; 2017. Available from: https://researchportal.bath.ac.uk/en/publications/european-cardiovascular-disease-statistics-2017 [Accessed: December 9, 2022]

[5] Béjot Y, Bailly H, Durier J, Giroud M. Epidemiology of stroke in Europe and trends for the 21st century. La Presse Médicale. 2016;**45**(12):e391–e398. DOI: 10.1016/j.lpm.2016.10.003

[6] Graham SH, Chen J. Programmed cell death in cerebral ischemia. Journal of Cerebral Blood Flow & Metabolism. 2001;**21**(2):99-109. DOI: 10.1097/00004647-200102000-00001

[7] Ross R. Atherosclerosis—An inflammatory disease. New England Journal of Medicine. 1999;**340**(2):115-126. DOI: 10.1056/nejm199901143400207

[8] Ferro JEM. Vasculitis of the central nervous system. Journal of Neurology. 1998;**245**(12):766-776. DOI: 10.1007/s004150050285

[9] Schievink WI. Spontaneous dissection of the carotid and vertebral arteries. New England Journal of Medicine. 2001;**344**(12):898-906. DOI: 10.1056/nejm200103223441206

[10] Neiman J, Haapaniemi HM, Hillbom M. Neurological complications of drug abuse: Pathophysiological mechanisms. European Journal of Neurology. 2000;**7**(6):595-606. DOI: 10.1046/j.1468-1331.2000.00045.x

[11] Murtagh B, Smalling RW. Cardioembolic stroke. Current Atherosclerosis Reports. 2006;**8**(4):310-316. DOI: 10.1007/s11883-006-0009-9

[12] Kamel H, Healey JS. Cardioembolic stroke. Circulation Research. 2017;**120**(3):514-526. DOI: 10.1161/circresaha.116.308407

[13] Del Brutto OH. Chapter 43 infections and stroke. Handbook of Clinical Neurology. 2008;**93**:851-872. DOI: 10.1016/S0072-9752(08)93043-8

[14] Berger JR. AIDS and stroke risk. The Lancet Neurology. 2004;**3**(4):206-207. DOI: 10.1016/s1474-4422(04)00704-5

[15] Masahiko K, Yuki H, Hitoshi S, Makoto I, Seiji Y. Serial magnetic resonance angiography in cerebral infarction after varicella infection. Psychiatry and Clinical Neurosciences. 2002;**56**(5):585-588. DOI: 10.1046/j.1440-1819.2002.01058.x

[16] Klingebiel R, Benndorf G, Schmitt M, von Moers A, Lehmann R.

Large cerebral vessel occlusive disease in Lyme neuroborreliosis. Neuropediatrics. 2002;**33**(1):37-40. DOI: 10.1055/s-2002-23589

[17] Sáez DM, de Ocariz M, Nader JA, Del Brutto H, OH, Santos Zambrano JA. Cerebrovascular complications of neurosyphilis: The return of an old problem. Cerebrovascular Diseases. 1996;**6**(4):195-201. DOI: 10.1159/000108021

[18] Pfister H-W, Borasio GD, Dirnagl U, Bauer M, Einhaupl KM. Cerebrovascular complications of bacterial meningitis in adults. Neurology. 1992;**42**(8):1497. DOI: 10.1212/wnl.42.8.1497

[19] Chen CH. Infective endocarditis with neurologic complications: 10-year experience. Journal of Microbiology, Immunology, and Infection. 2001;**34**(2):119-124

[20] Sarıer M, Duman İ, Göktaş Ş, Demir M, Kukul E. Results of multiplex polymerase chain reaction assay to identify urethritis pathogens. Journal of Urological Surgery. 2017;**4**(1):18-22. DOI: 10.4274/jus.1328

[21] Sarıer M. Prevalence of polymicrobial infection in urethritis. Journal of Urological Surgery. 2019;**6**(3):180-183. DOI: 10.4274/jus.galenos.2019.2405

[22] Sarier M, Kukul E. Classification of non-gonococcal urethritis: A review. International Urology and Nephrology. 2019;**51**(6):901-907. DOI: 10.1007/s11255-019-02140-2

[23] Sarier M, Demir M, Turgut H, Hizel A, Emek M, Kukul E, et al. New approach to microscopy of gramstained urethral smear: The kissing slide method. Sexually Transmitted Diseases. 2020;**47**(10):712-715. DOI: 10.1097/olq.0000000000001228

[24] Kuo CC, Jackson LA, Campbell LA, Grayston JT. Chlamydia pneumoniae (TWAR). Clinical Microbiology Reviews. 1995;**8**(4):451-461. DOI: 10.1128/CMR.8.4.451

[25] C-C K, Shor A, Campbell LA, Fukushi H, Patton DL, Grayston JT. Demonstration of chlamydia pneumoniae in atherosclerotic lesions of coronary arteries. Journal of Infectious Diseases. 1993;**167**(4):841-849. DOI: 10.1093/infdis/167.4.841

[26] Balin BJ, Gérard HC, Arking EJ, Appelt DM, Branigan PJ, Abrams JT, et al. Identification and localization of chlamydia pneumoniae in the alzheimer's brain. Medical Microbiology and Immunology. 1998;**187**(1):23-42. DOI: 10.1007/s004300050071

[27] Chlamydia Pneumonia—Statpearls—NCBI Bookshelf [Internet]. Available from: https://www.ncbi.nlm.nih.gov/books/NBK560874/. [Accessed: December 9, 2022]

[28] AbdelRahman YM, Belland RJ. The chlamydial developmental cycle: Figure 1. FEMS Microbiology Reviews. 2005;**29**(5):949-959. DOI: 10.1016/j.femsre.2005.03.002

[29] Redecke V, Dalhoff K, Bohnet S, Braun J, Maass M. Interaction of chlamydia pneumoniae and human alveolar macrophages: Infection and inflammatory response. American Journal of Respiratory Cell and Molecular Biology. 1998;**19**(5):721-727. DOI: 10.1165/ajrcmb.19.5.3072

[30] Krüll M, Maass M, Suttorp N, Rupp J. Chlamydophila pneumoniae. Mechanisms of target cell infection and

activation. Thrombosis and Haemostasis. 2005;**94**(2):319-326. DOI: 10.1160/TH05-04-0261

[31] Gieffers J, van Zandbergen G, Rupp J, Sayk F, Kruger S, Ehlers S, et al. Phagocytes transmit chlamydia pneumoniae from the lungs to the vasculature. European Respiratory Journal. 2004;**23**(4):506-510. DOI: 10.1183/09031936.04.00093304

[32] Kern JM, Maass V, Maass M. Molecular pathogenesis of chronic chlamydia pneumoniae infection: A brief overview. Clinical Microbiology and Infection. 2009;**15**(1):36-41. DOI: 10.1111/j.1469-0691.2008.02631.x

[33] Peters J, Wilson DP, Myers G, Timms P, Bavoil PM. Type III secretion à la chlamydia. Trends in Microbiology. 2007;**15**(6):241-251. DOI: 10.1016/j.tim.2007.04.005

[34] Azenabor AA, Muili K, Akoachere J-F, Chaudhry A. Macrophage antioxidant enzymes regulate chlamydia pneumoniae chronicity: Evidence of the effect of redox balance on host–pathogen relationship. Immunobiology. 2006;**211**(5):325-339. DOI: 10.1016/j.imbio.2005.12.001

[35] Fischer SF, Schwarz C, Vier J, Georg H. Characterization of antiapoptotic activities of chlamydia pneumoniae in human cells. Infection and Immunity. 2001;**69**(11):7121-7129. DOI: 10.1128/iai.69.11.7121-7129.2001

[36] Fischer SF, Vier J, Kirschnek S, Klos A, Hess S, Ying S, et al. Chlamydia inhibit host cell apoptosis by degradation of proapoptotic BH3-only proteins. Journal of Experimental Medicine. 2004;**200**(7):905-916. DOI: 10.1084/jem.20040402

[37] Campbell LA, C-Cho K. Chlamydia pneumoniae—An infectious risk factor for atherosclerosis? Nature Reviews Microbiology. 2004;**2**(1):23-32. DOI: 10.1038/nrmicro796

[38] Fryer RH, Schwobe EP, Woods ML, Rodgers GM. Chlamydia species infect human vascular endothelial cells and induce procoagulant activity. Journal of Investigative Medicine. 1997;**45**:168-174

[39] Dechend R, Maass M, Gieffers J, Dietz R, Scheidereit C, Leutz A, et al. Chlamydia pneumoniae infection of vascular smooth muscle and endothelial cells activates NF-KB and induces tissue factor and pai-1 expression. Circulation. 1999;**100**(13):1369-1373. DOI: 10.1161/01.cir.100.13.1369

[40] Netea MG, Selzman CH, Kullberg BJ, Galama JM, Weinberg A, Stalenhoef AF, et al. Acellular components of Chlamydia pneumoniae stimulate cytokine production in human blood mononuclear cells. European Journal of Immunology. 2000;**30**(2):541-549. DOI: 10.1002/1521-4141(200002)30:2<541::aid-immu541>3.0.co;2-x

[41] Gaydos CA. Growth in vascular cells and cytokine production bychlamydia pneumoniae. The Journal of Infectious Diseases. 2000;**181**(s3):S473-S478. DOI: 10.1086/315612

[42] Yang J, Hooper WC, Phillips DJ, Tondella ML, Talkington DF. Induction of proinflammatory cytokines in human lung epithelial cells during chlamydia pneumoniae infection. Infection and Immunity. 2003;**71**(2):614-620. DOI: 10.1128/iai.71.2.614-620.2003

[43] Krüll M, Kramp J, Petrov T, Klucken AC, Hocke AC, Walter C, et al. Differences in cell activation by chlamydophila pneumoniae and chlamydia trachomatis infection in human endothelial cells. Infection and

Immunity. 2004;**72**(11):6615-6621. DOI: 10.1128/iai.72.11.6615-6621.2004

[44] Krüll M, Klucken CA, Wuppermann FN. Signal transduction pathways activated in endothelial cells following infection with chlamydia pneumoniae. Journal of Immunology. 1999;**162**(8):4834-4841

[45] Gieffers J, Henriette F, Jürgen J, Klinger M, Dalhoff K, Katus HA, et al. Chlamydia pneumoniae infection in circulating human monocytes is refractory to antibiotic treatment. Circulation. 2001;**103**(3):351-356. DOI: 10.1161/01.cir.103.3.351

[46] Sakash JB, Byrne GI, Lichtman A, Libby P. Cytokines induce indoleamine 2,3-dioxygenase expression in human atheroma-associated cells: Implications for persistent chlamydophila pneumoniae infection. Infection and Immunity. 2002;**70**(7):3959-3961. DOI: 10.1128/IAI.70.7.3959-3961.2002

[47] Libby P. Inflammation in atherosclerosis. Arteriosclerosis, Thrombosis, and Vascular Biology. 2012;**32**(9):2045-2051. DOI: 10.1161/ATVBAHA.108.179705

[48] Gimbrone MA, García-Cardeña G. Endothelial cell dysfunction and the pathobiology of atherosclerosis. Circulation Research. 2016;**118**(4):620-636. DOI: 10.1161/CIRCRESAHA.115.306301

[49] Gimbrone MA. Vascular endothelium: An integrator of pathophysiologic stimuli in cardiovascular disease. Cardiovascular Disease. 1995;**2**:105-107. DOI: 10.1007/978-1-4615-1959-1_14

[50] Wentzel JJ, Chatzizisis YS, Gijsen FJ, Giannoglou GD, Feldman CL, Stone PH. Endothelial shear stress in the evolution of coronary atherosclerotic plaque and vascular remodelling: Current understanding and remaining questions. Cardiovascular Research. 2012;**96**(2):234-243. DOI: 10.1093/cvr/cvs217

[51] Michaela G, Myroni C, Noriaki K, Tucker C, Nitzan R. Vascular endothelium. Annals of the New York Academy of Sciences. 2006;**748**(1):122-131. DOI: 10.1111/j.1749-6632.1994.tb17312.x

[52] Shyy YJ, Hsieh HJ, Usami S, Chien S. Fluid shear stress induces a biphasic response of human monocyte chemotactic protein 1 gene expression in vascular endothelium. Proceedings of the National Academy of Sciences. 1994;**91**(11):4678-4682. DOI: 10.1073/pnas.91.11.4678

[53] Ohno M, Cooke JP, Dzau VJ, Gibbons GH. Fluid shear stress induces endothelial transforming growth factor beta-1 transcription and production. Modulation by potassium channel blockade. Journal of Clinical Investigation. 1995;**95**(3):1363-1369. DOI: 10.1172/jci117787

[54] Melaku L, Dabi A. The cellular biology of atherosclerosis with atherosclerotic lesion classification and biomarkers - bulletin of the National Research Centre [Internet]. Berlin, Heidelberg: SpringerOpen; 2021 [cited 2023 Jan 7]. DOI: 10.1186/s42269-021-00685-w

[55] Bentzon JF, Otsuka F, Virmani R, Falk E. Mechanisms of plaque formation and rupture. Circulation Research. 2014;**114**(12):1852-1866. DOI: 10.1161/CIRCRESAHA.114.302721

[56] Tabas I, Williams KJ, Jan B. Subendothelial lipoprotein retention as the initiating process in atherosclerosis. Circulation.

2007;**116**(16):1832-1844. DOI: 10.1161/circulationaha.106.676890

[57] Leitinger N, Schulman IG. Phenotypic polarization of macrophages in atherosclerosis. Arteriosclerosis, Thrombosis, and Vascular Biology. 2013;**33**(6):1120-1126. DOI: 10.1161/atvbaha.112.300173

[58] Clarke MC, Figg N, Maguire JJ, Davenport AP, Goddard M, Littlewood TD, et al. Apoptosis of vascular smooth muscle cells induces features of plaque vulnerability in atherosclerosis. Nature Medicine. 2006;**12**(9):1075-1080. DOI: 10.1038/nm1459

[59] Kolodgie FD, Gold HK, Burke AP, Fowler DR, Kruth HS, Weber DK, et al. Intraplaque hemorrhage and progression of coronary atheroma. New England Journal of Medicine. 2003;**349**(24):2316-2325. DOI: 10.1056/nejmoa035655

[60] Burke AP, Kolodgie FD, Farb A, Weber D, Virmani R. Morphological predictors of arterial remodeling in coronary atherosclerosis. Circulation. 2002;**105**(3):297-303. DOI: 10.1161/hc0302.102610

[61] Davies MJ. Coronary disease: The pathophysiology of acute coronary syndromes. Heart. 2000;**83**(3):361-366. DOI: 10.1136/heart.83.3.361

[62] Pelisek J, Eckstein H-H, Zernecke A. Pathophysiological mechanisms of carotid plaque vulnerability: Impact on ischemic stroke. Archivum Immunologiae et Therapiae Experimentalis. 2012;**60**(6):431-442. DOI: 10.1007/s00005-012-0192-z

[63] Kolodgie FD, Burke AP, Farb A, Gold HK, Yuan J, Narula J, et al. The thincap fibroatheroma: A type of vulnerable plaque: The major precursor lesion to acute coronary syndromes. Current Opinion in Cardiology. 2001;**16**(5):285-292. DOI: 10.1097/00001573-200109000-00006

[64] van der Wal AC, Becker AE, van der Loos CM, Das PK. Site of intimal rupture or erosion of thrombosed coronary atherosclerotic plaques is characterized by an inflammatory process irrespective of the dominant plaque morphology. Circulation. 1994;**89**(1):36-44. DOI: 10.1161/01.cir.89.1.36

[65] Virmani R, Burke AP, Farb A, Kolodgie FD. Pathology of the vulnerable plaque. Journal of the American college of. Cardiology. 2006;**47**(8):C13-C18. DOI: 10.1016/j.jacc.2005.10.065

[66] Schaar J. Terminology for high-risk and vulnerable coronary artery plaques. European Heart Journal. 2004;**25**(12):1077-1082. DOI: 10.1016/j.ehj.2004.01.002

[67] Stemme S, Faber B, Holm J, Wiklund O, Witztum JL, Hansson GK. T lymphocytes from human atherosclerotic plaques recognize oxidized low density lipoprotein. Proceedings of the National Academy of Sciences. 1995;**92**(9):3893-3897. DOI: 10.1073/pnas.92.9.3893

[68] Xu Q, Luef G, Weimann S, Gupta RS, Wolf H, Wick G. Staining of endothelial cells and macrophages in atherosclerotic lesions with human heat-shock protein-reactive antisera. Arteriosclerosis and Thrombosis: A Journal of Vascular Biology. 1993;**13**(12):1763-1769. DOI: 10.1161/01.atv.13.12.1763

[69] Epstein SE, Zhou YF, Zhu J. Infection and atherosclerosis. Circulation. 1999;**100**:4. DOI: 10.1161/01.cir.100.4.e20

[70] Danesh J, Appleby P. Persistent infection and vascular disease: A systematic review. Expert Opinion on

Investigational Drugs. 1998;7(5):691-713. DOI: 10.1517/13543784.7.5.691

[71] Kalayoglu MV, Byrne GI. Induction of macrophage foam cell formation bychlamydia pneumoniae. The Journal of Infectious Diseases. 1998;**177**(3):725-729. DOI: 10.1086/514241

[72] Ann Campbell L, Rosenfeld M. Pathogens and atherosclerosis: Update on the potential contribution of multiple infectious organisms to the pathogenesis of atherosclerosis. Thrombosis and Haemostasis. 2011;**106**(11):858-867. DOI: 10.1160/TH11-06-0392

[73] Kuo CC, Gown AM, Benditt EP, Grayston JT. Detection of chlamydia pneumoniae in aortic lesions of atherosclerosis by immunocytochemical stain. Arteriosclerosis and Thrombosis: A Journal of Vascular Biology. 1993;**13**(10):1501-1504. DOI: 10.1161/01.atv.13.10.1501

[74] Grayston JT, C-Chou K, Coulson AS, Campbell LA, Lawrence RD, Lee MJ, et al. Chlamydia pneumoniae (TWAR) in atherosclerosis of the carotid artery. Circulation. 1995;**92**(12):3397-3400. DOI: 10.1161/01.cir.92.12.3397

[75] Shi Y, Tokunaga O. Chlamydia pneumoniae (c. pneumoniae) infection upregulates atherosclerosis-related gene expression in human umbilical vein endothelial cells (huvecs). Atherosclerosis. 2004;**177**(2):245-253. DOI: 10.1016/j.atherosclerosis.2004.07.014

[76] Kreutmayer S, Csordas A, Kern J, Maass V, Almanzar G, Offterdinger M, et al. Chlamydia pneumoniae infection acts as an endothelial stressor with the potential to initiate the earliest heat shock protein 60-dependent inflammatory stage of atherosclerosis. Cell Stress and Chaperones. 2012;**18**(3):259-268. DOI: 10.1007/s12192-012-0378-7

[77] Coombes BK, Chiu B, Fong IW, Mahony JB. Chlamydia pneumoniaeinfection of endothelial cells in-duces transcriptional activation of platelet-derived growth factor–b: A potential link to intimal thickening in a rabbit model of atherosclerosis. The Journal of Infectious Diseases. 2002;**185**(11):1621-1630. DOI: 10.1086/340415

[78] Fazio G. Atherosclerosis, inflammation and chlamydia pneumoniae. World Journal of Cardiology. 2009;**1**(1):31. DOI: 10.4330/wjc.v1.i1.31

[79] Tuleta I, Reek D, Braun P, Bauriedel G, Nickenig G, Skowasch D, et al. Influence of intimal chlamydophila pneumoniae persistence on cardiovascular complications after coronary intervention. Infection. 2014;**43**(1):51-57. DOI: 10.1007/s15010-014-0694-1

[80] Chandra HR, Choudhary N, O'Neill C, Boura J, Timmis GC, O'Neill WW. Chlamydia pneumoniae exposure and inflammatory markers in acute coronary syndrome (CIMACS). The American Journal of Cardiology. 2001;**88**(3):214-218. DOI: 10.1016/s0002-9149(01)01628-9

[81] Maia IL, Nicolau JC, Mde M, Maia LN, Takakura IT, Rocha PR, et al. Prevalence of chlamydia pneumoniae and mycoplasma pneumoniae in different forms of coronary disease. Arquivos Brasileiros de Cardiologia. 2009;**92**(6):439-445. DOI: 10.1590/s0066-782x2009000600005

[82] Petyaev IM, Zigangirova NA, Petyaev AM, Pashko UP, Didenko LV, Morgunova EU, et al. Isolation of chlamydia pneumoniae from serum samples of the patients with acute coronary syndrome. International

Journal of Medical Sciences. 2010;7(4):181-190. DOI: 10.7150/ijms.7.181

[83] Baigent C, Pollicino C, Buck G, Blackwell L, Kearney PM, Keech A. Efficacy and safety of cholesterol-lowering treatment: Prospective meta-analysis of data from 90 056 participants in 14 randomised trials of statins. The Lancet. 2005;**366**(9493):1267-1278. DOI: 10.1016/s0140-6736(05)67394-1

[84] Cannon CP, Steinberg BA, Murphy SA, Mega JL, Braunwald E. Meta-analysis of cardiovascular outcomes trials comparing intensive versus moderate statin therapy. Journal of the American College of Cardiology. 2006;**48**(3):438-445. DOI: 10.1016/j.jacc.2006.04.070

[85] Albert MA, Danielson E, Rifai N, Ridker PM. Effect of statin therapy on C-reactive protein levels. The pravastatin inflammation/CRP evaluation (prince): A randomized trial and cohort study. ACC Current Journal Review. 2001;**10**(6):64-70. DOI: 10.1016/s1062-1458(01)00461-5

[86] Ridker PM. The jupiter trial. Circulation: Cardiovascular Quality and Outcomes. 2009;**2**(3):279-285. DOI: 10.1161/circoutcomes.109.868299

[87] Holstein SA, Hohl RJ. Isoprenoids: Remarkable diversity of form and function. Lipids. 2004;**39**(4):293-309. DOI: 10.1007/s11745-004-1233-3

[88] Lu Y, Peng W, Xu Y. Small gtpase and regulation of inflammation response in atherogenesis. Journal of Cardiovascular Pharmacology. 2013;**62**(4):331-340. DOI: 10.1097/fjc.0b013e3182a12eb3

[89] Sheridan A, Wheeler-Jones CPD, Gage MC. The immunomodulatory effects of statins on macrophages [Internet]. MDPI. Multidisciplinary Digital Publishing Institute; 2022 [cited 2023 Jan 7]. DOI: 10.3390/immuno2020021

[90] Kothe H, Dalhoff K, Rupp J, Müller A, Kreuzer J, Maass M, et al. Hydroxymethylglutaryl coenzyme a reductase inhibitors modify the inflammatory response of human macrophages and endothelial cells infected with chlamydia pneumoniae. Circulation. 2000;**101**(15):1760-1763. DOI: 10.1161/01.cir.101.15.1760

[91] Dechend R, Gieffers J, Dietz R, Joerres A, Rupp J, Luft FC, et al. Hydroxymethylglutaryl coenzyme a reductase inhibition reduces chlamydia pneumoniae -induced cell interaction and activation. Circulation. 2003;**108**(3):261-265. DOI: 10.1161/01.CIR.0000083367.93022.78

[92] Belland RJ, Ouellette SP, Gieffers J, Byrne GI. Chlamydia pneumoniaeand atherosclerosis. Cellular Microbiology. 2004;**6**(2):117-127. DOI: 10.1046/j.1462-5822.2003.00352.x

[93] Grayston JT, Kronmal RA, Jackson LA, Parisi AF, Muhlestein JB, Cohen JD, et al. Azithromycin for the secondary prevention of coronary events. New England Journal of Medicine. 2005;**352**(16):1637-1645. DOI: 10.1056/NEJMoa043526

[94] Elkind MS, Lin I-F, Grayston JT, Sacco RL. Chlamydia pneumoniae and the risk of first ischemic stroke. Stroke. 2000;**31**(7):1521-1525. DOI: 10.1161/01.str.31.7.1521

[95] Piechowski-Jóźwiak B, Mickielewicz A, Gaciong Z, Berent H, Kwieciński H. Elevated levels of anti-chlamydia pneumoniae IGA and IGG antibodies in young adults with ischemic stroke. Acta Neurologica Scandinavica. 2007;**116**(3):144-149. DOI: 10.1111/j.1600-0404.2007.00819.x

[96] Apfalter P. Chlamydia pneumoniae, stroke, and serological associations. Stroke. 2006;**37**(3): 756-758. DOI: 10.1161/01.STR.0000201970.88546.5e

[97] Su X, Chen H-L. Chlamydia pneumoniae infection and cerebral infarction risk: A meta-analysis. International Journal of Stroke. 2014;**9**(3):356-364. DOI: 10.1111/ijs.12248

[98] Sessa R, Di Pietro M, Schiavoni G, Santino I, Benedetti-Valentini F, Perna R, et al. Chlamydia pneumoniae DNA in patients with symptomatic carotid atherosclerotic disease. Journal of Vascular Surgery. 2003;**37**(5):1027-1031. DOI: 10.1067/mva.2003.200

[99] Gagliardi RJ, Caiaffa-Filho HH. Chlamydia pneumoniae and stroke: Is there a direct relationship? Arquivos de Neuro-Psiquiatria. 2009;**67**(3a):600-604. DOI: 10.1590/s0004-282x2009000400005

[100] Chen J, Zhu M, Ma G, Zhao Z, Sun Z. Chlamydia pneumoniae infection and cerebrovascular disease: A systematic review and meta-analysis. BMC Neurology. 2013;**13**(1). DOI: 10.1186/1471-2377-13-183

[101] Katsenis C, Kouskouni E, Kolokotronis L, Rizos D, Dimakakos P. The significance of chlamydia pneumoniae in symptomatic carotid stenosis. Angiology. 2001;**52**(9):615-619. DOI: 10.1177/000331970105200905

[102] LaBiche R, Koziol D, Quinn TC, Gaydos C, Azhar S, Ketron G, et al. Presence of chlamydia pneumoniae in human symptomatic and asymptomatic carotid atherosclerotic plaque. Stroke. 2001;**32**(4):855-860. DOI: 10.1161/01.str.32.4.855

[103] Heeringa J. Subclinical atherosclerosis and risk of atrial fibrillation. Archives of Internal Medicine. 2007;**167**(4):382. DOI: 10.1001/archinte.167.4.382

[104] Tang RB, Dong JZ, Liu XP, Ma CS. Inflammation and atrial fibrillation: Is chlamydia pneumoniae a candidate pathogen of atrial fibrillation? Medical Hypotheses. 2006;**67**(3):462-466. DOI: 10.1016/j.mehy.2006.03.017

[105] Gagliardi RJ, Silveira DR, Caffaro RA, Santos VP, Caiaffa-Filho HH. Chlamydia pneumoniae and symptomatic carotid atherosclerotic plaque: A prospective study. Arquivos de Neuro-Psiquiatria. 2007;**65**(2b):385-389. DOI: 10.1590/s0004-282x2007000300004

[106] Kaperonis EA, Liapis CD, Kakisis JD, Perrea D, Kostakis AG, Karayannakos PE. The association of carotid plaque inflammation and chlamydia pneumoniae infection with cerebrovascular symptomatology. Journal of Vascular Surgery. 2006;**44**(6):1198-1204. DOI: 10.1016/j.jvs.2006.08.029

[107] Clayton TC, Thompson M, Meade TW. Recent respiratory infection and risk of cardiovascular disease: Case-control study through a general practice database. European Heart Journal. 2007;**29**(1):96-103. DOI: 10.1093/eurheartj/ehm516

[108] Cristina ZM, Alonzo C, Laura B, Romano M, Alberto CL, Waisman G, et al. Recent respiratory infection predicts atherothrombotic stroke. Stroke. 2009;**40**(6):1986-1990. DOI: 10.1161/strokeaha.108.535559

[109] Grau AJ, Urbanek C, Palm F. Common infections and the risk of stroke. Nature Reviews Neurology. 2010;**6**(12):681-694. DOI: 10.1038/nrneurol.2010.163

[110] Puz P, Lasek–Bal A. Repeated measurements of serum concentrations of TNF-alpha, interleukin-6 and interleukin-10 in the evaluation of internal carotid artery stenosis progression. Atherosclerosis. 2017;**263**:97-103. DOI: 10.1016/j.atherosclerosis.2017.06.008

[111] Puz P, Lasek-Bal A, Ziaja D, Kazibutowska Z, Ziaja K. Inflammatory markers in patients with internal carotid artery stenosis. Archives of Medical Science. 2013;**2**:254-260. DOI: 10.5114/aoms.2013.34533

Section 4

Chlamydia as a Sexually Transmitted Disease

Chapter 14

Chlamydia trachomatis Infection in Women

Sibel Surmen Usta

Abstract

Chlamydia trachomatis infections are the most commonly encountered sexually transmitted disease worldwide. Multiple partners and failure to use condoms are the well-defined risk factors. A significant proportion of females are asymptomatic. Treatment modalities such as a single 1-g dose of azithromycin orally, or doxycycline 100 mg twice per day for 7 days have been widely used for noncomplicated genital infections. However, untreated *C. trachomatis* infections can cause late complications, including salpingitis, ectopic pregnancy, and female factor infertility. Screening is a possible strategy to control asymptomatic cases and women at increased risk of infection in a proportional group of women.

Keywords: *Chlamydia trachomatis*, sexually transmitted diseases, women genital infections, female infertility, screening

1. Introduction

Chlamydia trachomatis is the most commonly seen bacterial sexually transmitted infection worldwide. Studies have shown that women between 16 and 19 years have the highest prevalence of the infection [1]. On the other hand, it has also been reported that the true incidence and prevalence of the infection among women population is not well described [2] According to the WHO (World Health Organization) data, while annually about 100 million new cases have been registered, the majority of women with genital tract infections remains asymptomatic and undiagnosed [2]. Therefore, in a large group of women with chlamydia infection, treatment is neglected or delayed, which can lead to pelvic inflammatory disease (PID), ectopic pregnancy, preterm labor, infertility, and chronic pelvic pain. Additionally, untreated chlamydial infection during labor can be vertically transmitted, which may cause conjunctivitis and pneumonitis in infants [1, 3]. Obviously, it is very important to diagnose and identify chlamydial infection in women accurately and rapidly. Prompt and effective antibiotic treatment can prevent patients from the mentioned serious complications [3]. Moreover, it has been reported that the treatment of chlamydial infections and related complications has a tremendous impact on health services in several countries [2, 3].

All together this information clearly shows that it is essential to diagnose and properly treat infected women and their partners. Nowadays, screening programs performed by both gynecologists and urologist are strongly suggested. However, more importantly, physicians dealing with sexually transmitted diseases should have sufficient experience and knowledge to effectively treat chlamydial infection and associated complications.

2. General information: *C. trachomatis*

Chlamydial species have been described as gram-negative, aerobic, and obligate intracellular pathogens. Molecular studies have shown that they are unable to synthesize their ATP, and therefore they need to use their host cell's energy resources [1]. Due to this scientific fact, previously chlamydial species have been considered as viruses. *C. trachomatis* and Chlamydia pneumonia are pathogens causing infections in human. *C. trachomatis* has been divided into 19 serovars, according to the specificity of major outer protein membrane protein (MOPM) epitopes [4, 5]. It has been reported that while serovars A, B, Ba, and C are pathogens causing trachoma, serovars D, Da, E, F, G, Ga, H, I, Ia, J, and K are the most commonly encountered sexually transmitted agents. Furthermore, serovars L1, L2, L2a, and L3 are described as the bacteria, which are the pathogens of transmission of lymphogranuloma venereum (LGV) [4, 6].

Microbiological investigations provided that the chlamydial life cycle includes two different phases. The first phase is called the infectious phase, which occurs outside the target cells. During this phase, *chlamydia trachomatis* forms elementary forms, which cause the transmission of infection. After its transmission to the target cells, chlamydia forms the so-called reticulate forms, which are capable of replication. Basically, once the chlamydial elementary bodies infect non-ciliated columnar cells and macrophages, chlamydia induces its own endocytosis. Inside the host cell, the elementary bodies convert to reticulate bodies, which begin to replicate every 3 hours after an incubation of 7 to 21 days. Finally, after a certain production, the reticulate bodies change again into elementary bodies and shed off the cell membrane through exocytosis. It has been reported that because of its unique cell-wall structure chlamydial pathogens are able to survive against phagocytosis and destruction by lysosomal enzymes [4–6].

3. Epidemiology of *C. trachomatis* infection

C. trachomatis is the most common sexually transmitted infection causing cervicitis in female [2]. Chlamydial infections affect mainly young females between 16 and 24 years of age. According to the recent literature, a high number of sexual partners, unprotected sex, being unmarried, young age, low educational level, high-risk human papillomavirus (HPV) positivity, and black ethnicity increase the risk of chlamydial infections [4, 7]. Several studies have shown that the estimated prevalence of chlamydial infection vary between 1 and 12% [3–5]. Specifically, while the prevalence rate in the UK was reported as 10.3%, in Switzerland and France the prevalence rates were 2.8% and 3%, respectively. In a study group with a large number of individuals, the overall prevalence of chlamydial infection was 9.2%, with a peak of 12.2% among the 17-year-old women [8]. Ghazal-Aswad et al. investigated the prevalence of chlamydia infection in a middle eastern community and they reported that the estimated prevalence rate was about 2.6% and extremely higher in women screened in secondary care [9]. In a study from Brasil, the overall prevalence of *C. trachomatis* infection was reported as 11%, whit the highest prevalence seen in women between 16 and 20 years of age [10]. More recently, in a study from China, it has been shown that the overall prevalence of *C. trachomatis*, HPV, and *C. trachomatis*/HPV coinfection was 4.7%, 15.5%, and 1.2%, respectively, while the prevalence of asymptomatic infection of that was 3.8%, 10.8%, and 0.6%, respectively [11].

More importantly, studies have shown that prevalence rates range from 2 to 17% in asymptomatic women, which provides the importance of screening tests. In a screening study from France, it has been shown that there was a large difference between tested populations, ranging from 6 to 11% in women attending family planning centers, 1–3% in women attending preventive medical centers [4]. More recently in a study from India, prevalence of chlamydia infection was assessed among women visiting a gynecology outpatient clinic. In this study, the evaluation was performed by an in-house PCR assay. The authors reported 23% positive cases and chlamydial infection was predominantly seen between the ages of 18 and 33 years [12].

4. Clinical manifestation and diagnosis of *C. trachomatis* infection

Chlamydial infection of the lower genital tract, which causes endocervicitis in women, can be asymptomatic or may the patients complain of mucopurulent, odorless vaginal discharge, or postcoital bleeding. Additionally, edema and congestion of the cervix can also be observed. Urethritis can be concomitant with cervicitis. In such cases, a culture-negative leukocyturia is commonly suggestive for *C. trachomatis*. Furthermore, chlamydial infection in the lower genital tract does not cause vaginitis. Therefore, in the presence of vaginal findings, a different diagnosis should be considered. An ascending infection can lead to pelvic inflammatory disease (PID) [4, 13]. Endometritis is commonly related to an ascending infection and may cause irregular uterine bleeding. On the other hand, salpingitis and PID are usually asymptomatic. It has been shown that *C. trachomatis* is the cause of at least 60% of cases of acute PID [4, 14]. Some of the very well-known symptoms of PID include absent to severe abdominal pain with high fever, dyspareunia, prolonged menses, and intramenstrual bleeding. It has been shown that about 20% of women who developed PID become infertile, while 18% develop chronic pain and 9% eventually experience a tubal pregnancy (Ref. 13). Studies suggested that infertile women should be routinely tested for chlamydial infection. Moreover, specific anti-chlamydial antibodies are considered as valuable, noninvasive diagnostic methods [15, 16].

More recently, it has been reported that the estimated risk of post-chlamydial PID varies between 0.5 and 72%, depending on the study population and the definition criteria used in these investigations [16]. Subfertility and ectopic pregnancy occurred in 0.1–6% and 0–1% of women, respectively, after chlamydial infection [16]. Furthermore, studies have revealed that repeated diagnoses of *C. trachomatis* infections increased the risk of PID by 22% [16]. In another study from the UK, it has been reported that 20% of PIDs, 5% of ectopic pregnancies, and 30% of tubal factor subfertility pathologies are associated with post-chlamydial infections in women between the age of 16 to 44 years of age [16, 17].

In summary, studies suggest that several factors, including clinical symptoms, coinfections, reinfections, and sexual risk habits, probably affect the development of post-chlamydial complications in the female population. However, to definitely determine the risk and predisposing risk factors of the mentioned late complications, prospective studies are needed to provide robust data for prevention strategies related to *C. trachomatis* infections and complications [18, 19].

Nowadays, specific anti-chlamydial antibodies have been accepted as a valuable, noninvasive diagnostic tool. On the other hand, because *C. trachomatis* is an obligate intracellular bacteria, cell culture is considered as a reference method. However, various commercial non-culture-based diagnostic techniques are available [4]. Specimens for diagnosis can be obtained either by invasive or noninvasive approaches. While invasive approaches include endocervical and urethral swabs; self-collected specimens, such as first-void urine (FVU) and vulvovaginal swabs (VVS), are considered as noninvasive techniques [4].

Although cell culture has almost 100% specificity, it is not recommended for routine use, due to its pretty low sensitivity and its technical difficulty. Transport and storage difficulties of the specimens are additional drawbacks associated with the cell culture method. This technique should only be considered for medico-legal issues and for antibiotic susceptibility testing purposes [4].

While direct fluorescent staining with monoclonal antibodies (DFA) is a rapidly performed and specific test; it is subjective and not suitable for a large number of specimens [4]. Enzyme immunoassay (EIA) is an automated test and more usable than DFA, and the sensitivity is comparable to that of cell culture.

Nucleic acid hybridization tests, including DNA probing, have been described as the first molecular DNA test for *C. trachomatis*, which was widely used for a certain period. Studies showed that the performance of these tests is comparable to that of the DFA/EIA and cell culture [4].

Recently, nucleic acid amplification tests (NAATs) are suggested as the "Gold Standart" technique because of their high specificity and sensitivity, and their availability for a large range of sample types such as VVS and FVU in cases with chlamydial infections. There are various NAATs that use different technologies, including PCR and real-PCR, strand displacement amplification, transcription-mediated amplification, and nucleic acid sequence-based amplification. These measurement techniques are automated and can be used for screening programs and for the detection of *C. trachomatis* as well as *Neisseria gonorrhoeae* in the same sample [4].

5. Screening for *C. trachomatis* infections

Screening programs should be considered for mainly two approaches, including proactive, screening the entire target population, and opportunistic, targeting individuals attending a family planning or healthcare center. Studies have shown that opportunistic screening should target sexually active women under 25 years of age. Additionally, selective *C. trachomatis* screening of pregnant women according to risk factors can improve the benefit obtained from screening programs [18, 19].

6. Treatment of urogenital *C. trachomatis* infection

The treatment of *C. trachomatis* infection is exactly related to the localization of the infection, the age of the patient, and if the infection is complicated or noncomplicated. Additionally, the treatment of pregnant women differs from than of nonpregnant individuals.

For noncomplicated *C. trachomatis* infection cases; orally single doses of 1 g azithromycin or 100 mg doxycycline orally twice per day for 7 days are recommended. It has been reported that these treatment modalities have similar efficacy rates and adverse events profiles [13]. According to recent guidelines patients with urethritis need to be followed up if symptoms persist or in the presence of recurrence. In the case of a recurrence or persistent urethritis, treatment with 2 g metronidazole in a single dose combined with 500 mg erythromycin four times per day for 7 days, or 800 mg erythromycin orally four times per day for 7 days is recommended [13]. Importantly patients should be informed that they need to abstain from sexual intercourse for 7 days after starting the treatment. Of note, both patients and their sexual partners must be treated simultaneously.

While routine repeat testing for chlamydia after any treatment is not recommended, in pregnant cases or in patients with persisting symptoms, repeated test need to be performed. Because of the high rate of reinfection routine screening test need to be done 3 to 4 months after antibiotic treatment. The use of Postal testing kits PTK (partners post urine for testing) or patient-delivered partner therapy (PDPT) has been considered as novel intervention to reduce reinfection in women with chlamydia infection. In a controlled study, it has been described that these techniques do not reduce reinfection rates in women with chlamydia infection when compared with patient referral [20].

In PID cases treatment can be performed in a outpatient setting. However, in pregnant cases, in patients with severe illness, nausea or vomiting, in the presence of high fever concomitant with tuba-ovarian abscess hospitalization is mandatory. Additionally, hospitalization is indicated if there is a possibility of surgical emergencies. In patients who are unable to tolerate oral treatment regimens need also followed up on an inpatient basis.

Pregnant cases should not be treated with doxycycline and ofloxacin because their use is contradicted during pregnancy. Instead of these agents, erythromycin or amoxicillin should be the choice of treatment for chlamydia infection in pregnant women [13].

7. Prevention strategies

Recent guidelines suggest several main points for the prevention of the women population from genitourinary *C. trachomatis* infection. Primary prevention is mainly based on the change in sexual habits, which increase the risk of sexually transmitted diseases (STDs). In that issue, physicians should properly inform young women related to STDs and the importance of sexual behaviors.

Secondary prevention includes standard screening and treatment of STDs. Annual screening for chlamydial infection should be performed in all sexually active women 25 years and younger. Furthermore, women older than 25 years of age who have a new sex partner or have a history of multiple sex partners should be considered as high-risk cases, and need to be yearly screened for chlamydial infection [4, 13].

Author details

Sibel Surmen Usta
Vocational School of Health Sciences, Bilim University, Antalya, Turkey

*Address all correspondence to: drsibelsurmenustaotmail.com; mustafafarukustamail.com

References

[1] Stamm WE. Chlamydia trachomatis infections. Progress and Problems The Journal of Infectious Diseases. 1999;**179**(Supp 2):380-383. DOI: 10.1086/513844

[2] Land JA, Van Bergen JEAM, Morré SA, Postma MJ. Epidemiology of *chlamydia trachomatis* infection in women and the cost-effectiveness of screening. Human Reproduction Update. 2010;**16**(2):189-204. DOI: 10.1093/humupd/dmp035

[3] Su WH, Tsou TS, Chen CS, Ho TY, Lee WL, Yu YY, et al. Diagnosis of chlamydia infection in women. Taiwanese Journal of Obstetrics and Gynecology. 2011;**50**(3):261-267. DOI: 10.1016/j.tjog.2011.07.001

[4] Bébéar C, de Barbeyrac B. Genital *chlamydia trachomatis* infections. Clinical Microbiology and Infection. 2009;**15**(1):4-10. DOI: 10.1111/j.1469-0691.2008.02647.x

[5] Schachter J. Infection and disease epidemiology. In: Stephens RS, editor. Chlamydia. Washington, DC: ASM Press; 1999. pp. 139-169. DOI: 10.1128/9781555818203.ch6

[6] Papp JR, Schachter J, Gaydos CA, Van Der Pol B. Recommendations for the laboratory-based detection of chlamydia trachomatis and Neisseria gonorrhoeae — 2014. MMWR - Recommendations and Reports, 14. 2014;**63**:1-19

[7] Manavi K. A review on infection with *chlamydia trachomatis*. Best Practice & Research Clinical Obstetrics & Gynaecology. 2006;**20**(6):941-951. DOI: 10.1016/j.bpobgyn.2006.06.003

[8] Howell MR, , Gaydos JC, McKee JR. KT, Quinn TC, Gaydos CA: Control of chlamydia trachomatis infections in female Army recruits: Cost-effective screening and treatment in training cohorts to prevent pelvic inflammatory disease. Sexually Transmitted Diseases, 26 (9): 519-526,1999. https://www.jstor.org/stable/44965253

[9] Ghazal-Aswad S, Badrinath P, Osman N, Abdul-Khaliq S, Mc Ilvenny S, Sıdky I. Prevalence of *chlamydia trachomatis*infection among women in a middle eastern community. BMC Women's Health. 2004;**4**:3

[10] Brasiliense DM, Borges BN, Ferreira WAS. Genotyping and prevalence of chlamydia trachomatis infection among women in Belém, Pará, northern Brazil. The Journal of Infection in Developing Countries. 2016;**10**(2):134-137. DOI: 10.3855/jidc.6474

[11] Chen H, Luo L, Wen Y, He B, Ling H, Shui J, et al. *Chlamydia trachomatis* and human papillomavirus infection in women from southern Hunan Province in China: A large observational study. Frontiers in Microbiology, Section. Infectious Agents and Disease. 2020;**11**:1-8 DOI: 10.3389/fmicb.2020.00827

[12] Patel AL, Sachdev D, Nagpal P, Chaudry U, Sonkar SC, Mendiratta SL, et al. Prevalence of chlamydia infection among women visiting a gynaecology outpatient department: Evaluation of an in-house PCR assay for detection of *chlamydia trachomatis*. Annals of Clinical Microbiology and Antimicrobials. 2010;**9**(24):1-10

[13] Miller KE. Diagnosis and treatment of chlamydia trachomatis infection. American Family Physician. 2006;**73**(8):1411-1416

[14] Rogstadt K. Complications in the female and their management. In:

Moss T, editor. International Handbook of Chlamydia. 3rd ed. Haslemere, UK: Alden Press; 2008. pp. 111-121

[15] Malik A, Jain S, Rizvi M, Shukla I, Hakim S. *Chlamydia trachomatis* infection in women with secondary infertility. Fertility and Sterility. 2009;**91**(1):91-95. DOI: 10.1016/j.fertnstert.2007.05.070

[16] Wilkowska-Trojniel M, Zdrodowska Stefanow B, Ostazewska-Puchalska I, Zbucka M, Wolczynski S, Grygoruk C, et al. Chlamydia trachomatis urogenital infection in women with infertility. Advances in Medical Sciences. 2009;**54**(1):82-85

[17] Cleary RE. Jones RB,: Recovery of chlamydia trachomatis from the endometrium in infertile women with serum antichlamydial antibodies. Fertility and Sterility. 1985;**44**(2):233-235. DOI: 10.1016/S0015-0282(16)48743-1

[18] Chen MY, Fairley CK, De Guingand D, Hochking J, Tabrizi S, Wallace EM, et al. Screening pregnant women for chlamydia: What are the predictors of infection? Sexually Transmitted Infections. 2009;**85**:31-35. DOI: 10.1136/sti.2008.030700

[19] Macmillan S, McKenzie H, Templeton A. Which women should be tested for chlamydia trachomatis? British Journal of Obstetrics and Gynaecology. 2000;**107**:1088-1093. DOI: 10.1111/j.1471-0528.2000.tb11105.x

[20] Cameron ST, Glasier A, Scott G, Young H, Melvin L, Johnstone A, et al. Novel interventions to reduce re-infection in women with chlamydia: A randomized controlled trial. Human Reproduction. 2009;**24**(4):888-895. DOI: 10.1093/humrep/den475

Chapter 15

Chlamydia Infection from Androgical Perspective

Ibrahim Duman

Abstract

Chlamydia trachomatis is a microorganism known for years to cause ocular, urogenital, and neonatal infections in humans. It usually causes urogenital system infections. The pathogen, which is the most common cause of urethritis in males, is one of the sexually transmitted microorganisms. As most males are asymptomatic, they do not realize they are infected and act as reservoirs. This causes the incidence of urethritis due to chlamydia to increase day by day. Chlamydia urethritis, which poses a risk to sexual partners, can cause serious complications if left untreated. In this section, we assess the approach to male urethritis due to chlamydia, which is very common in urology practice and can cause serious problems if left untreated.

Keywords: Chlamydia, male urethritis, sexually transmitted disease, chlamydia trachomatis, treatment of chlamydial infection

1. Introduction

Urethritis is an inflammation of the urethra, a fibromuscular tube through which urine and semen pass. The main cause of urethral inflammation is infection by sexually transmitted bacteria. Bacterial agents associated with urethritis are classified as gonococcal and nongonococcal [1]. Nonspecific urethritis is a term used for urethritis caused by nongonococcal and nonchlamydial pathogens [2]. *Chlamydia trachomatis* is one of the leading causes of nongonococcal urethritis [3]. Together with the gonococcal pathogen *Neisseria gonorrhoeae*, they are the most common causes of sexually transmitted infections in men and women [4].

Other common pathogens of nongonococcal urethritis are *Mycoplasma genitalium*, *Ureaplasma urealyticum*, and *Trichomonas vaginalis* [5]. The role of *Ureaplasma parvum* and *Mycoplasma hominis* in urethritis is controversial. There is strong evidence that *M. hominis* can cause urethritis at high microbial loads. However, *U. parvum* is regarded more as a commensal bacterium of the normal microflora and is not considered a urethritis pathogen [6].

Pathogens that are occasionally detected in patients with urethritis but rarely identified as causes of infectious urethritis include herpes simplex virus, adenoviruses, *Treponema pallidum* (endourethral chancre), *Haemophilus influenzae*, *Candida*, *Neisseria meningitis*, *Escherichia coli*, and streptococci. These are transmitted by direct contact *via* the oral, anal, or vaginal route, depending on their location [7].

In some men with urethritis, no known pathogen can be detected. Some of these cases are noninfective. However, there may not be sufficient clinical and laboratory findings to clearly distinguish them from possible infective urethritis [8].

Rare causes of noninfectious urethritis include trauma caused by urethral catheterization and instrumentation, foreign body insertion, or cycling; friction due to tight clothing or sexual intercourse; and exposure to irritants such as soap, powder, and spermicide [9].

C. trachomatis is a small, gram-negative obligate intracellular microorganism in the chlamydial bacterial family. It preferentially infects squamocolumnar epithelial cells. *C. trachomatis* has many serotypes, and serovars D-K infect the genital tract [10].

Unlike other bacteria, *C. trachomatis* has a biphasic life cycle. During this life cycle, they assume two forms called the elementary body (EB) and reticular body (RB). The EB is a metabolically inactive, infective form that is resistant to environmental conditions. In contrast, the RB is a metabolically active form that is not infective but has the ability to multiply within host cells. Between 48 and 72 h after infection, the host cell ruptures and *C. trachomatis* returns to the EB form to infect other cells. Once inside the epithelial cells, there is a neutrophilic response followed by lymphocyte, macrophage, plasma cell, and eosinophilic invasion. Infected epithelial cells release cytokines and interferon, initiating an inflammatory cascade. Thus, *C. trachomatis* induces a humoral and cellular response and causes the symptoms of urethritis [10].

2. Epidemiology

C. trachomatis was first isolated in the genital tract in the 1950s. However, it was not assigned much importance until the 1990s because of the high asymptomatic rate in both genders [11]. Since the late 1990s, *C. trachomatis* has been the most frequently reported sexually transmitted disease in Europe and America. In 2017 in the United Kingdom (UK), 203,116 people were diagnosed with new *C. trachomatis* infections, while 44,676 were diagnosed with *N. gonorrhoeae* infections and 7137 were diagnosed with syphilis [12].

The actual number of people infected with *C. trachomatis* is believed to be much higher due to the fact that the disease is mostly asymptomatic and goes undiagnosed. Its prevalence is 1–40%, depending on the population [11]. In the UK, a screening of people aged 15–24 conducted by the National Chlamydia Screening Programme detected more than 126,000 genital chlamydia infections [12].

In 2018, the incidence of chlamydial urethritis was 381 per 100,000 men in the United States of America (USA), making *Chlamydia* the most commonly detected and reported urethritis pathogen. In the same study, the incidence of gonococcal urethritis was 213 per 100,000. Every year, 4 million Americans are affected by urethritis. About 600,000 of these are gonococcal, while 3 million are nongonococcal urethritis, half of which are caused by *Chlamydia* [9]. In one study, *N. gonorrhoeae* was detected in 127 (30%) of 424 male patients with acute urethritis, while *Chlamydia* was detected in approximately 143 (33%) [13]. The reported rate of urethritis increased by 36% between 2008 and 2018. This rising trend is also being observed in Europe according to a report from the European Centre for Disease Prevention and Control [14]. The rate of newly diagnosed chlamydial infections continues to rise. In a study conducted in the USA, the rate of newly diagnosed chlamydial infections increased by 4.7% between 2015 and 2016 [15].

This rapid increase in the prevalence of *Chlamydia* is also related to technological advances in diagnostic methods since the 1990s. Advancements in polymerase chain reaction technologies in particular led to the development of nucleic acid amplification tests (NAATs) [16]. With this method, extracted *Chlamydia* DNA fragments can be replicated to achieve sufficient samples for colorimetric evaluation, increasing the applicability and sensitivity of the test [17]. These assays are more effective than culture-based methods and could be used more widely in screening and diagnosis, resulting in a higher *Chlamydia* detection rate. However, the high rate of asymptomatic infection causes problems in the evaluation of infected individuals in health centers, leading to delays in diagnosis and treatment [18]. Therefore, the actual prevalence is much higher [19].

In a similar study, it was determined that the prevalence of *Chlamydia* infection peaked between the ages of 16 and 24 and was comparable in men and women [20]. The prevalence of *Chlamydia* infection was reported to be highest in women between the ages of 15 and 30, while in men it is seen between the ages of 20 and 29 [19]. The prevalence decreases rapidly after the age of 30 [20].

In a meta-analysis spanning 9 European countries, the prevalence of *Chlamydia* infection was found to be 2.7%, and there was no statistically significant difference in prevalence between men and women [19]. *Chlamydia* has been detected at a higher rate in African-Americans than in whites [15].

In a study conducted by Sonnenberg et al. on the British population, the rate of *Chlamydia* infection was found to be higher in those with gonorrhea. This was attributed to the fact that people with risky sexual behavior are more likely to encounter different pathogens. For this reason, gonococcal and nongonococcal infections can often occur concurrently [14]. There may be two pathogens in nongonococcal urethritis. The association of *M. genitalium* and *C. trachomatis* is not uncommon [7]. In some studies, dual infection was identified in up to 10% of cases [21].

In a study by Newbernet et al., adolescents with sexually transmitted diseases had twice the risk of contracting HIV infection compared to those without. Similarly, those who had a previous genital herpes infection were at increased risk of chlamydial, gonorrheal, and human papillomavirus (HPV) infection [14]. Other risk factors for urethritis include having multiple sexual partners at the same time, insufficient condom use, and having more than three different partners who are homosexual or bisexual. In addition, alcohol and other drug use can increase urethritis rates by contributing to risky sexual behaviors in young people [14].

3. History and physical examination

Chlamydial urethritis is asymptomatic in 75% of women and nearly 50% of men [11]. As men are more likely to be symptomatic than women, the diagnosis rate is reported to be higher in males [9]. The factors that determine whether the infection will be symptomatic or not remain unclear. The more common serovar E is known to cause more asymptomatic infections than other less common serotypes. For this reason, it is not uncommon for diagnosis and treatment to be delayed and the infection to persist for months or years. These patients are reservoirs for the disease [11]. In chronic chlamydial infection, RBs do not transform into EBs. When the environmental conditions change, *Chlamydia* can resume its life cycle [22].

Most patients are young and have history of unprotected sexual intercourse, previous urethritis, and antibiotic use. Transmission occurs through direct tissue contact during vaginal, anal, or oral intercourse. Symptoms begin 1–3 weeks after transmission [10] and generally include burning, urethral discharge, urethral itching, frequent urination, urgency, and/or lower abdominal and groin pain. The most common symptom of chlamydial urethritis is painful urination. More rarely, it may cause fever, testicular pain and tenderness, sore throat, and rectal pain and discharge. These must be differentiated from other infectious processes such as epididymitis, pharyngitis, and prostatitis [15].

Ideally, genital examination should be performed 2 h after last urination to detect urethral discharge. If discharge is not seen in the urethra, the clinician can attempt to express it by placing the thumb on the ventral root and the other four fingers on the dorsal surface of the penis and applying gentle pressure toward the urethral meatus. Although it is difficult to make a differential diagnosis based on clinical examination of discharge, a gray-white mucoid or clear discharge is more common in nongonococcal urethritis, whereas purulent discharge is typically seen in gonococcal infections. However, generalization is not reliable. Discharge may be seen continuously or only when the penis is milked, in the morning, or the form of underwear staining [15].

In addition, scrotum and testicle examination is performed to assess for epididymitis and orchitis. If prostatitis is suspected, rectal examination should be performed [7]. As it can also cause ulcers and lymphadenitis and coexist with other sexually transmitted diseases, the skin, pharynx, lymph nodes, and neurological system should also be evaluated in addition to the genital area in men with urethritis [23].

Urethritis is usually diagnosed based on history and physical examination, but laboratory tests should be used to confirm the diagnosis and identify the causative pathogen.

4. Evaluation

In patients whose history and physical examination suggest urethritis, Gram staining of urethral discharge is the first-line laboratory test, and detection of >5 white blood cells (WBC)/per oil immersion field allows a rapid diagnosis of urethritis. In some publications, >2 WBC/high power field (HPF) was used as the threshold value based on the argument that this would provide a more sensitive diagnosis. However, this has not been supported by other studies. The cut-off value accepted by the European Association of Urology (EAU) is >5 polymorphonuclear lymphocytes (PMNL)/HPF. This method has high specificity and sensitivity both for the diagnosis of urethritis and determining the presence or absence of gonococcal infection [24].

A positive leukocyte esterase test of first-void urine or >10 WBC/HPF in the sediment of first-void urine is also diagnostic criterion for urethritis [25].

Chlamydia is not detectable by Gram staining because it is a small obligate cell-borne parasitic bacteria. In a patient with pyuria and suspected urethritis based on history and physical examination, detecting no bacteria on Gram staining raises a strong suspicion of nongonococcal urethritis pathogens, most of which are *Chlamydia* [26].

All male patients with suspected urethritis should undergo NAATs, which are the gold standard for the diagnosis of *N. gonorrhoeae* and *C. trachomatis*, the most common urethritis pathogens. *N. gonorrhoeae* should be included in the NAAT panel even if it was not detected in Gram staining [25]. Even if gonococci were detected in Gram staining, there may be a concurrent chlamydial infection, so evaluation with NAATs should still be done [7].

Methods used in the diagnosis of *C. trachomatis* infection include cytological examination, cell culture, antigen quantification, direct fluorescent antibody tests, enzyme immunoassays, and NAATs if nucleic acid from the pathogen is detected. Among these, NAATs have the highest sensitivity [27]. This method has found widespread use worldwide [16]. Whereas, only urethral swab samples can be used for cultures and hybridization tests, NAATs can also be done using a first-void urine sample, with similar efficacy. NAATs work by amplifying and detecting chlamydial DNA from a very small number of organisms in clinical samples using specific primers and enzymes [10].

C. trachomatis culture is mostly used in treatment failure and to assess resistance to administered treatment [2]. As obligate intracellular parasites, *Chlamydia* cannot be grown in culture media. The living cell environment is necessary for their reproduction [28]. Therefore, as cell culturing requires an experienced team and a well-equipped laboratory, is difficult, and takes time, the use of this technique in the diagnosis of *C. trachomatis* has been replaced in recent years by nucleic acid screening tests, which are molecular techniques that provide faster results and have high specificity and sensitivity. NAAT is the gold standard diagnostic method for urogenital chlamydial infection and can be performed using urethral swab samples collected with a Dacron- or rayon-tipped plastic swab or cytobrush, or using first-void urine. Other swabs containing cotton may inhibit *C. trachomatis* [29]. Sampling is done by inserting a dry swab 3–4 cm into the anterior urethra and rotating it within the urethra before withdrawing. However, the patient should not have urinated in the last 1–2 h [20]. Likewise, for NAATs of first-void urine, the patient should not have urinated within the last 20–60 min. A sample of 10–20 mL is collected at the start of urination without cleaning the urethra. Some publications indicate that urethral swabs are less sensitive than urine in men but have the same specificity [10].

In men who have sex with men, samples for *Chlamydia* and *N. gonorrhoeae* testing should be obtained from the sites of possible sexual contact [2]. Although a normal urine sample is negative in these patients, it should not be forgotten that 70% of extragenital (oral and/or anal) sites may yield positive NAAT results [3].

If the urethral smear is normal and symptoms are inconclusive, repeating the smear in the morning with first-void urine is recommended. The patient should be advised to avoid excessive fluid intake the day before to ensure that urination is not urgent in the morning and they can give a first-void urine sample in the laboratory. If a symptomatic man has a negative smear, a positive leukocyte esterase test of first-void urine aids in the diagnosis of urethritis [2].

The EAU guideline also strongly recommends NAATs for chlamydia and gonorrhea before empirical treatment, if possible. However, treatment should be initiated immediately upon diagnosing urethritis in men with severe symptoms, without waiting for the results of chlamydia, gonorrhea, and *M. genitalium* tests. Patients with mild symptoms and microscopically low leukocyte counts (5–15 PMNL/HPF) are reevaluated after 3–7 days. A urethral smear is obtained early in the morning. NAAT and gonorrhea culture results are also examined when available. Urethritis can sometimes resolve spontaneously without treatment. If laboratory tests are positive and the urethritis persists according to microscopic findings, appropriate antibiotic treatment targeting the microorganism isolated at this second visit should be initiated, bearing local resistance patterns in mind [2]. If symptoms do not resolve in 3–4 weeks, urethritis is classified as persistent. In this case, evaluation with NAATs (including for *T. vaginalis*) should be repeated 4 weeks after the end of treatment [25]. Because men with chlamydial, gonorrheal, or trichomonal infections are at high risk of reinfection, they should be reevaluated by repeating the tests 3 months later. Although it is not an FDA-approved test for *Trichomonas* and *Mycoplasma*, NAAT is performed in many reference and commercial laboratories [7].

The immune response can affect the development of nongonococcal urethritis. A high microbial load (>1000/copies/mL in first-void urine) is a strong predictor of nongonococcal urethritis [2].

5. Treatment/management

The treatment of uncomplicated chlamydial infection aims to cure the patient and prevent complications and partner transmission. Sexual partners are also treated to prevent reinfection and transmission to other partners. Risk-reduction counseling should be provided and retesting performed to detect recurrent or persistent infection [10].

As *Chlamydia* is only metabolically active in host cells, it is treated with antibiotics that have intracellular activity. Antibiotics that accumulate intracellularly are tetracyclines, macrolides, and quinolones. Patients who are diagnosed and treated generally have a high cure rate and excellent prognosis [20].

For uncomplicated urethral chlamydial infection, single-dose azithromycin 1 g or doxycycline 100 mg twice daily for 1 week is recommended as the primary treatment and is reported to have a 95% cure rate [10]. However, a Cochrane study in 2019 indicated that 7-day doxycycline yielded higher cure rates than single-dose azithromycin [3]. However, because the use of azithromycin 1 mg causes resistance in *M. genitalium*, doxycycline 100 mg twice a day is now recommended as first-line treatment. If azithromycin is administered, it is recommended to give 500 mg on the first day, followed by 250 mg daily for 4 days [2]. However, no difference has been observed between single-dose azithromycin and 7-day doxycycline in terms of the resolution of persistent urethritis symptoms. Due to the worse adverse effect profile of doxycycline and better patient adherence to single-dose azithromycin, the latter continues to be used in clinical practice [3].

In two recent randomized controlled studies conducted in the USA, the efficacy of azithromycin and doxycycline in achieving a clinical cure was found to be less than 85% [2]. The use of lymecycline 300 mg twice daily for 10 days or tetracycline 500 mg twice daily for 10 days provided >95% clinical cure rate in *Chlamydia*-positive patients. In addition, these antibiotics did not increase photosensitivity, unlike doxycycline [2]. It seems that new approaches may emerge in this direction. Other alternative antibiotic regimens for *Chlamydia* are oral tetracycline 500 mg 4 times a day for 7 days, oral erythromycin 500 mg twice a day for 7 days, or oral ofloxacin 200–400 mg 2 times a day for 7 days [29].

Chlamydial infection is often accompanied by gonococcal infection [29]. If NAAT or Gram staining demonstrates the presence of gonococci, a single-dose 250 mg intramuscular injection of ceftriaxone is added to the 1 g of azithromycin [15].

Empirical therapy should not be initiated without clarifying a diagnosis of urethritis, because this can cause the symptoms to become permanent [2]. In addition, antibiotic resistance and urethritis caused by different microorganisms are other reasons to avoid empirical therapy [14]. Empirical treatment can only be given in exceptional cases. If the test cannot be performed or if a man with a high risk of infection is severely symptomatic, empirical therapy can be initiated based on a presumed diagnosis. Treatment should cover *Chlamydia* and gonorrhea [2].

It is difficult to evaluate the effectiveness of treatment because persistent inflammation does not equate to continuing infection. Detectable inflammation can persist for an unforeseeable period even if the causative pathogen is eliminated [2]. NAATs performed in the first 3 weeks after completing treatment may yield false positive results. Therefore, follow-up testing is not recommended in this period [3].

Men who have frequent unprotected sexual relations with men have a high risk of chlamydial urethritis and should be screened more frequently. In one study, it was found that single-dose doxycycline decreased the prevalence of chlamydial infection after suspicious intercourse between men without a condom [3]. However, this approach has not yet gained widespread acceptance. It may be beneficial to screen treated patients after 3 months and include patients in a follow-up program after discussing with them, by this has not been incorporated into routine care [10].

Partner therapy is recommended for patients with urethritis. The partners with whom the patient has had sexual intercourse within the last 60 days should be evaluated for sexually transmitted diseases and administered the same treatment regimen as the primary patient. The sexual partner should be treated in accordance with the principles of patient confidentiality [25].

Expedited treatment without examining the partner is legal in many countries and was found to be more effective than recommending partner treatment [3]. In chlamydial, gonorrheal, and trichomonal infections, partners should be called for follow-up testing after 3 months if possible because of the high reinfection rates [14].

Nevertheless, relapse and untreated reinfections from old or infected new partners are common [29]. Recurrent nongonococcal urethritis is defined as recurrence of symptoms within 30–90 days after acute treatment and occurs at a rate of 10–20% [2]. One study indicated that up to 20% of chlamydial infections were persistent or recurrent despite initial treatment [14].

Patients with recurrent or persistent symptoms should be reevaluated to determine whether they completed the full course of initial treatment and whether they were re-exposed to the pathogen. The same initial treatment should be repeated for untreated patients, received incomplete treatment, or encountered the pathogen again [7].

If only *Chlamydia* and gonorrhea were initially tested for in men with persistent nongonococcal urethritis, NAATs for *M. genitalium* and *T. vaginalis* should also be performed [2]. *M. genitalium* is the most common cause of recurrent and persistent nongonococcal urethritis. Therefore, a treatment regimen targeting this pathogen is important [15]. Coinfection and less common pathogens should also be investigated in persistent urethritis. The possibility of a persistent postinfectious immune response should be kept in mind. If a cause cannot be identified, underlying urinary tract anomalies and urethral pathologies should be evaluated [14].

6. Complications

Reinfection is common, and sequelae associated with complications are likely to increase with multiple infections. Untreated or inadequately treated patients may develop epididymitis and orchitis. These conditions can develop after urethritis or in the absence of urethritis. Symptoms are milder than with other causes of epididymitis [20]. It manifests with unilateral testicular pain, tenderness, and palpable swelling along with hydrocele and fever, whereas lymphogranuloma venereum presents clinically as a painless genital ulcer. The ulcer is typically small and star-shaped. After ulcer formation, inguinal lymphadenitis is also characteristic [29]. Testicular involvement can cause pyogranulomatous changes in the testicle. This may lead to testicular degeneration, resulting in serious andrological sequelae [20].

It can also cause serious complications such as chronic prostatitis/chronic pelvic pain and infertility. *C. trachomatis* has been the focus of attention in cases of chronic prostatitis/chronic pelvic pain of unclear etiology. Although the evidence is debatable, significantly more *Chlamydia* bacteria were reportedly detected in the urine, semen, and prostate fluid and tissue of patients with chronic prostatitis compared to the control group [10]. Studies on this subject are still ongoing, and its etiological role has not been fully clarified due to the diagnostic challenges.

Another serious complication of incomplete or untreated chlamydial infection is infertility. Asymptomatic persistent infection can negatively affect fertility in couples by causing chronic inflammation [11]. Studies evaluating the relationship between chlamydial infection and sperm quality have yielded conflicting results. Recent studies have generally demonstrated lower ejaculate quality in infected individuals. Persistent infection has been observed to cause scarring in the ejaculatory ducts and loss of stereocilia. In addition, some studies have associated infection with DNA fragmentation and sperm dysfunction, and death [10].

It should be kept in mind that chlamydial infections in women can also cause serious complications such as infertility, pelvic inflammatory disease, ectopic pregnancy, and Fitz-Hugh-Curtis syndrome [9]. *C. trachomatis* is also a common cause of symptomatic proctitis and proctocolitis in homosexual men [29].

7. Prevention and patient education

The high prevalence of asymptomatic chlamydial urethritis is gradually increasing the rate of undiagnosed or untreated infections. Therefore, screening is protective. At least annual follow-up of all sexually active women under 25 years of age and women over 25 years of age who are at risk for sexually transmitted infections is also recommended to reduce the rate of male infection. These screening programs have been shown to decrease the prevalence of infection and rates of complications. There is insufficient evidence for the efficacy and cost-effectiveness of routine *Chlamydia* screening in sexually active young men. However, in risky and high-prevalence areas, performing this screening to the extent allowed by clinical conditions is beneficial [29].

Risk groups include:

- people who have sex with people who have multiple sexual partners.
- people with new or multiple sexual partners.
- people in nonmonogamous relationships who have inconsistent condom use.
- people who pay for sex.
- people who have sex with people who are infected or have a history of infection.
- men who have sex with men.
- HIV carriers.
- women up to 35 years of age and men under 30 years of age who go to prison [29].

Patients with chlamydial infection should also be evaluated for other sexually transmitted diseases such as gonorrhea, syphilis, and HIV. The diagnosis and treatment of sexual partners are also important [29].

In many countries, notification of *C. trachomatis* infection is mandatory. The sexual partner must be informed, examined, and treated. Partner antibiotic therapy can also be performed in some cases without face-to-face contact with the patient to expedite treatment.

Patients should be informed about the serious risks of chlamydial infection and the importance of screening. Those who feel uneasy about urethral swap sampling for diagnosis should be tested using a first-void urine sample and prevented from leaving without being screened.

In the USA and other developed nations, the prevention of sexually transmitted genital infections and their complications is based on annual screening and treatment of nonpregnant women under the age of 25. In the presence of a risk factor, other women should also be screened. High-risk young men should also be screened if resources allow [29].

Health workers and nurses should educate patients about the importance of using condoms during sex and provide information about safe sex. Candid communication with the patient and helping them feel comfortable are essential in diagnosis, treatment, and follow-up [9].

Early treatment and full-dose antibiotics provide a near-perfect cure rate. Urethral infection with *C. trachomatis* produces a low-level immunological response [20]. The rise of chlamydial infections, for which there is not yet a vaccine, can be prevented by completed treatment, patient education, and screening.

The American Centers for Disease Control and Prevention (CDC) recommend that a sexual history should be obtained from patients and risk reduction strategies recommended when deemed necessary. In addition, the U.S. Preventive Services Task Force recommends that all sexually active adolescents and adults at risk of sexually transmitted infections be provided intensive counseling [3].

Patients should not engage in sexual intercourse for at least 7 days after the completion of treatment and sex should only be allowed after their partner has also completed treatment and symptoms have fully resolved [3].

Patients with urethritis should be vaccinated for other infectious diseases for which vaccines are available (hepatitis A/B, HPV).

The use of condoms reduces the risk. Selective sexual intercourse should be practiced and uncontrolled intercourse avoided. Circumcision was found to be beneficial in terms of genital ulcers and HPV, but ineffective in terms of transmission of *C. trachomatis* and gonorrhea [3].

When a sexually transmitted infection is detected, the patient should be educated by a team including physicians and trained healthcare professionals. Adequate sensitivity should be shown to patients regarding partner treatment and recurrence. An environment where patients feel safe and comfortable should be provided to enable the patient to ask questions and ensure accurate history-taking. If the patient does not feel safe, it will be difficult to obtain a detailed sexual history. This causes delays in diagnosis and treatment. Providing diagnosis and treatment with a professional approach will help curb the rapid rise of this disease [9].

8. Conclusion

Chlamydial urethritis involves difficulties in diagnosis and treatment [14]. *C. trachomatis* is an important pathogen in male urogenital system disease. There is robust evidence that the bacterium is a cause of epididymitis and orchitis, and also plays a role in the etiopathogenesis of chronic prostatitis and infertility. Early diagnosis, complete treatment, and prevention methods are essential for this infection, which also poses a serious risk for sexual partners. As its prevalence continues to rise substantially, a well-coordinated team approach has become imperative for patients infected with *C. trachomatis*.

Author details

Ibrahim Duman
Department of Urology, Medical Park Hospital, Antalya, Turkey

*Address all correspondence to: duman_ibrahim@hotmail.com

References

[1] Sarier M et al. Microscopy of Gram-stained urethral smear in the diagnosis of urethritis: Which threshold value should be selected? Andrologia. 2018;**50**(10):1. DOI: 10.1111/and.13143

[2] Horner PJ, Blee K, Falk L, van der Meijden W, Moi H. 2016 European guideline on the management of non-gonococcal urethritis. International Journal of STD AIDS. 2016;**27**(11):928-937. DOI: 10.1177/0956462416648585

[3] Sell J, Nasir M, Courchesne C. Uretritis rapid evidence. American Family Physician. 2021;**103**(9):553-558

[4] Burstein GR, Zenilman JM. Nongonococcal urethritis-A new paradigm. [Online]. Available from: https://academic.oup.com/cid/article/28/Supplement_1/S66/412243

[5] Jordan SJ et al. No pathogen-specific sign or symptom predicts the etiology of monomicrobial nongonococcal urethritis in men. Sex Transmitted Diseases. 2020;**47**(5):329-331. DOI: 10.1097/OLQ.0000000000001158

[6] Sarier M, Kukul E. Classification of non-gonococcal urethritis: A review. International Urology and Nephrology. 2019;**51**(6):901-907. DOI: 10.1007/s11255-019-02140-2

[7] Perkins MJ, Decker CF. Non-gonococcal urethritis. Disease-a-Month. 2016;**62**(8):274-279. DOI: 10.1016/j.disamonth.2016.03.011

[8] Sarıer M, Duman İ, Göktaş Ş, Kukul E. Results of multiplex polymerase chain reaction assay to identify urethritis pathogens. Journal of Urological Surgery. 2017;**4**(1):18-22. DOI: 10.4274/jus.1328

[9] Young A, Toncar A, Wray AA. Urethritis. Treasure Island (FL): StatPearls; 2022. Available from: https://www.ncbi.nlm.nih.gov/books/NBK537282/

[10] Murray PR, Baron EJ. Manual of Clinical Microbiology. 9th ed. Washington D.C: ASM Press; 2007

[11] Mackern-Oberti JP, Motrich RD, Breser ML, Sánchez LR, Cuffini C, Rivero VE. *Chlamydia trachomatis* infection of the male genital tract: An update. Journal of Reproduction Immunology. 2013;**100**(1):37-53. DOI: 10.1016/j.jri.2013.05.002

[12] Worboys M. Chlamydia: A Disease without a History. In: Szreter S, editor. The Hidden Affliction: Sexually Transmitted Infections and Infertility in History. Rochester (NY): University of Rochester Press; Oct 2019. Chapter Five. PMID: 31580630

[13] Bradshaw CS. et al. Etiologies of nongonococcal urethritis: Bacteria, viruses, and the association with orogenital exposure. 2006. [Online]. Available from: https://academic.oup.com/jid/article/193/3/336/2191545

[14] Bartoletti R et al. Management of urethritis: Is it still the time for empirical antibiotic treatments? European Urology Focus. 2019;**5**(1):29-35. DOI: 10.1016/j.euf.2018.10.006

[15] Territo H, Ashurst JV. Nongonococcal Urethritis. Treasure Island (FL): StatPearls; 2022. https://www.ncbi.nlm.nih.gov/books/NBK535411/

[16] Sarier M. Polymerase chain reaction assay in acute urethritis. Andrologia. 2019;**51**(8):1. DOI: 10.1111/and.13366

[17] Meyer T. Diagnostic Procedures to Detect Chlamydia trachomatis Infections. Microorganisms. 5 Aug 2016;**4**(3):25. DOI: 10.3390/microorganisms4030025. PMID: 27681919; PMCID: PMC5039585

[18] Sarier M et al. New approach to microscopy of gram-stained urethral smear: The Kissing Slide Method. Sex Transmitted Diseases. 2020;**47**(10):712-715. DOI: 10.1097/OLQ.0000000000001228

[19] Fischer N et al. Prevalence estimates of genital *Chlamydia trachomatis* infection in Belgium: Results from two cross-sectional studies. BMC Infected Diseases. 2021;**21**(1):2. DOI: 10.1186/s12879-021-06646-y

[20] Wagenlehner FME, Weidner W, Naber KG. Chlamydial infections in urology. World Journal of Urology. 2006;**24**(1):4-12. DOI: 10.1007/s00345-005-0047-x

[21] Sarıer M. Prevalence of polymicrobial infection in urethritis. Journal of Urological Surgery. 2019;**6**(3):180-183. DOI: 10.4274/jus.galenos.2019.2405

[22] Morrison RP. New insights into a persistent problem- Chlamydial infections. Journal of Clinical Investigation. 2003;**111**(11):1647-1649. DOI: 10.1172/JCI18770

[23] Barrow RY, Ahmed F, Bolan GA, Workowski KA. Recommendations for Providing Quality Sexually Transmitted Diseases Clinical Services, 2020. MMWR Recomm Rep. 2020;**68**(No. RR-5):1-20. DOI: 10.15585/mmwr.rr6805a1

[24] Moi H, Hartgill U, Skullerud KH, Reponen EJ, Syvertsen L, Moghaddam A. Microscopy of stained urethral smear in male urethritis; which cutoff should be used? Sex Transmitted Diseases. 2017;**44**(3):189-194. DOI: 10.1097/OLQ.0000000000000565

[25] Bonkat G, Bartoletti R, Bruyère F, Cai T, Geerlings SE, Köves B, et al. Guidelines on urological infections. European Association of Urology. 2022;**3**:30-34. Available from: http://uroweb.org/guideline/urological-infections

[26] Bachmann LH et al. Advances in the understanding and treatment of male urethritis. Clinical Infectious Diseases. 2015;**61**:S763-S769. DOI: 10.1093/cid/civ755

[27] Sarier M et al. Prevalence of sexually transmitted diseases in asymptomatic renal transplant recipients. Experiment in Clinical Transplantation. 2018;**2018**:1, 4. DOI: 10.6002/ect.2017.0232

[28] Mabey DCW, Solomon AW, Foster A. Trachoma. Lancet. 2003;**362**:223-229

[29] Mohseni M, Sung S, Takov V. Chlamydia. Treasure Island (FL): StatPearls; 2022. Available from: https://www.ncbi.nlm.nih.gov/books/NBK537286/

Chapter 16

Chlamydia trachomatis: A Tiny Being beyond the Nature

Esin Kasap

Abstract

Chlamydia trachomatis is the most common cause of sexually transmitted genital infections. Females are at high risk of cervix infections, and a significant proportion may also have urethral infections. Pelvic inflammatory disease (PID) can develop as a result of *C. trachomatis* ascending to the upper reproductive tract. *C. trachomatis* is an obligate intracellular bacterium that infects the genital tract and may cause chronic inflammation, damage to epithelial tissues, and pelvic inflammation. It has also been clinically associated with cervical atypia and metaplasia. *C. trachomatis* is the most prevalent sexually transmitted pathogen, and it can cause infertility if left undetected and untreated. Infertile women may be more susceptible to chlamydial infections due to their longer periods of active sexual life. Several diagnostic techniques are available to diagnose chlamydia, including DNA amplification testing (NAAT), culture, antigen detection, and genetic probes; microscopy is not useful for this purpose Chlamydia is treated with empiric therapy, which includes tetracyclines, macrolides, and some fluoroquinolones.

Keywords: chlamydial infection, gynecology, chlamydia trachomatis, chlamydial infections diagnosis, pelvic inflammatory disease (PID)

1. Introduction

1.1 A brief introduction

The most common cause of sexually transmitted genital infections is *Chlamydia trachomatis* [1]. Almost all the affected individuals are asymptomatic, thus providing an ongoing reservoir of infection. Conjunctivitis and pneumonia can occur in infants born through an infected birth canal. The rectum and conjunctivae are common epithelial sites where males and females can develop clinical syndromes due to infection. There is an incubation period of 5–15 days following infection before symptomatic disease develops. The infection may remain active in asymptomatic individuals for an indefinite period before they become symptomatic.

Among 10 studies of untreated, uncomplicated genital chlamydial infections, 56–89% detected the presence of chlamydia over the short term (weeks to months after diagnosis), and 46–57% detected the presence of chlamydia over the long term [2]. There is, however, a lack of documentation of the date of infection or evaluation of whether the infection was persistent or recurrent. This limits our understanding of the duration of untreated chlamydial infections. According to subsequent modeling studies, chlamydial infections are less likely to establish. In contrast, once established, the disease progresses slowly and more slowly in males than in females (mean undetected durations of 2.84 and 1.35 years, respectively, in males and females [3, 4]. The treatment of all patients with Chlamydia is recommended, despite the possibility of spontaneous resolution.

1.2 A clinical analysis of female syndromes

The majority of females who are infected with *C. trachomatis* are asymptomatic, but the pathogen is a significant contributor to several clinical syndromes that are common among women.

1.2.1 Genitourinary tract infection

Females are at high risk of cervix infections [5], and a significant proportion may also have urethral infections. When left untreated, cervical cavity infections may progress into the upper genital tract, resulting in pelvic inflammatory disease, infertility, and chronic pain. Pregnant women with genital chlamydial infections are also at risk for complications.

An increased risk of chlamydial infection has been associated with cervical ectropion (columnar epithelium on the outer surface of the cervix in addition to the endocervical canal). Furthermore, some studies have linked cervical neoplasia to the infection [6, 7], but the extent of this effect remains unknown.

1.2.2 Cervicitis

In most cases (at least 85%) of females with cervicitis, no symptoms are observed, which is why young, sexually active females should undergo routine annual screenings. There was only 6–14% of females who developed a new infection within a year of testing who had symptoms of genital chlamydial infection in four out of five sites in a multinational study that looked at women at high risk for genital chlamydial infection using polymerase chain reaction testing of vaginal swabs [8]. Some of the symptoms that can be confused with vaginitis or genital tract pathology are a change in vaginal discharge, intermenstrual vaginal bleeding, and post-coital bleeding. These symptoms can present in many ways, such as an increase in release, a change in color or odor, an increase in itching or burning, or an increase in pain or discomfort during intercourse. The discharge may also have an abnormally high pH, indicative of an infection. Abnormal exam findings are found in approximately 10–20% of females with genital chlamydial infection. When signs of cervicitis are present, they include mucopurulent discharge from the endocervical cavity, easily induced bleeding from the endocervical cavity, and edematous ectopy.

It has been observed that some of these females report symptoms of urinary tract infections, such as frequency and dysuria, but they do not report symptoms specific to the urethra. If not subjected to specific tests for C trachomatis, these females may be mistaken for cystitis [9, 10]. Despite pyuria in the urine analysis, no organisms are detected in the Gram stain or bacterial culture. Therefore, it is reasonable to suspect that sexually active females with pyuria and no bacteriuria may have a chlamydial infection of the urethra based on the combination of symptoms described above.

As a result of these conditions, several possible diagnoses are available, including low-colony urinary tract infections (such as *Staphylococcus saprophyticus*), which cannot be confirmed by culture or detected by urinalysis, or urethritis caused by another STI, such as *Neisseria gonorrhoeae*, Trichomonas vaginalis, or herpes simplex.

1.2.3 Pelvic inflammatory disease

As a result of C trachomatis ascending to the upper reproductive tract (uterus, fallopian tubes, and ovaries), pelvic inflammatory disease (PID) can develop [16–20]. The prevalence of clinical PID in females presenting to STI clinics ranged from 2 to 4.5% between the diagnosis of chlamydia infection and the follow-up visit [2]. Following the administration of ineffective antibiotics against Chlamydia, a small study of 20 females with *N. gonorrhoea* and *C. trachomatis* coinfection reported a 30% incidence of PID [11]. As a result, no cases of clinical PID have been reported in studies of females at low risk of exposure to chlamydia after a year without treatment. As many cases of PID do not cause symptoms and are only detected later in cases of tubal infertility, these studies may underestimate the incidence of PID in chlamydial infection.

Most commonly, abdominal and pelvic pain is present with symptoms of PID. Infection with chlamydia in conjunction with cervicitis should raise a significant suspicion that the upper genital tract is involved. PID is characterized by cervical motion and tenderness in the uterus or adnexa. PID caused by C trachomatis is associated with a higher rate of subsequent tubal infertility, ectopic pregnancy, and chronic pelvic pain as compared with PID caused by gonorrhea, which typically presents in an acute manner [12].

1.2.4 Invasive cervical carcinoma (ICC)

Invasive cervical carcinoma (ICC) is most likely caused by the human papillomavirus (HPV). Research investigating the etiology of cervical neoplasia and invasive cervical carcinoma has recently examined factors that may affect susceptibility to or progression of HPV infection [13]. *C. trachomatis* may be a significant HPV cofactor for cervical cancer among sexually transmitted diseases other than HPV. As well as HPV, *C. trachomatis* may play an important role in cervical cancer development. *C. trachomatis* is an obligate intracellular bacterium that infects the genital tract [14]. Genital *C. trachomatous* infection may cause chronic inflammation, damage to epithelial tissues, and pelvic inflammation in some cases. In addition, it has been clinically associated with cervical atypia and metaplasia, increasing women's risk of cervical neoplasia [15].

A case-control study from England and a pooled analysis of cohort studies from Finland, Norway and Sweden have found positive associations between *C. trachomatis* microimmunofluorescence (MIF) seropositivity and ICC [16, 17]. According to a Swedish cohort study, *C. trachomatis* DNA is highly predictive of the development of ICC [18].

Squamous cell ICC may also be increased by infections with *C. trachomatis* by increasing a host's susceptibility to HPV and enhancing its effects. Infection with C trachomatis may lead to inflammation, which can produce reactive oxygen species, which can damage DNA and increase the risk of HPV-associated cancer [19]. According to in vitro experiments, Chlamydia-infected cells are also less likely to undergo the normal process of programmed cell death [19, 20]. The cadherin-catenin junction structure in cervical epithelial cells is altered by C trachomatis, increasing the risk of infection with HPV. As opposed to cellular mechanisms, humoral mechanisms (Th2) may mediate the immune response to a particular antigen [21]. The symptoms of cervical neoplasia may be difficult to control in women with C trachomatis infection. An increase in HPV persistence after 12 months was associated with a previous history of C trachomatis, according to a study conducted among Swedish women aged 32–38 years old [22].

1.2.5 Infertility

Worldwide, infertility is becoming an increasingly prevalent health issue [12]. *C. trachomatis* is becoming a more prominent sexually transmitted disease as a result of the increase in cases [23]. Currently, *C. trachomatis* is the most prevalent sexually transmitted pathogen. The symptoms of chlamydial infection are less severe than those of other sexually transmitted diseases. A patient may be unaware of the infection until secondary or tertiary symptoms develop due to these deceptively mild symptoms. Infections such as acute salpingitis and pelvic inflammatory disease that go undetected and untreated can result in not only significant morbidity but also infertility [24].

Infertility associated with *C. trachomatis* can be prevented if detected early [25]. Infertile women are estimated to be infected with chlamydial infections by 18–20%, according to a WHO study [23].

It is reported that infertility is reported to last between 2 and 4 years in chlamydia-positive women [26]. Women with secondary infertility were more likely to contract *C. trachomatis* infection. Due to their long period of active sexual life, they may be more susceptible to chlamydial infections. There was a surprisingly high percentage of infertile women (38%) who were positive for *C. trachomatis*. There was no history of previous upper genital tract infection in the majority of these women [23].

1.2.6 Complications of pregnancy

Furthermore, the chlamydial genital infection may increase the risk of premature rupture of the membranes during labor, preterm delivery, and low birth weight infants in addition to the risk of future ectopic pregnancy [27]. According to a study of 3913 pregnant Dutch women screened for *C. trachomatis*, those with chlamydial infection had a higher risk of preterm delivery (adjusted odds ratio 4.35, 95% CI 1.3–15.2). However, the chlamydial infection did not predict miscarriage or perinatal death [24].

1.2.7 Perihepatitis (Fitz-Hugh-Curtis syndrome)

Perihepatitis is an inflammation of the liver capsule and adjacent peritoneal surfaces that may occur in patients with chlamydia infection. An acute PID is more likely to result in perihepatitis, which occurs in 5–15% of cases. In most cases, there is no abnormality in liver enzymes, but there can be a pain in the right upper part of the rig or pleuritic pain. We do not fully understand the pathogenesis of this condition. An immunological mechanism may be involved, or the infected material could be directly transmitted from the cul-de-sac to the lymphatics and peritoneum [28, 29].

1.2.8 Reactive arthritis/reactive arthritis triad (RAT)

STIs can trigger reactive arthritis. There is a small percentage of patients with sexually acquired reactive arthritis who develop the complete reactive arthritis triad, consisting of arthritis, conjunctivitis, uveitis, and urethritis. It has been shown that *C. trachomatis* causes sexually acquired reactive arthritis most frequently.

Detection of chlamydial nucleic acids in synovial tissue further supports the association between chlamydia and reactive arthritis. Seven out of nine patients with RAT had a positive in situ hybridization for chlamydial RNA in synovial tissue samples compared to three out of thirteen patients without RAT (the cause of arthritis was not otherwise determined). In addition, five of eight sexually acquired reactive arthritis patients and one control patient with another form of arthritis had stored synovial tissues that contained chlamydial DNA found by polymerase chain reaction.

1.2.9 Conjunctivitis

Serovars D through K of *C. trachomatis* can cause genital disease in the conjunctival epithelium. The most common method for achieving this goal is directly inoculating infected genital secretions. Inclusion conjunctivitis, which may appear cobbled, is a typical presentation of sexually acquired chlamydial conjunctivitis. Serovars A through C cause endemic trachoma, but this type of infection differs.

1.2.10 Pharyngitis

There is no evidence that *C. trachomatis* is a significant cause of pharyngitis. However, nucleic acid amplification testing has detected C trachomatis in the pharynx, and some investigators believe this site serves as a reservoir for the infection.

1.2.11 L serovars

In European and North American MSM, particularly those living with HIV, lymphogranuloma venereum (LGV) has been reported to be caused by *C. trachomatis* L1, L2, and L3 serovars [30]. Symptoms occur in most cases. It has been reported in case studies that anorectal pain, discharge, tenesmus, rectal bleeding, and constipation are among the symptoms reported. It is also possible to experience systemic symptoms such as fever and malaise as well as local symptoms. Several anatomic findings can be observed under anesthesia, including mucopurulent exudate, internal lesions, masses, or polyps. As a result of this presentation, it is sometimes mistaken for an inflammatory bowel disease [31]. Rectal infections caused by the L1, L2, and L3 serovars can result in fistulas and strictures if left untreated [32].

1.2.12 D through K serovars

In addition to causing genital infection in MSM, these non-LGV serovars are also capable of causing rectum infection. This infection, however, is usually asymptomatic, unlike LGV. For example, according to a study of MSM screened for rectal chlamydial infection, only 16% (49 of 301 cases) of non-LGV infections were symptomatic compared to 95% (58 of 62 cases) of rectal LGV infections [32, 33].

Infected females with rectal C trachomatis usually have D through K serovars and are generally asymptomatic. It is also possible for females to develop symptomatic proctitis [33], but this occurs less frequently than in MSM.

2. Diagnosis of chlamydial infections

Several diagnostic techniques are available to diagnose chlamydia, including DNA amplification testing (NAAT), culture, antigen detection, and genetic probes; microscopy is not useful for this purpose. Nevertheless, NAAT is the preferred diagnostic technique due to its superior sensitivity, specificity, and wide availability [34, 35].

2.1 Nucleic acid amplification testing (test of choice)

DNA or RNA sequences from *C. trachomatis* are amplified using polymerase chain reaction (PCR), transcription-mediated amplification (TMA), or strand displacement amplification (SDA). The "gold standard" of diagnostics is to use these sensitive, specific tests if they are available [34, 36].

2.2 The preferred testing specimen for diagnosis varies by syndrome

2.2.1 Genitourinary infection or screening in females

A vaginal swab is the most appropriate specimen that the patient can collect. NAAT can be performed on either endocervical specimens (for example, cervical specimens collected into liquid cytology medium for Pap testing) or vaginal swabs for females undergoing speculum exams (for example, to evaluate symptoms of cervicitis). Compared to vaginal and endocervical swab samples, first-catch urine samples detect up to 10% fewer infections in females [36, 37].

2.2.2 Test performance

The NAATs can collect specimens without a pelvic examination in females [38]. The most sensitive specimen for diagnosing chlamydial infection in females is a swab of vaginal fluid [38, 39]. Compared with urine and, in some cases, endocervical swabs, NAAT on vaginal swab fluid on females had higher sensitivity than urine and, in some cases, endocervical swabs. Several studies have shown that NAAT on rectal specimens can detect rectal chlamydia more accurately than culture and still have high specificity [40]. Men who have sex with men (MSM) can also self-collect these samples to facilitate screening [41].

2.3 Other diagnostic techniques

2.3.1 Rapid tests for chlamydia

Even though NAAT has replaced culture as the new "gold standard," same-day results have not been available traditionally. NAAT-based rapid tests have been developed. Their use will likely be influenced by practical issues, such as waivers for non-laboratory use and cost, as they become more available [41].

2.3.2 The XPert C trachomatis/N gonorrhea (CT/NG) assay

A NAAT, the XPert C trachomatis/N gonorrhea (CT/NG) test provides results for chlamydia (and gonorrhea) within 90 minutes [42]. It is FDA-approved for use on vaginal and endocervical swabs. Using electrochemical detection technology, the Binx io CT/NG NAAT assay produces results within 30 min [43]. It is FDA-approved for use on vaginal swabs. 96, 99, 91, and 100% were the sensitivity, specificity, positive, and negative predictive values for CT. **Culture methods** for detecting chlamydiosis are now limited to research and reference laboratories due [44]. **Serology for C trachomatis** (complement fixation titers >1:64) is usually performed infrequently, is non-standardized, and requires a high level of expertise for interpretation. Furthermore, it may not perform as well as a test to diagnose rectal infections in males as in females with upper genital tract infections [45–47]. **Testing for antigens requires** invasive methods such as cervix swabs or urethral swabs. Compared to culture, this method has an 80–95% sensitivity. Currently available **genetic probe methods** require invasive testing with a direct cervix or urethral swab since they do not amplify genetic targets. This assay is 80% more sensitive than culture. Although these tests are relatively inexpensive, their sensitivity is significantly lower than NAAT, and NAAT has become more cost-competitive, so they are no longer as commonly used.

Adolescent girls and young women may no longer be required to visit their doctors annually since there is no longer a need for annual cervical cancer screening. A young woman's annual visit is an important opportunity to obtain advice and information regarding her reproductive health, access contraception, receive counseling regarding sexually transmitted diseases (STDs), and to be screened for these diseases.

2.4 Who are the candidates to test for chlamydial infections

2.4.1 Symptomatic and at-risk asymptomatic patients

The diagnosis of *C. trachomatis* should be based on the clinical signs and symptoms associated with chlamydia in sexually active individuals. There is a high risk of infection and complications associated with chlamydia in sexually active patients. Most of these infections are asymptomatic because most chlamydial infections do not present any symptoms. Furthermore, chlamydia should also be tested on patients who have a history of documented gonococcal infection. Moreover, patients treated for chlamydia should be rescreened around 3 months after treatment, regardless of whether they think their sexual partners have been treated as well [44]. In the months following an initial infection with chlamydia, a high rate of reinfection has been documented as well [43, 48].

2.4.2 Patients with persistent symptoms

Symptoms that persist after appropriate treatment and good adherence to confirmed chlamydial infection are usually not the results of primary treatment failure. NAAT testing and ompA genotyping were used to characterize the reinfection or persisting infection rates in a longitudinal cohort of adolescent females assessed every 3 months [49]. There were 478 infections observed among 210 participants. Of these females, 121 experienced repeated infections. Only 2.2% were infections that persisted without documented treatment. Most of these infections (84%) were likely reinfections, 14% were probable or possible treatment failures, and 14% persisted without documented treatment.

2.4.3 Recurrence of symptoms

When chlamydia, gonorrhea, bacterial vaginosis, and other sexually transmitted diseases that cause urethritis or cervicitis have resolved after a first evaluation, a repeat evaluation is recommended for the prior treatment; NAAT remains the test of choice to diagnose reinfection in symptom recurrence [37]. Repeat diagnosis of chlamydia in previously treated patients usually indicates reinfection, as noted above [37].

Diagnosing *C. trachomatis* should also prompt testing for *N. gonorrhoeae* since both pathogens cause similar clinical syndromes and coexist in a significant proportion of patients with chlamydial infection [36].

3. Treatment of *Chlamydia trachomatis* infection

Males and females alike are most at risk for bacterial sexually transmitted infections (STIs) caused by *C. trachomatis*, a small gram-negative bacterium.

Preventing complicated infections caused by chlamydia and its sequelae are the primary goals of management (e.g., pelvic inflammatory disease, infertility, chronic pelvic pain, ectopic pregnancy, and epididymitis). The screening and treatment of young females for *C. trachomatis* infection, for example, has been shown to reduce the risk of subsequent PID [50]; however, early treatment of PID, particularly when *C. trachomatis* is detected, reduces the risk of ectopic pregnancy and infertility compared to delayed treatment [51]. Treatment with doxycycline or azithromycin results in clinical improvement in 83 and 86 per cent of symptomatic patients with cervicitis and urethritis, respectively [51, 52]. The risk of reinfection is high for persons who have previously contracted chlamydia. Persons with symptoms such as cervicitis, PID, urethritis, epididymitis, and acute proctitis may benefit from empiric therapy for chlamydial infection.

Empiric therapy should also be offered to patients recently exposed to chlamydia. A patient with documented gonococcal infection should also receive empiric chlamydia treatment unless the nucleic acid amplification test (NAAT) is negative [51].

3.1 Antimicrobial susceptibility of C trachomatis

Tetracyclines, macrolides, and some, but not all, fluoroquinolones are uniformly effective against *C. trachomatis* [53]. The in vitro persistence of *C. trachomatis* is associated with penicillins [53, 54], but amoxicillin has also been effective. The aminoglycosides and sulfonamides have limited activity against *C. trachomatis*, but antibiotic resistance is sporadic for those agents [55].

Moreover, the extracellular elementary body of *C. trachomatis*, an infectious organism, is metabolically inert and resistant to killing, so the breadth of active agents is limited [56]. Therefore, antibiotics need to target the sequestered intracellular and intravacuolar phases of this pathogen's life cycle, which is why antibiotics with good intracellular penetration are vital [57].

Maintaining antibiotic concentrations throughout the organism's life cycle, ranging from 36 to 48 hours, is also necessary. To ensure adequate levels of antibiotics, either a prolonged course of therapy or the selection of an antibiotic with a long half-life is required [57, 58].

Moreover, the elementary body is relatively inert, limiting replication opportunities and resulting in antibiotic-resistant mutations [59].

3.2 Defining antibiotic efficacy

As part of its four primary outcomes of recommending antimicrobial regimens for treating sexually transmitted infections (along with symptom resolution, prevention of sequelae, and prevention of transmission), the Center for Disease Control and Prevention explicitly incorporated microbial eradication (along with symptom resolution, prevention of sequelae, and prevention of transmission) to one of four outcomes. The effectiveness of a drug can be more reliably predicted by its ability to cure bacteria than by its ability to cure the patient for two reasons: many patients have other coinfections that are not responsive to treatment [59], and most patients are not manifesting clinical symptoms at the beginning of the treatment.

3.3 Comprehensive treatment approach

The complete care of C trachomatis-infected patients includes antibiotic treatment, evaluation, and treatment of other sexually transmitted diseases (STIs, such as gonorrhea and HIV), counseling on adherence and sexual activity, follow-up testing, and managing sex partners. Females and males are more likely to have asymptomatic infections that can only be detected on screening; however, these should also be treated promptly [56].

3.4 Antibiotic treatment of chlamydia

3.4.1 Doxycycline as the preferred agent

For optimal outcomes, patients should be counseled to adhere to the prescribed dosage of 100 mg twice daily for 7 days [60]. It is safe and effective to administer delayed-release doxycycline (200 mg daily for 7 days) compared with twice-daily doxycycline. However, it is more costly and may not be accessible to all patients [60]. Previously, azithromycin was considered an alternative option, but mounting evidence indicates that doxycycline is a more effective microbial agent, especially for rectal infections and possibly pharyngeal infections [61]. Azithromycin is now considered an alternative. For this reason, azithromycin is reserved for individuals who are unlikely to be able to complete the seven-day doxycycline course (e.g., patients with adherence issues) and is administered as a single, directly observed dose of 1 g. It is also the preferred antibiotic for pregnant women [62].

3.4.2 Levofloxacin (500 mg orally once daily for 7 days)

Levofloxacin and ofloxacin (300 mg twice daily for 7 days) are highly effective against *C. trachomatis*. There may be limited availability of this alternative fluoroquinolone. They are more expensive than doxycycline, and neither offers a significant advantage. Fluoroquinolones should not be used for uncomplicated infections since they are associated with severe adverse effects. Therefore, fluoroquinolones as a treatment for *C. trachomatis* is rare. Then, levofloxacin (or ofloxacin) can be used as an antichlamydial agent. Before, these fluoroquinolones were utilized primarily for treating coexisting gonococcal and chlamydial infections. Despite this, due to drug resistance, fluoroquinolones no longer provide adequate protection against *N. gonorrhoeae* [63, 64].

Fluoroquinolones are less well-studied for targeted therapy for *C. trachomatis* than doxycycline or azithromycin. Studies comparing fluoroquinolones (e.g., ofloxacin) to doxycycline have failed to demonstrate any difference in microbiologic cure rates. Fluoroquinolones are inappropriate; ciprofloxacin has poor microbiologic outcomes. Alternatively, moxifloxacin has not been studied as a targeted therapy for

C. trachomatis, it has shown promising efficacy in treating PID and is recommended as an alternative treatment regimen for select females with PID [65, 66].

Penicillins and erythromycin are significantly less effective than penicillin, resulting in a microbial cure, with cure rates ranging from 85 to 89%. Therefore, penicillins (such as amoxicillin) are primarily prescribed to pregnant women who cannot tolerate other antibiotics [67, 68].

Author details

Esin Kasap
Department of Gynecology and Obstetrics, Health Sciences University, Tepecik Education and Research Hospital, İzmir, Turkey

*Address all correspondence to: dresincelik@windowslive.com

References

[1] Workowski KA, Berman SM. Centers for Disease Control and Prevention sexually transmitted disease treatment guidelines. Clinical Infectious Diseases. 2011;**53**(suppl_3):S59-S63

[2] Geisler WM. Duration of untreated, uncomplicated chlamydia trachomatis genital infection and factors associated with chlamydia resolution: A review of human studies. The Journal of Infectious Diseases. 15 Jun 2010;**201**(Supplement_2):S104-S113

[3] Lewis J, Price MJ, Horner PJ, White PJ. Genital *Chlamydia trachomatis* infections clear more slowly in men than women, but are less likely to become established. The Journal of Infectious Diseases. 2017;**216**(2):237-244

[4] Price MJ, Ades A, Angelis DD, Welton NJ, Macleod J, Soldan K, et al. Mixture-of-exponentials models to explain heterogeneity in studies of the duration of *Chlamydia trachomatis* infection. Statistics in Medicine. 2013;**32**(9):1547-1560

[5] Dunne EF, Gift TL, Stamm WE. What about the men? Sexually Transmitted Diseases. Nov 2008;**35**(11 Suppl)S:1-2

[6] Jensen KE, Thomsen LT, Schmiedel S, Frederiksen K, Norrild B, van den Brule A, et al. *Chlamydia trachomatis* and risk of cervical intraepithelial neoplasia grade 3 or worse in women with persistent human papillomavirus infection: A cohort study. Sexually Transmitted Infections. 2014;**90**(7):550-555

[7] Vriend HJ, Bogaards JA, van Bergen JE, Brink AA, van den Broek IV, Hoebe CJ, et al. Incidence and persistence of carcinogenic genital human papillomavirus infections in young women with or without *Chlamydia trachomatis* co-infection. Cancer Medicine. 2015;**4**(10):1589-1598

[8] Detels R, Green AM, Klausner JD, Katzenstein D, Gaydos C, Handsfield HH, et al. The incidence and correlates of symptomatic and asymptomatic *Chlamydia trachomatis* and *Neisseria gonorrhoeae* infections in selected populations in five countries. Sexually Transmitted Diseases. 2011;**38**(6):503

[9] Shipman SB, Risinger CR, Evans CM, Gilbertson CD, Hogan DE. High prevalence of sterile pyuria in the setting of sexually transmitted infection in women presenting to an emergency department. Western Journal of Emergency Medicine. 2018;**19**(2):282

[10] Tomas ME, Getman D, Donskey CJ, Hecker MT. Overdiagnosis of urinary tract infection and underdiagnosis of sexually transmitted infection in adult women presenting to an emergency department. Journal of Clinical Microbiology. 2015;**53**(8):2686-2692

[11] Lamontagne DS, Baster K, Emmett L, Nichols T, Randall S, McLean L, et al. Incidence and reinfection rates of genital chlamydial infection among women aged 16-24 years attending general practice, family planning and genitourinary medicine clinics in England: A prospective cohort study by the Chlamydia Recall Study Advisory Group. Sexually Transmitted Infections. 2007;**83**(4):292-303

[12] den Heijer CD, Hoebe CJ, Driessen JH, Wolffs P, van den Broek IV, Hoenderboom BM, et al. *Chlamydia trachomatis* and the risk of pelvic inflammatory disease, ectopic

pregnancy, and female infertility: A retrospective cohort study among primary care patients. Clinical Infectious Diseases. 2019;**69**(9):1517-1525

[13] Moreno V, Bosch FX, Muñoz N, Meijer CJ, Shah KV, Walboomers JM, et al. Effect of oral contraceptives on risk of cervical cancer in women with human papillomavirus infection: The IARC multicentric case-control study. The Lancet. 2002;**359**(9312):1085-1092

[14] Schachter J, Hill EC, King EB, Heilbron DC, Ray RM, Margolis AJ, et al. *Chlamydia trachomatis* and cervical neoplasia. JAMA. 1982;**248**(17):2134-2138

[15] Moscicki AB, Grubbs Burt V, Kanowitz S, Darragh T, Shiboski S. The significance of squamous metaplasia in the development of low grade squamous intraepithelial lesions in young women. Cancer. 1999;**85**(5):1139-1144

[16] Anttila T, Saikku P, Koskela P, Bloigu A, Dillner J, Ikäheimo I, et al. Serotypes of *Chlamydia trachomatis* and risk for development of cervical squamous cell carcinoma. JAMA. 2001;**285**(1):47-51

[17] Jha P, Beral V, Pike M, Hermon C, Peto J, Deacon J, et al. Antibodies to human papillomavirus and to other genital infectious agents and invasive cervical cancer risk. The Lancet. 1993;**341**(8853):1116-1119

[18] Wallin KL, Wiklund F, Luostarinen T, Ångström T, Anttila T, Bergman F, et al. A population-based prospective study of *Chlamydia trachomatis* infection and cervical carcinoma. International Journal of Cancer. 2002;**101**(4):371-374

[19] Castle PE, Hillier SL, Rabe LK, Hildesheim A, Herrero R, Bratti MC, et al. An association of cervical inflammation with high-grade cervical neoplasia in women infected with oncogenic human papillomavirus (HPV). Cancer Epidemiology Biomarkers & Prevention. 2001;**10**(10):1021-1027

[20] Fan T, Lu H, Hu H, Shi L, McClarty GA, Nance DM, et al. Inhibition of apoptosis in chlamydia-infected cells: Blockade of mitochondrial cytochrome c release and caspase activation. The Journal of Experimental Medicine. 1998;**187**(4):487-496

[21] Eckert L, Hawes S, Wölner-Hanssen P, Money D, Peeling R, Brunham R, et al. Prevalence and correlates of antibody to chlamydial heat shock protein in women attending sexually transmitted disease clinics and women with confirmed pelvic inflammatory disease. The Journal of Infectious Diseases. 1997;**175**(6):1453-1458

[22] Morris BJ, Rose BR. Cervical screening in the 21st century: The case for human papillomavirus testing of self-collected specimens. Clinical Chemistry and Laboratory Medicine. 2007;**45**(5):577-591

[23] Tubal infertility: serologic relationship to past chlamydial and gonococcal infection. World Health Organization Task Force on the Prevention and Management of Infertility. Sexually Transmitted Diseases. Mar-Apr 1995;**22**(2):71-77

[24] Hoenderboom BM, Van Benthem BH, Van Bergen JE, Dukers-Muijrers NH, Götz HM, Hoebe CJ, et al. Relation between *Chlamydia trachomatis* infection and pelvic inflammatory disease, ectopic pregnancy and tubal factor infertility in a Dutch cohort of women previously tested for chlamydia in a chlamydia screening trial. Sexually Transmitted Infections. 2019;**95**(4):300-306

[25] Akande V, Turner C, Horner P, Horne A, Pacey A, Society BF. Impact of *Chlamydia trachomatis* in the reproductive setting: British Fertility Society Guidelines for practice. Human Fertility. 2010;**13**(3):115-125

[26] Shi X, Liu F, Zhang H. Study of *Chlamydia trachomatis* infection on cervical secretion of women with early pregnancy and secondary sterility. Hunan yi ke da xue xue bao= Hunan yike daxue xuebao= Bulletin of Hunan Medical University. 2001;**26**(2):169-170

[27] Bender N, Herrmann B, Andersen B, Hocking JS, van Bergen J, Morgan J, et al. Chlamydia infection, pelvic inflammatory disease, ectopic pregnancy and infertility: Cross-national study. Sexually Transmitted Infections. 2011;**87**(7):601-608

[28] Peter NG, Clark LR, Jaeger JR. Fitz-Hugh-Curtis syndrome: A diagnosis to consider in women with right upper quadrant pain. Cleveland Clinic Journal of Medicine. 2004;**71**(3):233-241

[29] Theofanakis CP, Kyriakidis A. Fitz-Hugh–Curtis syndrome. Gynecological Surgery. 2011;**8**:129-134

[30] de Vrieze NH, de Vries HJ. Lymphogranuloma venereum among men who have sex with men. An epidemiological and clinical review. Expert Review of Anti-Infective Therapy. 2014;**12**(6):697-704

[31] Høie S, Knudsen LS, Gerstoft J. Lymphogranuloma venereum proctitis: A differential diagnose to inflammatory bowel disease. Scandinavian Journal of Gastroenterology. 2011;**46**(4):503-510

[32] Stoner BP, Cohen SE. Lymphogranuloma venereum 2015: Clinical presentation, diagnosis, and treatment. Clinical Infectious Diseases. 2015;**61**(Suppl 8):S865-S873

[33] Rank RG, Yeruva L. An alternative scenario to explain rectal positivity in Chlamydia-infected individuals. Clinical Infectious Diseases. 2015;**60**(10):1585-1586

[34] Meyer T, Buder S. The laboratory diagnosis of *Neisseria gonorrhoeae*: Current testing and future demands. Pathogens. 2020;**9**(2):91

[35] Sarier M, Duman İ, Göktaş Ş, Demir M, Kukul E. Results of multiplex polymerase chain reaction assay to identify urethritis pathogens. Journal of Urological Surgery. 2017;**1**:18-22. DOI: 10.4274/jus.1328)

[36] Malhotra M, Sood S, Mukherjee A, Muralidhar S, Bala M. Genital chlamydia trachomatis: An update. The Indian Journal of Medical Research. 2013;**138**(3):303

[37] Rodríguez-Granger J, López BE, Cobo F, Morente GB, Martinez AS, Sánchez JT, et al. Update on the diagnosis of sexually transmitted infections. Actas Dermo-Sifiliográficas (English Edition). 2020;**111**(9):711-724

[38] Schachter J, McCormack WM, Chernesky MA, Martin DH, Van Der Pol B, Rice PA, et al. Vaginal swabs are appropriate specimens for diagnosis of genital tract infection with *Chlamydia trachomatis*. Journal of Clinical Microbiology. 2003;**41**(8):3784-3789

[39] Davies B, Turner KM, Benfield T, Frølund M, Andersen B, Westh H, et al. Pelvic inflammatory disease risk following negative results from chlamydia nucleic acid amplification tests (NAATs) versus non-NAATs in Denmark: A retrospective cohort. PLoS Medicine. 2018;**15**(1):e1002483

[40] Geisler WM. Diagnosis and management of uncomplicated *Chlamydia trachomatis* infections in adolescents and adults: Summary of evidence reviewed for the 2010 Centers for Disease Control and Prevention sexually transmitted diseases treatment guidelines. Clinical Infectious Diseases. 2011;**53**(Suppl 3):S92-S98

[41] Cook RL, Hutchison SL, Østergaard L, Braithwaite RS, Ness RB. Systematic review: Noninvasive testing for *Chlamydia trachomatis* and *Neisseria gonorrhoeae*. Annals of Internal Medicine. 2005;**142**(11):914-925

[42] Gaydos CA, Van Der Pol B, Jett-Goheen M, Barnes M, Quinn N, Clark C, et al. Performance of the cepheid CT/NG Xpert rapid PCR test for detection of *Chlamydia trachomatis* and *Neisseria gonorrhoeae*. Journal of Clinical Microbiology. 2013;**51**(6):1666-1672

[43] Hosenfeld CB, Workowski KA, Berman S, Zaidi A, Dyson J, Mosure D, et al. Repeat infection with chlamydia and gonorrhea among females: A systematic review of the literature. Sexually Transmitted Diseases. 2009;**36**(8):478-489

[44] Verkooyen R, Willemse D, Hiep-van Casteren S, Mousavi Joulandan S, Snijder R, Van den Bosch J, et al. Evaluation of PCR, culture, and serology for diagnosis of *Chlamydia pneumoniae* respiratory infections. Journal of Clinical Microbiology. 1998;**36**(8):2301-2307

[45] Keltz MD, Gera PS, Moustakis M. Chlamydia serology screening in infertility patients. Fertility and Sterility. 2006;**85**(3):752-754

[46] Meyer T. Diagnostic procedures to detect *Chlamydia trachomatis* infections. Microorganisms. 2016;**4**(3):25

[47] Tuuminen T, Palomäki P, Paavonen J. The use of serologic tests for the diagnosis of chlamydial infections. Journal of Microbiological Methods. 2000;**42**(3):265-279

[48] Rose SB, Garrett SM, Stanley J, Pullon SRH. Retesting and repeat positivity following diagnosis of *Chlamydia trachomatis* and *Neisseria gonorrhoea* in New Zealand: A retrospective cohort study. BMC Infectious Diseases. 2017;**17**(1):526

[49] Batteiger BE, Tu W, Ofner S, Van Der Pol B, Stothard DR, Orr DP, et al. Repeated *Chlamydia trachomatis* genital infections in adolescent women. The Journal of Infectious Diseases. 2010;**201**(1):42-51

[50] Lanjouw E, Ouburg S, De Vries H, Stary A, Radcliffe K, Unemo M. 2015 European guideline on the management of *Chlamydia trachomatis* infections. International Journal of STD & AIDS. 2016;**27**(5):333-348

[51] Mishori R, McClaskey EL, WinklerPrins V. *Chlamydia trachomatis* infections: Screening, diagnosis, and management. American Family Physician. 2012;**86**(12):1127-1132

[52] Wyrick PB. *Chlamydia trachomatis* persistence in vitro: An overview. The Journal of Infectious Diseases. 2010;**201**(Suppl 2):S88-S95

[53] Wang SA, Papp JR, Stamm WE, Peeling RW, Martin DH, Holmes KK. Evaluation of antimicrobial resistance and treatment failures for *Chlamydia trachomatis*: A meeting report. The Journal of Infectious Diseases. 2005;**191**(6):917-923

[54] Suchland R, Geisler W, Stamm WE. Methodologies and cell lines used for antimicrobial susceptibility testing of

Chlamydia spp. Antimicrobial Agents and Chemotherapy. 2003;**47**(2):636-642

[55] Nwokolo NC, Dragovic B, Patel S, Tong CW, Barker G, Radcliffe K. 2015 UK national guideline for the management of infection with *Chlamydia trachomatis*. International Journal of STD & AIDS. 2016;**27**(4):251-267

[56] Workowski KA, Berman S; Centers for Disease Control and Prevention (CDC). Sexually transmitted diseases treatment guidelines, 2010. MMWR Recommendations and Reports. 17 Dec 2010;**59**(RR-12):1-110

[57] Hsu K. Treatment of *Chlamydia trachomatis* infection. In: Post TW, editor. UpToDate. Waltham, MA: UpToDate; 2020

[58] Hafner L, Timms P. Development status and future prospects for a vaccine against Chlamydia trachomatis infection. Vaccine. 20 Mar 2014;**32**(14):1563-1571

[59] Morré SA, Peña AS. An integrated approach to the understanding of Chlamydia infections: Introduction to the 2009 update. Drugs of Today. 2009;**45**(11):3

[60] Geisler WM, Uniyal A, Lee JY, Lensing SY, Johnson S, Perry RC, et al. Azithromycin versus doxycycline for urogenital chlamydia trachomatis infection. New England Journal of Medicine. 2015;**373**(26):2512-2521

[61] Bhengraj AR, Vardhan H, Srivastava P, Salhan S, Mittal A. Decreased susceptibility to azithromycin and doxycycline in clinical isolates of *Chlamydia trachomatis* obtained from recurrently infected female patients in India. Chemotherapy. 2010;**56**(5):371-377

[62] Dukers-Muijrers NH, Wolffs PF, De Vries H, Götz HM, Heijman T, Bruisten S, et al. Treatment effectiveness of azithromycin and doxycycline in uncomplicated rectal and vaginal *Chlamydia trachomatis* infections in women: A multicenter observational study (FemCure). Clinical Infectious Diseases. 2019;**69**(11):1946-1954

[63] Mikamo H, Sato Y, Hayasaki Y, Hua YX, Tamaya T. Adequate levofloxacin treatment schedules for uterine cervicitis caused by *Chlamydia trachomatis*. Chemotherapy. 2000;**46**(2):150-152

[64] Mikamo H, Sato Y, Hayasaki Y, Tamaya T. Adequate macrolide treatment schedules for uterine cervicitis caused by *Chlamydia trachomatis*. Chemotherapy. 1999;**45**(5):396-398

[65] Deguchi T, Hatazaki K, Ito S, Kondo H, Horie K, Nakane K, et al. Macrolide and fluoroquinolone resistance is uncommon in clinical strains of *Chlamydia trachomatis*. Journal of Infection and Chemotherapy. 2018;**24**(8):610-614

[66] Yokoi S, Yasuda M, Ito S-I, Takahashi Y, Ishihara S, Deguchi T, et al. Uncommon occurrence of fluoroquinolone resistance-associated alterations in GyrA and ParC in clinical strains of *Chlamydia trachomatis*. Journal of Infection and Chemotherapy. 2004;**10**(5):262-267

[67] Cramers M, Kaspersen P, From E, Møller B. Pivampicillin compared with erythromycin for treating women with genital *Chlamydia trachomatis* infection. Sexually Transmitted Infections. 1988;**64**(4):247-248

[68] How SJ, Hobson D, Hart CA, Webster RE. An in-vitro investigation of synergy and antagonism between antimicrobials against *Chlamydia trachomatis*. Journal of Antimicrobial Chemotherapy. 1985;**15**(5):533-538

Chapter 17

Organizational and Socio-Psychological Difficulties of Management of Patients with Chlamydia Infection

Anna Fedorova

Abstract

Lack of detection of chlamydia infection does not correspond to the high prevalence of its clinical manifestations. It is associated with a frequent asymptomatic course, the prevalence of persistent forms of infection and difficulties in their diagnosis. Unification of approaches to diagnosis and therapy of chlamydial infections without taking into account the topical diagnosis leads to insufficient therapy. It is difficult to find a balance between the need for long-term antibiotic therapy for chlamydial persistence and the dangers of its consequences. Difficulties in the treatment of chlamydia infection are also associated with socio-psychological factors: low efficiency and even inexpediency of etiotropic therapy of chlamydia in polygamous relationships, promiscuous behavior; poor synchronization of partner therapy, often treating only one partner in a couple; orientation of patients towards short-term "pill" therapy, which is not sufficiently effective for chronic persistent chlamydia with significant morphological changes in the genitals; low compliance of male partners to therapy in a couple "by contact" in the absence of clinically apparent manifestations; peculiarities of public consciousness regarding chlamydia infection. As a result, therapy often only stops exacerbations of inflammation and does not eliminate the infection completely.

Keywords: chlamydiosis, persistent form of chlamydia infection, biopsychosocial approach to chlamydia, management of patients, socio-psychological problems

1. Introduction

Genital infection caused by Chlamydia trachomatis is considered one of the most common sexually transmitted infections in the world. C. trachomatis is an obligate intracellular parasite with a unique intracellular development cycle. The peculiarities of the pathogen itself, the imperfection of the immune response to it, and the characteristic course of the disease determine the difficulties of its diagnosis and treatment.

Chlamydia infection is asymptomatic in most cases, more than 2/3 of women and men. Symptoms of the acute form of the disease (short-term urethritis, moderate discharge) often go unnoticed. This is the reason for the late visit to the doctor and the widespread spread of infection. Without timely and adequate therapy, the infection becomes a chronic persistent form.

Persistent chlamydia infection is widespread and presents the greatest difficulties for doctors. It is associated with a large number of diseases accompanied by chronic inflammation and fibrosis—chronic cervicitis and salpingitis, chronic recurrent urethritis, including "postcoital" urethritis in women, chronic prostatitis, chronic epididymitis, and orchoepididymitis. Clinical manifestations are poorly expressed, or absent altogether, or appear only with exacerbations. As the infection exists, fibrosis processes occur with the formation of adhesions in the appendages of the uterus and pelvis, intrauterine synechiae, and sclerosing processes of the male genital sphere. Pronounced dysfunctional changes in the anti-infective protection system can lead to the translocation of chlamydia from the genitourinary tract to the extra-genital areas of the body. Fibrous changes can hinder the development of the acute phase of inflammation, but lead to infertility in both women (violation of the patency of the fallopian tubes, miscarriage of pregnancy) and men (violations of the morphology and function of sperm), to the formation of chronic pelvic pain syndrome.

Chronic endometritis is also a frequent cause of infertility. Nowadays, it is a widespread disease. It is thought to occur in ¼ of women [1]. Currently, there is no definitive opinion on the role of bacterial factor and chlamydia inclusive in the development and maintenance of chronic endometritis. However, clinical practice gives us some evidence of their important role. Some evidence-based studies show an increase in the frequency of implantation and an improvement in reproductive outcomes in assisted reproductive technology programs after antibiotic therapy [2, 3].

Patients' subjective underestimation of their condition is one of the reasons for the late detection of chlamydia infection. Often, it is diagnosed only when a woman applies for infertility, miscarriage, or other chronic conditions, and men are examined as a partner. As a result, most men and women with chlamydia infection go to the doctor already with the development of deep lesions of the genital area, pronounced adhesive processes, with decompensation of the body's defense mechanisms. The detection of chlamydia infection by routine methods may be difficult at this stage, and it remains unrecognized.

In clinical practice, the physician is faced with a mismatch between the widespread clinical and anatomical manifestation characteristic of chlamydia and its low detectability [4–6]. It can be assumed that this occurs against the background of an increase in the frequency of persistent species C. trachomatis, which develops primarily due to irrational antibiotic therapy [6].

2. Diagnostic methods and detectability of chlamydia infection in the light of a socio-psychological approach

Laboratory diagnostic method of chlamydia infection is of paramount importance due to the frequent absence of specific clinical manifestations. The gold standard for the diagnosis of chlamydia infection is currently considered to be the nucleic acid amplification test (NAAT), which is positioned as highly sensitive (99%) and specific (WHO 2016). Its undoubted advantages are accessibility, speed, and the possibility of mass examination of a large group of patients. The quality of diagnostics depends on the quality of test systems used, the quality of sampling, and storage of biomaterial.

Other diagnostic methods are culture, direct fluorescence of antibodies, enzyme immunoassay, and immunohistochemical assays.

The cultural method, previously considered a reference due to its high specificity, has receded into the background. This is due to the labor intensity, high cost, strict rules for the transportation of clinical samples, high requirements for the qualification of medical personnel, as well as low sensitivity (33–85%). The detection rate of chlamydia is low in inactive stage and chronic ascending infection. Currently, it is not used in routine diagnostics, but is carried out mainly for special indication.

The method of direct immunofluorescence of antibodies is highly specific, fast, but "good in the right hands." It depends on the quality of the test systems used, the quality of biomaterial sampling, and requires high professionalism of a specialist in luminescent microscopy. This method is highly sensitive and highly specific mainly when performed correctly by an experienced laboratory technician. Otherwise, it is impossible to exclude both false-positive and false-negative results of the study.

Enzyme immunoassay determines the presence and titer in the blood of antibodies to chlamydia—Ig G, Ig M, Ig A. It allows us to find out the stages and nature of the course of infection, its activity. However, chlamydia antigens have weak immunogenicity, so the production and accumulation of antibodies to them occur in small quantities. Antibodies to chlamydia are found only in about half of patients. The absence of immunoglobulins does not allow us to talk about the absence of chlamydia infection in the body. If only Ig G to chlamydia is detected, it is impossible to diagnose an existing disease, but only to assert that the body has met with the pathogen. Enzyme immunoassay may be appropriate for verification of persistent infection.

All these methods are among the additional ones and in most countries are not included in the most common health insurance programs. The clinical guidelines recommend a single method, nucleic acid amplification test (NAAT), for suspected chlamydial urogenital infections. It is positioned as highly sensitive and highly specific, and available and adequate. Has the problem of diagnosis of chlamydia infection been solved?

Unfortunately, it is not that simple. The detectability of chlamydia infection has sharply decreased with the transition exclusively to the NAAT method. This is particularly true in cases of ascending infection, chronic persistent course, and fibrosis processes in women (chronic cervicitis and endometritis, adhesions in the pelvis, obstruction of the fallopian tubes, reproductive losses). Many researchers note the difficulties when diagnosing widespread forms of chlamydia infection with a prolonged, recurrent nature of the course. Persistent forms of chlamydia are difficult to verify by microbiological methods due to changes in metabolism and antigenic structure. The pathogen is often inaccessible for diagnosis in complicated ascending infection. In these cases, in order to reliably verify the pathogen, it is necessary to expand the list of clinical specimens obtained not only from the cervical canal and urethra, but also from other organs.

An important diagnostic criterion may be an enzyme immunoassay that determines antibodies to chlamydia in the blood. Unfortunately, a suppressed immune response may also limit the possibilities of serodiagnosis. Against this background, the focus of specialists has shifted toward viruses, bacterial films, and non-specific opportunistic flora identified in such patients. However, the possibility of a chronic persistent chlamydial infection undetected by NAAT cannot be excluded. The latter assumption may be supported by cases of C. trachomatis isolation in such patients using a culture method and its detection also by a culture method in partners. In clinical practice, patients with recurrent exacerbations of chronic genital inflammatory diseases and negative NAAT of urethral and cervical duct material are often found to have C. trachomatis Ig A, indicating an active course of chlamydial infection,

C. trachomatis Ig G, and C. trachomatis heat shock protein Ig G (cHSP60) in their blood by enzyme immunoassay [6, 7].

The problems of diagnosing chlamydia infection are related to the fact that there is currently no unified algorithm for examining patients with suspected chronic, persistent chlamydia infection. It is this form that occurs most often. A comprehensive competent approach to the diagnosis of chlamydia using several methods and a scientifically based assessment of the results obtained may be optimal. Detection of chlamydia, determination of the nature of the infectious and inflammatory process, and the extend of the lesion are important for the correct choice of therapy.

What happens in practice? The possibilities of using the entire set of tests for the diagnosis of chlamydia infection are small. This is expensive, not covered by health insurance programs. Doctors who work in insurance medicine cannot use additional tests if the NAAT test is negative. Ethical and financial problems are also important. Is it ethical to offer patients additional tests if they are not included in clinical guidelines, there are no other approved algorithms of examination in chronic ascending processes, and NAAT methods are positioned as highly effective?

It is also worth noting the psychological problems of patients. When several diagnostic tests are used and a chlamydial infection is found in only one of them or in only one of the partners, questions almost always arise. Why focus on tests that show the presence of a chlamydial infection and not those that do not? Why was one partner diagnosed with chlamydia, and the other did not? What does all this mean? These questions cause patients to doubt the correctness of the diagnosis, the competence of the physician and medicine in general, and difficulties in achieving compliance with the physician about the therapy. The result can be refusal of therapy, violation of doctor's recommendations, development of stress and anxiety disorders in patients, conflicts between partners (each may have his own opinion and his own motivation for treatment), and lack of faith in the cure.

3. Problems of therapy of chlamydia infection

Research in recent years recommends that in the treatment of chronic inflammatory diseases of the genitals, efforts should be directed toward the elimination of pathogens instead of the classical empirical prescription of broad-spectrum antibiotics [8]. This is especially true for chlamydial infections. Analysis of the problems of diagnosis of chlamydia infection clearly shows that the prevalence of chlamydia infection, especially chronic persistent forms of it, is much wider than the results of the NAAT examination show. This is reflected in the choice of therapy and its results. Patients with chronic inflammatory diseases of the genital area and undiagnosed chlamydia infection either do not receive therapy or receive insufficiently adequate therapy. The use of broad-spectrum antibiotics capable of penetrating cells in the treatment of such cases to a certain extent makes it possible to compensate for diagnostic deficiencies. However, antibiotic therapy is not sufficiently effective in cases of persistent forms of chlamydia. Other factors are also important.

Chlamydiosis is a sexually transmitted disease. It requires the treatment of both partners, the use of protection during sexual intercourse until both partners are tested negative for chlamydia. There are no such requirements for the treatment of genital inflammatory processes caused presumably by viruses and opportunistic microorganisms. In undiagnosed chlamydial infections, renewed sexual contact with a previous partner or partners leads to reinfection after therapy.

DOI: http://dx.doi.org/10.5772/intechopen.109748

Another problem of chlamydia therapy is associated with the tendency to unify therapeutic approaches without taking into account the topical diagnosis, and pathoanatomic and clinical features of the course of the disease. The Clinical Guidelines for the treatment of chlamydia indicates the sufficiency of prescribing 1 g of azithromycin once or 200 mg of doxycycline for 7–10 days. The efficacy of such therapy in a long-standing chlamydial process with chronic inflammation and fibrosis is unlikely, and diagnostic problems often do not allow this to be seen.

Analysis of the clinical studies shows that researchers pay little attention to the comparison of the choice of an antibacterial drug, the duration and regimen of its administration, and the possibility of reinfection in the treatment of chlamydial infection [9]. The difficulties of such a comparative analysis can be explained not only by the different clinical course of chlamydial infections, but also by various socio-psychological factors.

The sexually transmissible nature of chlamydial infections dictates that sexual partners must be examined and treated. Examination of partners is necessary regardless of the presence or absence of complaints and clinical symptoms. It is optimal not only to try to identify the pathogen, but also to clarify the clinical form, the presence of structural changes, and assess the duration of persistence of the infection. This is necessary for the correct choice of the duration and composition of therapy. Treatment of sexual partners is advisable even in cases where chlamydia is not detected ("contact therapy"). It is highly probable that in these cases there is a chronic ascending infection, a persistence of chlamydia, which requires more attention. Often, however, the partners are examined formally or not at all. They are given a short course of antibiotics without regard to the nature of the process. Such treatment "by contact" may not be effective enough. It does not eliminate the chronic infection, but rather turns it into a chronic form.

4. Socio-psychological and partner problems of chlamydia infection therapy

The most difficult and intractable are the socio-psychological and partnership problems of chlamydia infection therapy. Therapy of chlamydial infection is carried out on the principle of voluntariness. Patients may not follow the recommendations. Sexual partners often shy away from examination and treatment, especially if they have no clinically expressed complaints, they are not interested in therapy and have other sexual contacts.

Many patients have their own understanding of the disease and its impact on health, their own past individual experiences of sexuality and treatment, and their own vision of therapy. It is purely subjective and often determined by motives other than maintaining health. Chlamydia infection is widely discussed on the Internet and everyone can find confirmation of their views. The notion that today's evolving pharmacotherapy can easily and quickly solve any problem is strong. There is a lot of information about the negative impact of antibacterial therapy on the immune system, liver function. As a result, many patients are focused on a short course of antibacterial therapy and expect a guaranteed cure. The need for a deeper examination and long-term treatment for fibrotic processes is not understood by either patients or health care organizers. In the current situation, doctors have to find a satisfactory balance in each case among the expediency of a full-fledged examination, the duration of antibacterial therapy for chlamydia persistence, and the widely discussed negative consequences of antibiotic therapy, between their professional views and perceptions and fears of the patient to achieve compliance.

It may be difficult to cooperate with a specialist who is treating a sexual partner due to individual differences in views on the clinical situation. Unified approaches to the diagnosis and therapy of chlamydia infection, on the one hand, help when working with a partner couple (e.g., they position the mandatory treatment of a partner when a chlamydia infection is detected) and, on the other hand, limit the possibilities of an individual approach. For example, complex treatment of a patient with chronic long-term chlamydia infection may be useless if the partner is not examined, receives only a short course of antibiotics, does not take medications, or does not use protection against STIs.

Etiotropic therapy of chlamydia infection is not very effective in polygamous relationships. Promiscuity behavior is quite widespread among young people. The search for a variety of sexual experiences, the constant change of partners, and the predominance of relaxation motives often precede the establishment of a partner sexual relationship. During this period, the correct and consistent use of protective equipment (condoms) is important. Unfortunately, condoms are often used from time to time or incorrectly [10]. The main focus of the partners is on HIV prevention, everything else is considered irrelevant. If a man or woman is subjectively convinced that his or her partner is not HIV-positive, condoms can stop being used.

Men are often not interested in the examination and treatment of STIs, which are asymptomatic. There is an opinion that chlamydia infection is widespread, there is a high probability of infection when changing partners, so it is inexpedient to be examined and treated only after establishing monogamous partnerships and planning a pregnancy. This pattern is supported by the common notion that a chlamydial infection can be easily cured by taking 1 g of azithromycin.

Therapy of chronic chlamydia infection is difficult in couples in which at least one partner has other sexual contacts and plans to keep them. A full-fledged examination and therapy of all patients from the chain of contacts, as a rule, is unrealistic.

It is necessary to take into account some features of public consciousness regarding chlamydia infection. Among them are two opposing views "chlamydia cannot be completely cured, chlamydia remains" and "a short course of antibiotics is enough to guarantee a cure." Both of these views prevent the responsible implementation of the doctor's recommendations.

Chlamydia is a common cause of reproductive dysfunction. Traditionally, concern for reproductive health is more characteristic of women. They visit a gynecologist more often than men visit an urologist, conduct examinations more often, and are more focused on conducting therapy. Less interest of men and their resistance can nullify the therapeutic efforts of a couple.

5. Conclusion

Successful management of chlamydia is possible only with its timely and complete detection.

The peculiarities of the clinical course of chlamydia infection, the difficulties of its diagnosis, and therapy in chronic persistent forms determine the difficulties of patient curation.

The prevalence of chlamydial infection, especially its persistent forms, is probably much higher than its detection rate.

A standardized approach to diagnosis and therapy is optimal for acute chlamydia infection.

The tactics of examination and treatment of patients with chronic persistent forms are not systematized, not generalized, and require a personalized approach. The latter is complicated, associated with high material costs, and may be insufficiently effective due to a number of socio-psychological and partner factors. The current practice of managing patients is aimed more at controlling exacerbations of chlamydial infection than at eliminating it.

The affective control of the spread of chlamydia infection requires raising public awareness about its nature, clinical manifestations, consequences, diagnostic capabilities, and preventive measures.

Simple educational activities about the importance and rules of condom use—counseling, broader educational programs aimed at individuals or couples—are appropriate. These can raise awareness and promote consistent use. Communication training on sex education and teaching young people and adolescents how to resist provocative offers of sex without a condom can also be useful [9].

An important direction may be the reorientation of the doctor-patient interaction model from a biomedical health model to a biopsychosocial one, in which the patient is informed and consciously makes decisions regarding his health. This will require improving the communication competence of health care workers to achieve the necessary result.

Author details

Anna Fedorova
Mechnikov North-Western State Medical University, Saint Petersburg, Russia

*Address all correspondence to: feanna@inbox.ru

References

[1] Song D, Feng X, Zhang Q, et al. Prevalence and confounders of chronic endometritis in premenopausal women with abnormal bleeding or reproductive failure. Reproductive Biomedicine Online. 2018;**36**:78-83. DOI: 10.1016/j.rbmo.2017.09.008

[2] Puente E, Alonso L, Laganà AS, et al. Chronic Endometritis: Old problem, novel insights and future challenges. Int J Fertil Steril. 2020;**13**(4):250-256. DOI: 10.22074/ijfs.2020.577921

[3] Di Speizio SA, Palma F, Calagna G, et al. Chronic Endometritis. In: Genital Infections and Infertility. London: IntechOpen; 2016. DOI: 10.5772/63023

[4] Fedorova AI, Novikov EI, Grin EA, Myagkov AE, Koptelova AI. The role of chronic cervicitis and disorders of local immunity of the cervix in the etiology of undeveloped pregnancy. Gynecology. 2021;**23**(6):509-515. DOI: 10.26442/20795696.2021.6.201259

[5] Bradshaw CS, Tabrizi SN, Read TR, Garland SM, Hopkins CA, Moss LM, et al. Etiologies of nongonococcal urethritis: Bacteria, virus- es, and the association with orogenital ex- posure. The Journal of Infectious Diseases. 2006;**193**(3):336-345. DOI: 10.1086/499434

[6] Molochkov VA, Aleshkin VA, Skirda TA, Karaulov AV, Molochkova JV, Antonova EV, et al. On the assessment and the treatment of patients in persistent urogenital chlamydiosis. Almanac of Clinical Medicine. 2016;**44**(1):114-120. DOI: 10.18786/2072-0505-2016-44-1-114-120

[7] Witkin SS, Jeremias J, Toth M, Ledger WJ. Proliferative response to conserved epitopes of the *chlamydia trachomatis* and human 60-kilodalton heat-shock proteins by lymphocytes from women with salpingitis. American Journal of Obstetrics and Gynecology. 1994;**171**:455-460

[8] Sarier M, Kukul E. Classification of non-gonococcal urethritis: A review. International Urology and Nephrology. 2019;**51**:901-907. DOI: 10.1007/s11255-019-02140-2

[9] Páez-Canro C, Alzat JP, González LM, Rubio-Romero JA, Lethaby A, Gaitan HG. Antibiotics for treating urogenital *chlamydia trachomatis* infection in men and non-pregnant women. Cochrane Database of Systematic Reviews. 2019;**1**:CD010871. DOI: 10.1002/14651858.CD010871.pub2

[10] Lopez LM, Otterness C, Chen M, Steiner M, Gallo MF. Behavioral interventions for improving condom use for dual protection. Cochrane Database of Systematic Reviews. 2013;**2013**:CD010662

Chapter 18

Chlamydia: The Female Reproductive System and Infertility

Alev Özlem Özdemir-Karabağ

Abstract

Chlamydial infection can cause diseases in many organs, including the genitourinary system. It is the most reported sexually transmitted bacterial infection throughout the world and one of the leading cause of female infertility. Chlamydia affects columnar epithelium, so adolescent women are particularly at risk since the squamocolumnar junction is located on the ectocervix until early adulthood. The bacterium is usually transmitted through sexual activity. Genital tract infection is the most common clinical picture but 50% of infected men and 80% of infected women are asymptomatic. This is the most important reason for the infection's being unrecognized and untreated. The most significant morbidity related to infection is partial or total sterility due to obstruction and scarring of the fallopian tubes. *Chlamydia trachomatis* infection, even if it does not present clinical symptoms, has been shown to be associated with increased tubal factor infertility, implantation failure, and disruption of embryo development.

Keywords: *Chlamydia trachomatis* infection, sexually transmitted diseases, PID, female infertility, tubal factor infertility

1. Introduction

Chlamydias are small gram-negative, obligate intracellular living microorganisms, preferably infecting squamocolumnar epithelial cells. The microorganisms can be divided into two subtypes as Chlamydia (e.g., *C. trachomatis*) and Chlamydophila (e.g., *Chlamydophila pneumoniae* and *Chlamydophila psittaci*). *C. trachomatis* is divided into 19 different serological variants (A, B/Ba, C, D/Da, E, F, G/Ga, H, I/Ia, J, K, L1, L2, L2a, and L3) according to monoclonal antibody-based analyses and variants that are classified according to ompA genotyping. Of these, types A, B, Ba, and C are the causative agents of Trachoma, an endemic serious eye disease in Africa and Asia; D-C strains lead to genital tract infections. L1-L3 strains cause Lymphogranuloma venereum disease, which is especially seen in tropical countries and is characterized by genital ulcers [1].

Chlamydia can affect various organs, and the genitourinary system is one of the major sites of this infection. It can cause clinical conditions in nasopharynx, epididymis, urethra, cervix, uterus, and salpinx [2–4]. It is the most reported sexually transmitted bacterial infection and one of the major causes of female infertility. This infection also leads to conjunctivitis, pneumonia, afebrile pneumonia syndrome (in vaginally born babies from infected mothers), and trachoma, a leading cause of

 IntechOpen

acquired blindness in the world and perihepatitis condition also known as Fitz-Hugh-Curtis syndrome [5].

There are one million sexually transmitted disease transmissions every day in the world [6]. The annual number of *C. trachomatis* genital infections reached 4 million annually in 2018, up from about 2.86 million cases in 2008 [7]. Research shows similar incidences in Germany [8], France [9], the Netherlands [10], New Zealand [11], and Australia [12]. In a report by the World Health Organization (WHO) Initiative for Vaccine Research (IVR) it is estimated that there are more than 140 million cases of *C. trachomatis* infection worldwide [13]. Chlamydia carrier rates in the sexually active female population are around 20%. This ratio is 2–3 times higher than the N. gonorrhea incidence.

2. Pathophysiology

Chlamydia affects columnar epithelium, so adolescent women are particularly at risk since the squamocolumnar junction is located on the ectocervix until early adulthood. Chlamydia has extraordinary features regarding its life cycle. It has two different forms in the course of infection in both intracellular and extracellular environments. The elementary body (EB) is the infectious form existing in the extracellular space; it is a spore-like, inactive structure that enters the host cell. Inside the cell, it turns into an active form called a reticulate body (RB). The RB uses the host cell's amino acids and the energy sources in the form of ATP to synthesize its own DNA, RNA, and proteins to replicate and after enough RBs have formed, some of them turn back to the EB form, which can then exit the initial host cell and infect others. This cycle is then repeated in the adjacent cells [14, 15]. Thus, this process creates an immunogenic environment around the infection. However, there are ways for *C. trachomatis* to escape and evade the immune system. For example, by preventing T-cell immune recognition, it down-regulates the major histocompatibility complexes I and II; it modulates some specific cytokines, such as beta interferon, type 1 interferons, interleukin 18 and, inhibits apoptosis by the secretion of Chlamydial protease-like activity factor proteins and enhancing cell survival signals. By this way, it creates a chronic inflammation that allows the infection to become persistent. Replication mechanisms that adapt to the environment during the biphasic development cycle and evolutionary defense mechanisms that allow to escape from the immune system and environmental inflammatory stress are also challenging obstacles to infection treatment and vaccine development [16]. Still, with advances *in silico* studies using bioinformatics tools and machine learning-based modeling, Shiragannavar and his colleagues, have succeeded in developing a candidate vaccine that stimulates T and B cells in a way that provides long-term immunity [17]. There are also other vaccine candidates that use immune and proteomic approaches as well as *in silico* methods [18].

The bacterium is usually transmitted through sexual activity. The risk of an infected man infecting an uninfected woman with each sexual contact is 25%. Chlamydia can also spread vertically. The risk of transmission from the infected mother to the newborn is around 50–60%, and in most cases, the neonatal infection is in the form of conjunctivitis or pneumonia. (In 10–20% of cases, in the form of Afebrile Pneumonia Syndrome).

Genital tract infection is the most common clinical picture. The incubation period is around 1–3 weeks. In total, 50% of infected men and 80% of infected women are asymptomatic. But the infection can cause mucopurulent cervicitis in women, and it can lead to urethritis in men [19]. Ascending infection can result in the development of PID in women and is the most common cause of epididymitis in men under 35 years of age. In total, 5–10% of women who have had PID may progress to perihepatitis also known as Fitz-Hugh-Curtis syndrome.

Although the presence of any STD in one patient increases the likelihood of coinfection with another STD, the most common coinfection in such a case is the combination of Chlamydia and Gonorrhea. In total, 40% of women and 20% of men with chlamydia infection are coinfected with gonorrhea [20, 21]. Other pathogens that can cause coinfection with Chlamydia are *Mycoplasma genitalium* [22, 23] and HPV [24, 25] possibly causing an association between cervical intraepithelial neoplasia and Chlamydia [26]. The frequency of Reiter's syndrome (reactive arthritis, conjunctivitis, and urethritis) in patients with chlamydia is also increased compared to the normal population. LGV cases are the reason for 10% of genital ulcers in tropical countries. In the course of a LGV case, localized inguinal lymphadenopathy and ulceration develop within 2–12 hf after exposure to infection. In untreated cases, proctitis, rectal strictures, and elephantiasis secondary to lymphatic obstruction may occur.

3. Etiology

C. trachomatis transmission occurs with direct contact, this includes the vaginal, anal, or oral sexual routes and vertical transmission to the newborn from an infected mother during vaginal birth.

Specific risk factors for the chlamydial infection are 15–24 years of age, poor socioeconomic conditions, multiple sexual partners, exchange of sex for money, intercourse without a barrier contraceptive, current coinfection with another STD, or a history of previous STD, certain cytokine polymorphisms that are related to severe disease and the risk of tubal factor infertility [27], specific variants in Toll-like receptor 1 and 4 genes creating infection predisposition [28].

4. Prognosis

Antibiotic therapy is 95% effective as a first-line treatment. If treatment is started early and fully completed, the prognosis is good. Although treatment failure with first-line treatments is quite rare, recurrences may occur with alternative treatments. Reinfection is very frequent, either because the partner is not treated or because it is reacquired from a new partner. Therefore, treatment of all possible sexual partners is mandatory.

Abscess rupture due to salpingitis and progression to tubo-ovarian abscess and death due to peritonitis are rare. Chlamydia is an indirect cause of ectopic pregnancy-related deaths. Death due to ectopic pregnancy caused by chlamydia is more likely than deaths due to tubo-ovarian abscess.

5. Clinic considerations

In Chlamydia, due to the asymptomatic course of the infection, diagnosis can usually be delayed until discovery of a symptomatic partner or a positive screening result. Therefore, the chlamydia screening programs, which have been shown to reduce PID rates [29, 30], can be claimed to be necessary for the timely diagnosis and treatment of this infection.

Despite this mostly asymptomatic course, *C.trachomatis* can cause a broad range of urogenital diseases, including cervicitis, endometritis, salpingitis, pelvic inflammatory disease, urethritis, prostatitis, epididymitis, lymphogranuloma venereum; and extragenital diseases like conjunctivitis, pharyngitis, reactive arthritis, proctitis, and neonatal pneumonia. Asymptomatic men and women act as reservoirs for the infection. In a previous study, the rate of transmission was estimated to be 68% both for women and men [31].

In the symptomatic patients, clinical signs and symptoms depend on the infection site, and local mucosal inflammation with a subsequent discharge can lead to vaginitis, cervicitis, and urethritis in females and urethritis in males.

Symptoms are felt with different severity in different anatomic regions, depending on the bacterial variants that vary according to the specific epitopes encoded by ompA [32, 33]. There is a link between the genotype of *C.trachomatis* and its pathogenicity and the severity of infection [34, 35]. Chen et al. showed in their study that patients infected with genotype D, the most prevalent type in their study, had a lower risk of both coinfection with other pathogens and cervical cancer. Genotype F was found to be the most associated with bacterial coinfections, and serovar G was also the type at risk for coinfection. Genotype E was associated with mucopurulent cervicitis and cervical dysplasia [36]. Extensive studies of *C. trachomatis* serovars have found that variant prevalence show marked geographic distributions and differ by studied region, gender, ethnicity, and sexual orientation [34, 37–40].

The most common signs, symptoms, and history issues can be listed as follows:

These can be encountered in both sexes:

- Possible history of STDs.
- Dysuria.
- Urethral mucopurulent discharge.

These can be seen in females:

- History of sexual activity without a barrier contraceptive method or with the failure of the method.
- Vaginal discharge.
- Dyspareunia.
- Dysuria.
- Abnormal vaginal bleeding (postcoital or intermenstrual).
- In case of receptive anal intercourse; rectal discharge, proctitis, or both.
- Lower abdominal pain.
- Fever (in PID).
- No symptoms (in 80%).

DOI: http://dx.doi.org/10.5772/intechopen.111756

Signs of chlamydial infection in women may include the following:

- Mucopurulent cervical or vaginal discharge.
- Cervical friability (easy bleeding on manipulation).
- Cervical motion tenderness.
- Urethral discharge (usually thin and mucoid).
- Mucopurulent rectal discharge.
- Adnexal or lower abdomen fullness or tenderness (progression to PID).
- Upper right quadrant abdominal tenderness (Fitz-Hugh-Curtis syndrome).

Signs of lymphogranuloma venereum (LGV) may include the following:

- Genital ulceration.
- Localized inguinal adenopathy or buboes.
- "Groove sign" – Separation of the inguinal and femoral lymph nodes by the inguinal ligament (seen in 15–20% of patients).

6. Complications

Chlamydial infections are one of the most important causes of female infertility. Since infertility is one of the most significant issues to focus on chlamydia, it will be discussed in a separate section.

C.trachomatis is also the leading cause of PID. PID is a serious condition that may require hospitalization, intravenous antibiotic therapy, and tests to rule out a tubo-ovarian abscess. The risk of ectopic pregnancy is 7–10 times higher in women who have had PID than in those who have not. Pelvic adhesions involving the ovaries and tubes in 15% of women after PID may cause chronic pelvic pain in the long term. The case of perihepatitis, also known as Fitz-Hugh-Curtis syndrome, is a rare complication of PID, which is five times more common in chlamydia than in N. gonorrhea. Especially with serotype G infection, the risk of developing cervical cancer increases by about 6.5 times. Chlamydia infection also increases genital mucosal inflammation, facilitating HIV transmission.

A pregnant woman with a chlamydia infection can pass the infection to the baby during childbirth, and this can lead to pneumonia or conjunctivitis in the baby. Neonatal conjunctivitis, if remains untreated, can lead to blindness. Reiter's syndrome, reactive arthritis that may develop secondary to the immune response after primary chlamydia infection, is manifested by asymmetrical polyarthritis, urethritis, uveitis, mouth ulcers, circinate balanitis, and keratoderma blennorrhagica. The etiology is uncertain, but it usually follows an infectious attack and 80% of patients are HLA B27 positive. Other serious potential complications that can be related to chlamydia infection are miscarriage [41] and preterm birth [42].

There is no known association between chlamydia and tumor development in men, according to the evidence to date. However, this relationship in women has been reported by some authors. Paavonen et al. showed that the presence of enhanced antibodies to heat shock protein-60 is a high risk for cervical cancer; this also suggests that persistent *C. trachomatis* infection is associated with the development of cervical tumors [43]. One of the possible molecular mechanisms explaining the association of chlamydial infection with increased cervical cancer risk is that the infection generates an inflammatory response that triggers releases of ROS, cytokines, chemokines, growth, and angiogenic factors, leading to genetic instability and abnormal mitosis [44, 45]. *C. trachomatis* also affects beta-catenin and N-cadherin proteins, which have significant structural and regulatory roles [46]. In addition, there is evidence that CT infection increases HPV transmission and persistence. This coinfection increases the risk of cervical cancer as the epithelial destruction caused by the bacterium facilitates the entry of the virus; at the same time, with the weakening of the immune system, a microenvironment is formed that prepares the ground for the development of cancer [47, 48]. Anttila et al. found that the type of bacteria which bears the highest risk of developing cancer is the G serotype [49].

Since persistent inflammation is known to be related with tumor development, the ovaries may also be affected by chlamydia infection, as expected [50]. Shanmughapriya and colleagues showed that about 80% of ovarian cancer patients are infected with chlamydia [51]. Correspondingly, several studies have shown that the anti-Hsp60 protein is increased in ovarian cancer patients [52]. But despite these evidence, there are different consequences related to this issue, so more studies are needed to shed light on this topic [53].

7. Differential diagnosis and diagnostic workup

Since *Chlamydia trachomatis* can cause a wide spectrum of clinical presentations and manifestations, differential diagnosis of various signs and symptoms are also broad. Similar clinical manifestations affecting each body part should be considered carefully for other etiologies. The most common diseases that should be considered in differential diagnosis can be listed as: vaginal candidiasis, bacterial vaginosis, gonorrhea,*Trichomonas vaginalis*, *Ureaplasma* or *Mycoplasma genitalium* infection, foreign body, genital herpes, urinary tract infection, appendicitis, constipation, ovarian cysts, endometriosis adenomyosis, inflammatory bowel disease, allergy, cervical or endometrial polyp, cervical cancer, cervical ectropion, syphilis, chancroid, granuloma inguinale, leiomyoma, and pregnancy.

Considering the *C. trachomatis* infections, trachoma is the only one that can be diagnosed based upon clinical findings. All other chlamydial infections require laboratory confirmation. All patients with any sexually transmitted disease (STD) should also be evaluated for chlamydial infection because of the possibility of coinfection. Based on the patient's sexual practices achieved from history; endocervical, urethral, rectal, or oropharyngeal specimens should be collected and evaluated for *C. trachomatis* infection in both males and females [54]. Today, the gold standard for the diagnosis of urogenital chlamydia infections is nucleic acid amplification testing (NAAT) [55, 56]. A voided urine sample, whether first-void or midstream can be used to detect the chlamydial organism for nucleic acid amplification testing (NAAT). Self-collected vaginal swab specimens are shown to be equivalent in sensitivity and specificity to those collected by a clinician using NAATs [55, 57, 58]. If the newly mother had a documented untreated chlamydial infection during pregnancy, the infant should be treated doubtlessly without a need for confirmation.

7.1 Basic laboratory tests

A complete blood count (CBC) must be done if pelvic inflammatory disease (PID) is suspected. HIV testing, testing sexual partners for Chlamydia and a Pap smear test should also be considered. A pregnancy test is essential for females when determining the treatment because pregnancy is a contraindication for some treatment options.

7.2 Cytology and cell culture

Cytologic diagnosis is used to evaluate endocervical scrapings in genitourinary infection, but cultures are difficult to gather, not easy to analyze, and their sensitivity is low, many false-negative results are encountered. Because of the need for expert laboratory skills, they are also expensive. They may be incompatible when trying to assess a large number of patients. But they are still mandatory in certain clinical situations such as legal indications like rape or sexual abuse because of their high specificity (100%). Cell culture can also be the choice for rectal specimens because of the confounding effect of the stool microorganisms in other tests when interpreting the results.

C. trachomatis can be grown well in cell lines like McCoy and HeLa cells. Incubation time is 40–72 hours, depending on the cell type and specific biovar. Intracytoplasmic inclusions can be captured either by Giemsa stains or by immunofluorescent staining with monoclonal antibodies.

7.3 Molecular techniques for detecting antigen, DNA, or RNA/rapid tests

Since *C.trachomatis* only grows within columnar cells, it is essential to gather a specimen directly from the cervix or urethra that will involve cells. When trying to obtain cells from vaginal or urethral discharge, it should be tried to apply pressure to the inside of the cervix or urethra. In males, after the urethra is milked down for secretions, collection swabs should be inserted 1–2 cm inside to urethra or "kissing slide" method can be used for sample collection [59]. Transport and kit's manufacturer instructions should always be fulfilled.

Enzyme-linked immunosorbent assay (ELISA) is the most preferred test for Chlamydia in outpatient clinics and emergency departments for large number of patients since it is cost-effective and mostly automatized. It has 40–60% sensitivity and a 99% specificity.

Direct fluorescent antibody (DFA) testing for *C. trachomatis* has a sensitivity of 50–80% and a specificity of 99%. It is often preferred to confirm other assays but, labor and skilled personnel are needed to perform.

7.4 Nucleic acid amplification tests

Non-culture tests for the detection of *C. trachomatis* have been substantially replaced by higher-performing NAATs. These tests show high performance even in noninvasive samples. NAATs have recently become the test of choice to effectively screen and diagnose infection because of their high sensitivity and their ability to perform noninvasive testing that does not require pelvic examination or urethral swab [60–62]. NAATs target and amplify nucleic acid sequences found in almost every clinical strain of *C. trachomatis*, including genital, LGV, and ocular serovars. The APTIMA Combo 2 Assay used for ribosomal RNA can be used on liquid-based Pap smear samples [63]. The gold-standard method for bacterium genotyping is DNA sequencing of the ompA gene, encoding the major outer membrane protein (MOMP) [64]. This method is relatively simple and inexpensive. Most studies have reported sensitivity of more than 70% and specificity of 97–99% in populations where the prevalence of infection in men and women is 5% or more. The FDA-approved NAATs are recommended for the detection of infections caused by *C.trachomatis* and *N.gonorrhoeae* in men and women with or without symptoms [56]. Multiplex polymerase chain reaction assays are now started to be used widely, especially for polymicrobial infections and simultaneously testing the possible STDs from a single specimen [65, 66]. Older non-culture or non-NAAT tests with lower sensitivity are not recommended anymore. The Centers for Disease Control and Prevention (CDC) recommend NAATs for extragenital sites such as rectal and oropharyngeal infections because of their higher sensitivity and ease of sample handling and processing. Routine repeat testing is not recommended for NAAT-positive genital tract infections because repeated testing does not increase the positive predictive value of the test. Cultures of *C. trachomatis* and *N. gonorrhoeae* may still be necessary for the detection of sexual abuse in boys and extragenital infections in girls [56].

While NAATs are sensitive, they also have some drawbacks. Primarily, they are expensive, and so healthcare units may not be able to use them for comprehensive screening due to cost [67]. Another disadvantage of FDA-approved NAATs is that they cannot distinguish LGV strains from others. This is an important point because the duration of treatment in LGV infections needs to be extended. In addition, NAATs detect the DNA or RNA of the bacterium rather than the live microorganism, and it is common for control tests 3 weeks after the end of treatment to still show positivity [68]. For this reason, NAATs should not be used as a cure-determination test except in pregnant women, who must be shown to have a cure 3–4 weeks after the end of treatment to prevent infection in the infant.

In studies to shorten test result times, a prototype developed by TwistDx (prototype TwistDx RPA assay, Cambridge, UK) with an isothermal recombinant polymerase amplification approach shows promise. CT detection with this method takes 15 minutes. Validation studies of this prototype are still ongoing. But if this test is approved and made commercially available, it will mark a milestone in CT infection control, allowing doctors to diagnose and treat it in the same session [69, 70].

7.5 Serology

Antichlamydia immunoglobulin M (IgM) positivity is not common in adults with genital tract infections. Antichlamydial immunoglobulin G (IgG) positivity is high in sexually active adults, even if there is no active infection, and this most likely indicates a previous infection. Although there is a statistically significant relationship between chlamydia-specific serum immunoglobulin A (IgA) and active infection, none of the serological tests are sufficient to detect active disease in terms of clinical sensitivity, specificity, and predictive values. Therefore, it is not recommended for the diagnosis of genital tract infections. Nevertheless, they are still being used for research purposes and appear to be useful, especially for the detection of past infections using IgG.

7.6 CT, radiography, and ultrasonography

Imaging techniques are usually not necessary for uncomplicated genital chlamydia infections. However, CT and ultrasonography may be useful in complicated upper genital tract infections. For example, Fitz-Hugh-Curtis syndrome (perihepatitis) can be diagnosed with CT, and ultrasound can be used to investigate the presence of a tubo-ovarian abscess.

8. Screening

The social and financial burdens imposed by chlamydia are quite numerous. For this reason, some states such as the UK, Australia, the Netherlands, and Sweden have established a national chlamydia screening program. Each of these programs aimed to reduce the transmission of infection and its overall prevalence in the community with different strategies [71, 72]. Such a program should cover all sexually active individuals who are at an age where clinical intervention can alter long-term outcomes [73]. Evidence supports that screening should be available to those under 25 years old [74]. Studies on the subject have shown that because it is less invasive and easier, the postal screening method, in which people take samples on their own instead of the traditional way in the medical setting, increases screening rates [75, 76]. As Hoenderboom et al. points out, these samples may not be blood, but urine or vaginal swab samples [77].

Despite different opinions on the cost-effectiveness of screening programs, some authors argue that the screening program in the UK should be supported in this respect as well [78–80]. Retrospective studies of the chlamydia screening program in Sweden have shown that even in the first phase, the number of new cases has decreased. However, this reduction was achieved by using a more precise testing method, such as PCR, instead of more traditional methods such as culture. It was therefore concluded that faster, easier and more sensitive methods should be used for the diagnosis of chlamydia [37, 80]. Some other studies reported that the number of chlamydia infections was higher than expected, so screening should be done regardless of the estimated prevalence [81, 82]. In addition, several studies report that the prevalence of infection is high in adolescents and young women due to both their biological and behavioral predispositions, so a screening program should be established for at least 15–24 years of age [83]. All this evidence shows that it is important to establish screening programs to cover all sexually active individuals and to repeat tests for possible recurrent infections at regular intervals in order to prevent the spread of chlamydia and possible morbidity in the community by treating infected people in a timely manner. For such a screening program to be successful, noninvasive screening methods must be used. In this way, more people will be reached and the real incidence in the population will be determined, the measures to be taken for the control of the infection will be planned in a healthier way and the society will be made aware of the risk factors through prevention campaigns [84].

Recently, Huai and colleagues published a meta-analysis to estimate the prevalence of chlamydia infection worldwide and found that rates varied widely in the regions they studied, with the lowest prevalence in Southeast Asia. The authors then concluded, based on previous studies on the cost-effectiveness of screening programs, that it is critical to establish *Chlamydia trachomatis* screening programs using different guidelines in Latin America and Africa [85].

The US Preventive Services Task Force also recommends routine *Chlamydia* screening for sexually active young women to prevent consequences of undiagnosed and untreated chlamydial infection and has made the following recommendations: [86, 87].

- Screen for chlamydial infection in all sexually active nonpregnant young women aged 24 years or younger and for older nonpregnant women who are at increased risk.

- Screen for chlamydial infection in all pregnant women aged 24 years or younger and in older pregnant women who are at increased risk.

- Do not routinely screen for chlamydial infection in women aged 25 years or older, regardless of whether they are pregnant, or if they are not at increased risk.

9. Treatment

The most important points in the treatment of chlamydia infection are to make the correct diagnosis and to ensure the patient's compliance with the treatment. Undiagnosed chlamydia infection can progress to PID and result in partial or complete infertility. It is undesirable for this to happen early in life, before childbearing. STIs can often be confused with a urinary tract infection. Therefore, those with a history of recurrent urinary tract infections should be evaluated for STDs. Adolescents are a high-risk group for noncompliance with treatment, especially if they are trying to keep secret from their parents. In this group, single-dose, in-office treatment is increasingly used to ensure compliance and confidentiality. Partner treatment is vital for the prevention of reinfection. The development of PID in an adolescent should be considered as an absolute indication for hospitalization due to noncompliance with prolonged treatment regimens and the possibility of developing infertility. Before starting treatment, samples should be taken from the infection area for laboratory or culture examination, and a pregnancy test should be performed as it may change the treatment and follow-up plan. Antibiotic therapy should be started as soon as possible. Compliance with treatment, cost and potential side effects should be considered in the selection of treatment, and the possibility of coinfection of gonorrhea should be kept in mind. It should be reminded that sexual intercourse should be avoided until treatment is complete and all sexual partners have been tested for infection.

Treatment should be started as soon as genitourinary chlamydial infection is diagnosed or suspected. Chlamydias are sensitive to antibiotics that affect DNA and protein synthesis; these include tetracyclines, macrolides, and quinolones [88]. The CDC recommends azithromycin and doxycycline as first-line drugs for the treatment of chlamydia [55, 60]. Medical treatment with these agents is 95% effective. Alternative medicines include erythromycin, levofloxacin, and ofloxacin [55]. Since the FDA issued a warning in 2013 that azithromycin can cause life-threatening arrhythmias, doxycycline should be preferred in patients with QT-interval anomalies or taking antiarrhythmic drugs. There is no need to retest for a cure after treatment, but a reevaluation is recommended after 3 months due to the high probability of reinfection [60].

In cases where compliance to treatment may decrease due to reasons such as cost, age, and confidentiality, it is recommended to apply single-dose treatment under observation for lower genital infections.

Due to the severity of potential complications, the presence of a condition affecting the upper genital tract should be carefully and meticulously investigated, especially in adolescents. Improper and inadequately treated PID can result in chronic pelvic pain, infertility, and sepsis. Monitoring of hospital treatment and response to treatment is especially important when PID is suspected, as adolescents may have trouble ignoring symptoms and continuing follow-ups.

In the treatment of PID, even if it is known gonorrhea to be present, treatment against C.trachomatis and anaerobic bacteria should always be included. Oral and parenteral regimens have shown similar efficacy in mild or moderate PID [60]. Patients treated in the hospital should not be discharged until significant clinical improvement is seen and confirmation that the patient will complete medical treatment. The recommended parenteral regimens are a continuation of doxycycline with cefoxitin or cefotetan for 14 days. Alternatively, clindamycin-gentamicin or doxycycline plus ampicillin-sulbactam may be given.

Out-of-hospital treatment for PID; following a single dose intramuscular administration of a second or third-generation cephalosporin, administration of doxycycline for 14 days, with or without metronidazole 500 mg for 14 days. After the emergence of quinolone-resistant cases of *N. gonorrhoeae*, treatments containing quinolone are no longer recommended for the treatment of PID. For sexual partners of the index case, treatment should also be given if the last sexual intercourse was within the last 60 days. Patients undergoing treatment for gonorrhea should also be treated for chlamydial infection.

Regarding treatment during pregnancy, CDC guidelines recommend a single dose, 1 g of azithromycin. Alternatively, amoxicillin 500 mg or erythromycin three times a day for 7 days can be used. Doxycycline, ofloxacin, and levofloxacin are contraindicated in pregnancy. To demonstrate eradication of chlamydia in pregnancy, it is recommended to test 3–4 weeks after the end of treatment, preferably by the NAAT method.

9.1 Treatment failure and novel approaches

The main causes of treatment failure are noncompliance with treatment, early testing for cure, and reinfection as a result of sexual partners not being adequately informed and adequately treated. In addition, treatment failure can be caused by antibiotic resistance caused by gene mutations in the bacterium or by the bacterium becoming insufficiently cleaned and persistent due to its natural characteristics [89]. In an *in vitro* study of antibiotic resistance, which included Croatia, the country with the highest azithromycin consumption in Europe, resistance was not shown to either azithromycin or doxycycline [90]. However, an experimental study in the UK comparing azithromycin with doxycycline found that treatment failure with azithromycin was higher in nongenital infections [91]. Multidrug-resistant CT serovars may be the reason for the ineffectiveness of azithromycin therapy. Some *in vitro* studies show that point mutations in the ribosomal proteins of the bacterium L genotype are responsible for azithromycin resistance [92]. There is also *in vitro* evidence that previous penicillin exposure may lead to azithromycin resistance in *C. trachomatis* [93].

Based on this evidence, it is clear that new drugs are needed to be developed to successfully combat *C. trachomatis* infection. Some researchers have studied Corallopyronin A, an antimicrobial compound synthesized by *Corallococcus coralloides*, and have shown that it inhibits CT proliferation [94] Shima et al. have also found promising results with this compound and have proposed it as an alternative to CT treatment in the future [94, 95]. A nanoparticle developed by Yang et al. successfully prevented vaginal CT infection by stimulating autophagy in human cells [96].

Recently, Nunez-Otero and his team demonstrated the role of a second-generation 2-pyridone amide molecule (KSK213) in the control of CT infection, in which they reduced its toxicity without damaging the commensal flora. This molecule acts through transcription inhibition in critical genes responsible for the conversion of EB to RB, the key point in the CT infection cycle [97].

In addition to all these, natural anti-chlamydia treatments derived from herbal extracts are also emphasized. Hamarsheh et al. studied the effect of Artemisia Inculta Delile extract and showed that it effectively inhibits infection in Hela cells [98]. As the issue of antibiotic resistance remains critical since 2020, some researchers have studied potential nonantibiotic agents. Lam et al. published their findings on cyclic peptomers that inhibit gram-negative bacteria and recommended 4EpDN cyclic peptomer as a prophylactic treatment against chlamydia [99].

Drug repurposing, which has been researched mostly in cancer treatment, has also been tried in this regard. Itoh et al. have shown that Bortezomib, an anticancer drug, may also be effective in treating CT infection through the induction of apoptosis [100]. More comprehensive studies are needed to be able to apply all these new strategies in the treatment of CT infection and to put the results of research into clinical practice. In order to eradicate this infection worldwide, the development of an effective vaccine in addition to all treatment strategies is critical.

9.2 Posttherapy care

Due to the high incidence of reinfection, retesting is recommended in the third month after treatment of chlamydia, gonorrhea, and trichomonas. In pregnancy, control testing after amoxicillin and erythromycin treatment should be considered. Due to the positive results from nonviable organisms, it would be better not to use non-culture methods in control tests.

Patients should be reminded to refrain from sexual activity for 7 days after a single dose treatment, and for longer treatments until the end of treatment and all sexual partners have been treated.

10. Prevention

Sexually active people should be aware of all other STDs, not just genital chlamydia infection. Diagnosed patients should be checked for all other STDs as much as possible. If possible, all sexual partners should be referred for diagnosis and treatment. Patients should also be informed that the most important way to prevent these infections, other than avoiding sexual activity, is to practice safe sex, that is, to use an appropriate barrier method such as a latex condom in every sexual relationship.

The American College of Obstetricians and Gynecologists (ACOG) has released guidelines about expedited partner therapy for chlamydial and gonorrheal infections [101, 102]. Although developed to prevent reinfection of chlamydia and gonorrhea, the recommendations may also be used for other STDs.

The ACOG recommendations can be listed as follows:

- Expedited partner therapy to prevent reinfection, with the legalization of expedited partner therapy.

- Counsel partners to undergo screening for HIV infection and other STDs.

- Expedited partner therapy is contraindicated in cases of suspected abuse or compromised patient safety, pretreatment evaluation for abuse potential is recommended.

- Expedited partner therapy medications and protocols based on CDC, state, and/or local guidelines.

11. WHO guidelines on the treatment of *Chlamydia trachomatis* infection

11.1 Uncomplicated genital chlamydia

WHO recommendations for the treatment of uncomplicated genital chlamydia are as follows [103]:

- Azithromycin 1 g orally as a single dose or.

- Doxycycline 100 mg orally twice a day for 7 days or one of these alternatives: tetracycline 500 mg orally four times a day for 7 days, erythromycin 500 mg orally twice a day for 7 days, or ofloxacin 200–400 mg orally twice a day for 7 days.

11.2 Anorectal chlamydial infection

In anorectal chlamydial infection, the WHO recommends doxycycline 100 mg orally twice a day for 7 days over azithromycin 1 g orally as a single dose.

11.3 Chlamydial infection in pregnant women

WHO recommendations for the treatment of chlamydial infection in pregnancy are as follows:

- Azithromycin recommended over erythromycin,

- Azithromycin recommended over amoxicillin,

- Amoxicillin recommended over erythromycin,

- Azithromycin 1 g orally as a single dose or,

- Amoxicillin 500 mg orally three times a day for 7 days or,

- Erythromycin 500 mg orally twice a day for 7 days.

11.4 Lymphogranuloma Venereum

WHO recommendations for the treatment of lymphogranuloma venereum (LGV) are as follows:

- In adults and adolescents with LGV, the guidelines suggest doxycycline 100 mg orally twice daily for 21 days over azithromycin 1 g orally weekly for 3 weeks.

- Good practice dictates the treatment of LGV, particularly for men who have sex with men and for people with HIV infection.
- When doxycycline is contraindicated, azithromycin should be provided.
- When neither treatment is available, erythromycin 500 mg orally four times a day for 21 days is an alternative.
- Doxycycline should not be used in pregnant women.

12. Infertility: a major complication of *C. trachomatis* infection

Potential factors affecting the association between chlamydia infection and infertility in women can be summarized in four categories; [1].

1. Host factors: Behavior, prevalence, genotype, microbiome.
2. Immunological factors: Cellular pathology, cHSP60 antibodies, suppressed immunity, IFN-gamma production.
3. Epidemiological factors: Age, sexual behavior, smoking, recurrent infection.
4. Pathogenic factors: Serovar, infectious burden, persistence, genotype, treatment failure, ability to ascend.

As stated in a review examining the sexually transmitted disease and infertility association, tubal factor infertility (TFI) is one of the most common causes of infertility. While it is responsible for up to 33% of female infertility cases worldwide, this rate is disproportionately high in developing countries. In sub-Saharan Africa, for example, it is more than 85%. The vast majority of TFI cases are caused by salpingitis and subsequent pelvic-peritoneal adhesions due to previous or persistent infections. Bacteria climb up the cervix along mucosal surfaces to reach the endometrium and eventually the fallopian tubes. This pathway manifests itself clinically as PID and it has a significant association with subsequent TFI. About 15% of women who have PID end up with TFI, and if the number of PID attacks increases, the likelihood of infertility also increases. However, most women with TFI do not have a clinically diagnosed PID history, but instead have minimally symptomatic or totally asymptomatic salpingitis as a result of an upper genital tract infection. Studying the effects of such infections, especially those without clinical PID, is necessary to explain TFI because of the mostly asymptomatic course of *C. trachomatis*. To date, evidence has shown that ascending *C. trachomatis* infection causes irreversible damage to the fallopian tubes, leading to obstructions and thus, infertility. Heat shock protein (HSP60) synthesized by *C. trachomatis* produces a proinflammatory immune response in the human fallopian tube epithelium, causing scarring and obstruction in the tube [104, 105].

In a series of sero-epidemiological studies examining antibodies to *C. trachomatis* and chlamydial hsp60 in laparoscopic or HSG-confirmed fallopian tube injury and ectopic pregnancies, previous *C. trachomatis* infection has been shown to significantly increase tubal infertility in women, regardless of whether it presents clinical symptoms or not. Patients with PID are also more likely to develop infertility later in the presence of a history of *C. trachomatis* than those without a history of chlamydia [106, 107].

A cohort study, involving 1250 women with demonstrated tubal patency undergoing fertility treatment, examined *C. trachomatis* seropositivity using IgG1 and IgG3 antibody subtypes [108]. The presence of IgG3 from these two antibody subtypes was shown to be a strong indicator of both failure to conceive and ectopic pregnancy outcomes. This is because IgG3 is related to the inflammatory response in the early phase of the infection and its detection may indicate that either a recent or persistent infection has caused tube damage, although it has not yet caused tubal obstruction [108]. Another study of subfertile women without visible tubal pathology found 33% lower rates of spontaneous pregnancies in the presence of chlamydial antibodies [107, 108]. Coppus et al. suggest that this decline in pregnancy rates may not only be related to the known chronic inflammatory response but also to the fact that persistent CT infection impairs implantation and embryo development due to the autoimmune response to human heat shock proteins [108, 109]. Therefore, chlamydial antibody tests are likely to continue to be an important predictor both in the evaluation of tubal patency and in the evaluation of ectopic pregnancy, intrauterine insemination failure, and embryo and pregnancy loss independent of tubal damage.

In another systematic review investigating the effect of CT infection on female infertility, a positive correlation between infection and infertility was found in 76.47% of the included studies [110]. The study by Menon et al., which included 239 women, showed that up to half of the subfertile women may have CT infection as a concomitant factor [111]. den Heijer et al. also found that CT-positive women were 70% more likely to experience infertility [112]. Davies [113], Ramadhani [114], and Kayiira [115] also showed results that reinforce this relationship in different countries and populations, noting that routine chlamydia screening, along with interventions to prevent initial and recurrent infections, is extremely important to protect women's long-term reproductive health.

Considering PID, which causes significant adhesions and severe tubal damage, it is easy to conclude that these anatomical causes are detrimental to fertility. However, there are some cases where there is no apparent damage, suggesting that some molecular mechanisms are also involved. Since CT is an intracellular pathogen that disrupts endothelial and tubal muscle structure, it is highly likely to lead to impaired tubal motility and endothelial cilia function. This explains the changes observed in the form of constrictions in the intrauterine and tubal structure after the application of a saline solution to the female reproductive tract during the laparoscopy procedure. Even if CT remains in the female reproductive organs for a short time, it facilitates the settlement of other microorganisms in the area, leads to changes in the structure of the microbiota, and affects gametes and their conjunction by antigenic stimulation [116, 117]. These immunological changes also explain the state of mild endometriosis in women who have had a preliminary CT infection; once an immunological imbalance has occurred, lymphocyte activity becomes insufficient and, which leads to the retention of viable endometrial cells in the pelvic environment [118]. Thus, as well as the endometriosis, CT infection and the mechanical and biochemical damage it creates, induce a hostile environment for gametes in the female reproductive pathway. A significant point here to emphasize is that as age progresses, *C. trachomatis* is eliminated from the host and can no longer be detected by PCR. Therefore, a more accurate approach would be using long-standing IgG-specific antibodies to detect past infections that may be responsible for infertility [1].

Author details

Alev Özlem Özdemir-Karabağ
Obstetrics and Gynecology Private Clinic, Eskişehir, Türkiye

*Address all correspondence to: alevozdem@gmail.com

References

[1] Rodrigues R, Sousa C, Vale N. Chlamydia trachomatis as a current health problem: Challenges and opportunities. Diagnostics. 2022;**12**:1795

[2] CDC Grand Rounds. Chlamydia prevention: Challenges and strategies for reducing disease burden and sequelae. MMWR. Morbidity and Mortality Weekly Report. 2011;**60**(12):370-373

[3] [Guideline] Geisler WM. Diagnosis and management of uncomplicated chlamydia trachomatis infections in adolescents and adults: Summary of evidence reviewed for the 2010 Centers for Disease Control and Prevention sexually transmitted diseases treatment guidelines. Clinical Infectious Diseases. 2011;**53**(Suppl 3):S92-S98

[4] Hammerschlag MR. Chlamydial and gonococcal infections in infants and children. Clinical Infectious Diseases. 2011;**53**(Suppl. 3):S99-S102

[5] Keenan JD, Lakew T, Alemayehu W, Melese M, Porco TC, Yi E, et al. Clinical activity and polymerase chain reaction evidence of chlamydial infection after repeated mass antibiotic treatments for trachoma. The American Journal of Tropical Medicine and Hygiene. 2010;**82**(3):482-487

[6] WHO. WHO FACTSHEET. WHO; 2015

[7] Satterwhite CL, Torrone E, Meites E, Dunne EF, Mahajan R, Ocfemia MC, et al. Sexually transmitted infections among US women and men: Prevalence and incidence estimates, 2008. Sexually Transmitted Diseases. 2013;**40**(3):187-193

[8] Schmidt AJ, Marcus U. Self-reported history of sexually transmissible infections (STIs) and STI-related utilization of the German health care system by men who have sex with men: Data from a large convenience sample. BMC Infectious Diseases. 2011;**11**:132

[9] Goulet V, de Barbeyrac B, Raherison S, Prudhomme M, Semaille C, Warszawski J. Prevalence of chlamydia trachomatis: Results from the first national population-based survey in France. Sexually Transmitted Infections. 2010;**86**(4):263-270

[10] van Bergen JE, Fennema JS, van den Broek IV, Brouwers EE, de Feijter EM, Hoebe CJ, et al. Rationale, design, and results of the first screening round of a comprehensive, register-based, chlamydia screening implementation programme in the Netherlands. BMC Infectious Diseases. 2010;**10**:293

[11] Morgan J, Colonne C, Bell A. Trends of reported chlamydia infections and related complications in New Zealand, 1998-2008. Sexual Health. 2011;**8**(3):412-418

[12] Guy RJ, Kong F, Goller J, Franklin N, Bergeri I, Dimech W, et al. A new national chlamydia sentinel surveillance system in Australia: Evaluation of the first stage of implementation. Communicable Diseases Intelligence. 2010;**34**(3):319-328

[13] World Health Organization. Chlamydia Trachomatis. Initiative for Vaccine Research. World Health Organization;

[14] Witkin SS, Minis E, Athanasiou A, Leizer J, Linhares IM. Chlamydia trachomatis: The persistent pathogen. Clinical and Vaccine Immunology. 2017;**24**:e00203-e00217

[15] Gottlieb SL, Brunham RC, Byrne GI, Martin DH, Xu F, Berman SM. Introduction: The natural history and immunobiology of chlamydia trachomatis genital infection and implications for chlamydia control. The Journal of Infectious Diseases. 2010;**201**(Suppl. 2):S85-S87

[16] Poston TB, Darville T. Chlamydia trachomatis: Protective adaptive responses and prospects for a vaccine. Current Topics in Microbiology and Immunology. 2018;**412**:217-237

[17] Shiragannavar S, Madagi S, Hosakeri J, Barot V. In silico vaccine design against chlamydia trachomatis infection. Network Modeling and Analysis in Health Informatics and Bioinformatics. 2020;**9**:39

[18] Aslam S, Ahmad S, Noor F, Ashfaq UA, Shahid F, Rehman A, et al. Designing a multi-epitope vaccine against chlamydia trachomatis by employing integrated Core proteomics, Immuno-informatics and In Silico approaches. Biology. 2021;**10**:997

[19] Sarıer M, Kukul E. Classification of non-gonococcal urethritis:A review. International Urology and Nephrology. 2019;**5**:4

[20] Lim RBT, Wong ML, Cook AR, Brun C, Chan RKW, Sen P, et al. Determinants of chlamydia, gonorrhea, and coinfection in heterosexual adolescents attending the National Public Sexually Transmitted Infection Clinic in Singapore. Sexually Transmitted Diseases. 2015;**42**:450-456

[21] Seo Y, Choi KH, Lee G. Characterization and trend of Co-infection with Neisseria gonorrhoeae and chlamydia trachomatis from the Korean National Infectious Diseases Surveillance Database. World Journal of Mens Health. 2021;**39**:107-115

[22] Harrison SA, Olson KM, Ratliff AE, Xiao L, Van Der Pol B, Waites KB, et al. Mycoplasma genitalium coinfection in women with chlamydia trachomatis infection. Sexually Transmitted Diseases. 2019;**46**:e101-e104

[23] Borgogna J-LC, Shardell MD, Yeoman CJ, Ghanem KG, Kadriu H, Ulanov AV, et al. The association of chlamydia trachomatis and mycoplasma genitalium infection with the vaginal metabolome. Scientific Reports. 2020;**10**:3420

[24] Bellaminutti S, Seraceni S, De Seta F, Gheit T, Tommasino M, Comar M. HPV and chlamydia trachomatis co-detection in young asymptomatic women from high incidence area for cervical cancer. Journal of Medical Virology. 2014;**86**:1920-1925

[25] Escarcega-Tame MA, López-Hurtado M, Escobedo-Guerra MR, Reyes-Maldonado E, Castro-Escarpulli G, Guerra-Infante FM. Co-infection between genotypes of the human papillomavirus and chlamydia trachomatis in Mexican women. International Journal of STD & AIDS. 2020;**31**:1255-1262

[26] Lima LM, Hoelzle CR, Simões RT, Lima MIM, Fradico JRB, Mateo ECC, et al. Sexually transmitted infections detected by multiplex real time PCR in asymptomatic women and association with cervical intraepithelial neoplasia. Revista Brasileira de Ginecologia e Obstetrícia. 2018;**40**:540-546

[27] Ohman H, Tiitinen A, Halttunen M, Lehtinen M, Paavonen J, Surcel HM. Cytokine polymorphisms and severity of tubal damage in women with chlamydia-associated infertility. The Journal of Infectious Diseases. 2009;**199**(9):1353-1359

[28] Taylor BD, Darville T, Ferrell RE, Kammerer CM, Ness RB, Haggerty CL.

Variants in toll-like receptor 1 and 4 genes are associated with chlamydia trachomatis among women with pelvic inflammatory disease. The Journal of Infectious Diseases. 2012;**205**(4):603-609

[29] Scholes D, Stergachis A, Heidrich FE, Andrilla H, Holmes KK, Stamm WE. Prevention of pelvic inflammatory disease by screening for cervical chlamydial infection. The New England Journal of Medicine. 1996;**334**(21):1362-1366

[30] Kamwendo F, Forslin L, Bodin L, Danielsson D. Decreasing incidences of gonorrhea- and chlamydia-associated acute pelvic inflammatory disease. A 25-year study from an urban area of Central Sweden. Sexually Transmitted Diseases. 1996;**23**(5):384-391

[31] Quinn TC, Gaydos C, Shepherd M, Bobo L, Hook EW 3rd, Viscidi R, et al. Epidemiologic and microbiologic correlates of chlamydia trachomatis infection in sexual partnerships. Journal of the American Medical Association. 1996;**276**(21):1737-1742

[32] Lesiak-Markowicz I, Schötta A-M, Stockinger H, Stanek G, Markowicz M. Chlamydia trachomatis serovars in urogenital and ocular samples collected 2014-2017 from Austrian patients. Scientific Reports. 2019;**9**:18327

[33] Morré SA, Rozendaal L, van Valkengoed IG, Boeke AJ, van Voorst Vader PC, Schirm J, et al. Urogenital chlamydia trachomatis serovars in men and women with a symptomatic or asymptomatic infection: An association with clinical manifestations? Journal of Clinical Microbiology. 2000;**38**:2292-2296

[34] Chen Y, Chen J, Yang L, Jiang Y, Li L, Yi W, et al. Distribution of chlamydia trachomatis genotypes in infective diseases of the female lower genital tract. Medical Science Monitor. 2017;**23**:4477-4481

[35] Abdelsamed H, Peters J, Byrne GI. Genetic variation in chlamydia trachomatis and their hosts: Impact on disease severity and tissue tropism. Future Microbiology. 2013;**8**:1129-1146

[36] Balasubramaniam SD, Balakrishnan V, Oon CE, Kaur G. Key molecular events in cervical cancer development. Medicina. 2019;**55**:384

[37] Sylvan SPE, Von Krogh G, Tiveljung A, Siwerth B-M, Henriksson L, Norén L, et al. Screening and genotyping of genital chlamydia trachomatis in urine specimens from male and female clients of youth-health centers in Stockholm County. Sexually Transmitted Diseases. 2002;**29**:379-386

[38] Sabbatucci M, Salfa MC, Regine V, Pezzotti P, Suligoi B. Estimated burden of chlamydia trachomatis female infection and consequent severe pelvic inflammatory disease, Italy, 2005-2016. Annali dell'Istituto Superiore di Sanità. 2019;**55**:217-223

[39] Borrego MJ, Gomes JP, Lefebvre JF, Eb F, Orfila J, Catry MA. Genotyping of Portuguese chlamydia trachomatis urogenital isolates. Sexually Transmitted Infections. 1997;**73**:561-563

[40] Casillas-Vega N, Morfín-Otero R, García S, Llaca-Díaz J, Rodríguez-Noriega E, Camacho-Ortiz A, et al. Frequency and genotypes of chlamydia trachomatis in patients attending the obstetrics and gynecology clinics in Jalisco, Mexico and correlation with sociodemographic, behavioral, and biological factors. BMC Women's Health. 2017;**17**:83

[41] Baud D, Goy G, Jaton K, Osterheld MC, Blumer S, Borel N, et al.

Role of chlamydia trachomatis in miscarriage. Emerging Infectious Diseases. 2011;**17**(9):1630-1635

[42] Rours GI, Duijts L, Moll HA, Arends LR, de Groot R, Jaddoe VW, et al. Chlamydia trachomatis infection during pregnancy associated with preterm delivery: A population-based prospective cohort study. European Journal of Epidemiology. 2011;**26**(6):493-502

[43] Paavonen J, Karunakaran KP, Noguchi Y, Anttila T, Bloigu A, Dillner J, et al. Serum antibody response to the heat shock protein 60 of chlamydia trachomatis in women with developing cervical cancer. American Journal of Obstetrics and Gynecology. 2003;**189**:1287-1292

[44] Zhu H, Shen Z, Luo H, Zhang W, Zhu X. Chlamydia trachomatis infection-associated risk of cervical cancer: A meta analysis. Medicine. 2016;**95**:e3077

[45] Yang X, Siddique A, Khan AA, Wang Q, Malik A, Jan AT, et al. Chlamydia trachomatis infection: Their potential implication in the etiology of cervical cancer. Journal of Cancer. 2021;**12**:4891-4900

[46] Prozialeck WC, Fay MJ, Lamar PC, Pearson CA, Sigar I, Ramsey KH. Chlamydia trachomatis disrupts N-cadherin-dependent cell-cell junctions and sequesters beta-catenin in human cervical epithelial cells. Infection and Immunity. 2002;**70**:2605-2613

[47] Jensen KE, Thomsen LT, Schmiedel S, Frederiksen K, Norrild B, van den Brule A, et al. Chlamydia trachomatis and risk of cervical intraepithelial neoplasia grade 3 or worse in women with persistent human papillomavirus infection: A cohort study. Sexually Transmitted Infections. 2014;**90**:550-555

[48] Simonetti AC, Melo JH, de Souza PR, Bruneska D, de Lima Filho JL. Immunological's host profile for HPV and chlamydia trachomatis, a cervical cancer cofactor. Microbes and Infection. 2009;**11**:435-442

[49] Anttila T, Saikku P, Koskela P, Bloigu A, Dillner J, Ikäheimo I, et al. Serotypes of chlamydia trachomatis and risk for development of cervical squamous cell carcinoma. JAMA. 2001;**285**:47-51

[50] Xie X, Yang M, Ding Y, Chen J. Microbial infection, inflammation and epithelial ovarian cancer. Oncology Letters. 2017;**14**:1911-1919

[51] Shanmughapriya S, Senthilkumar G, Vinodhini K, Das BC, Vasanthi N, Natarajaseenivasan K. Viral and bacterial aetiologies of epithelial ovarian cancer. European Journal of Clinical Microbiology & Infectious Diseases. 2012;**31**:2311-2317

[52] Bodzek P, Partyka R, Damasiewicz-Bodzek A. Antibodies against Hsp60 and Hsp65 in the sera of women with ovarian cancer. Journal of Ovarian Research. 2014;**7**:30

[53] Hosseininasab-nodoushan S-A, Ghazvini K, Jamialahmadi T, Keikha M, Sahebkar A. Association of chlamydia and mycoplasma infections with susceptibility to ovarian cancer: A systematic review and meta-analysis. Semin. Cancer Biol. 2021;**86** (Pt 2):923-928

[54] Peters RPH, Nijsten N, Mutsaers J, Jansen CL, Morré SA, van Leeuwen AP. Screening of oropharynx and Anorectum increases prevalence of chlamydia trachomatis and Neisseria gonorrhoeae infection in female STD clinic visitors. Sexually Transmitted Diseases. 2011;**38**(9):783-787

[55] Centers for Disease Control and Prevention. Chlamydial Infections. CDC

[56] Centers for Disease Control and Prevention. Recommendations for the laboratory-based detection of chlamydia trachomatis and Neisseria gonorrhoeae--2014. MMWR - Recommendations and Reports. 2014;**63**(RR-02):1-19

[57] Knox J, Tabrizi SN, Miller P, Petoumenos K, Law M, Chen S, et al. Evaluation of self-collected samples in contrast to practitioner-collected samples for detection of chlamydia trachomatis, Neisseria gonorrhoeae, and trichomonas vaginalis by polymerase chain reaction among women living in remote areas. Sexually Transmitted Diseases. 2002;**29**(11):647-654

[58] Masek BJ, Arora N, Quinn N, Aumakhan B, Holden J, Hardick A, et al. Performance of three nucleic acid amplification tests for detection of chlamydia trachomatis and Neisseria gonorrhoeae by use of self-collected vaginal swabs obtained via an internet-based screening program. Journal of Clinical Microbiology. 2009;**47**(6):1663-1667

[59] Sarıer M, Demir M, Turgut H, Hizel A, Emek M, Kukul E, et al. New approach to microscopy of gram-stained urethral smear: The kissing slide method. Sexually Transmitted Diseases. 2020;**47**(10):712-715

[60] Workowski KA, Bolan GA. Centers for Disease Control and Prevention. Sexually transmitted diseases treatment guidelines, 2015. MMWR - Recommendations and Reports. 2015;**64**(RR-03):1-137

[61] Harkins AL, Munson E. Molecular diagnosis of sexually transmitted chlamydia trachomatis in the United States. ISRN Obstetrics and Gynecology. 2011;**2011**:279149

[62] Gaydos CA, Ferrero DV, Papp J. Laboratory aspects of screening men for chlamydia trachomatis in the new millennium. Sexually Transmitted Diseases. 2008;**35**(Suppl. 11):S45-S50

[63] Chernesky M, Freund GG, Hook E 3rd, Leone P, D'Ascoli P, Martens M. Detection of chlamydia trachomatis and Neisseria gonorrhoeae infections in north American women by testing SurePath liquid-based pap specimens in APTIMA assays. Journal of Clinical Microbiology. 2007;**45**(8):2434-2438

[64] Schillinger JA, Katz BP, Markowitz LE, Braslins PG, Shrier LA, Madico G, et al. Genotype-specific concordance of chlamydia trachomatis genital infection within heterosexual partnerships. Sexually Transmitted Diseases. 2016;**43**:741-749

[65] Sarıer M. Prevalance of Polymicrobial infection in urethritis. Journal of Urological Surgery. 2019;**6**(3):180-183

[66] Sarıer M, Duman İ, Göktaş Ş, Demir M, Kukul E. Results of multiplex polymerase chain reaction assay to identify urethritis pathogens. Journal of Urological Surgery. 2017;**1**:18-22

[67] Hadgu A, Sternberg M. Reproducibility and specificity concerns associated with nucleic acid amplification tests for detecting chlamydia trachomatis. European Journal of Clinical Microbiology & Infectious Diseases. 2009;**28**(1):9-15

[68] Dukers-Muijrers NH, Morré SA, Speksnijder A, van der Sande MA, Hoebe CJ. Chlamydia trachomatis test-of-cure cannot be based on a single highly sensitive laboratory test taken at least 3 weeks after treatment. PLoS One. 2012;**7**(3):e34108

[69] Adamson PC, Loeffelholz MJ, Klausner JD. Point-of-care testing for sexually transmitted infections: A review of recent developments. Archives of Pathology & Laboratory Medicine. 2020;**144**:1344-1351

[70] Harding-Esch EM, Fuller SS, Chow SC, Nori AV, Harrison MA, Parker M, et al. Diagnostic accuracy of a prototype rapid chlamydia and gonorrhoea recombinase polymerase amplification assay: A multicentre cross-sectional preclinical evaluation. Clinical Microbiology and Infection. 2019;**25**(380):e1-380.e7

[71] Sheringham J, Baraitser P, Simms I, Hart G, Raine R. Chlamydia screening in England: A qualitative study of the narrative behind the policy. BMC Public Health. 2012;**12**:317

[72] Low N, Hocking JS, van Bergen J. The changing landscape of chlamydia control strategies. Lancet. 2021;**398**:1386-1388

[73] Kretzschmar M, Welte R, van den Hoek A, Postma MJ. Comparative model-based analysis of screening programs for chlamydia trachomatis infections. American Journal of Epidemiology. 2001;**153**:90-101

[74] van Aar F, de Moraes M, Morré SA, van Bergen JE, van der Klis FR, Land JA, et al. Chlamydia trachomatis IgG seroprevalence in the general population of the Netherlands in 1996 and in 2007: Differential changes by gender and age. Sexually Transmitted Infections. 2014;**90**:434-440

[75] Chernesky M, Jang D, Martin I, Arias M, Shah A, Smieja M, et al. Mycoplasma genitalium, chlamydia trachomatis, and Neisseria gonorrhoeae detected with aptima assays performed on self-obtained vaginal swabs and urine collected at home and in a clinic. Sexually Transmitted Diseases. 2019;**46**:e87-e89

[76] Graseck AS, Shih SL, Peipert JF. Home versus clinic-based specimen collection for chlamydia trachomatis and Neisseria gonorrhoeae. Expert Review of Anti-Infective Therapy. 2011;**9**:183-194

[77] Hoenderboom BM, van Ess EF, van den Broek IVF, van Loo IHM, Hoebe C, Ouburg S, et al. Chlamydia trachomatis antibody detection in home-collected blood samples for use in epidemiological studies. Journal of Microbiological Methods. 2018;**144**:164-167

[78] Batteiger BE, Tu W, Ofner S, Van Der Pol B, Stothard DR, Orr DP, et al. Repeated chlamydia trachomatis genital infections in adolescent women. The Journal of Infectious Diseases. 2010;**201**:42-51

[79] Ditkowsky J, Shah KH, Hammerschlag MR, Kohlhoff S, Smith-Norowitz TA. Cost-benefit analysis of chlamydia trachomatis screening in pregnant women in a high burden setting in the United States. BMC Infectious Diseases. 2017;**17**:155

[80] LaMontagne DS, Fenton KA, Randall S, Anderson S, Carter P. Establishing the National Chlamydia Screening Programme in England: Results from the first full year of screening. Sexually Transmitted Infections. 2004;**80**:335-341

[81] Yuguero O, Fernández-Armenteros JM, Vilela Á, Aramburu J, Laín R, Godoy P. Preliminary results of a screening Programme for chlamydia in an asymptomatic young population in Spain. Frontiers in Public Health. 2021;**9**:615110

[82] Low N, Cassell JA, Spencer B, Bender N, Martin Hilber A, van Bergen J, et al. Chlamydia control activities in Europe: Cross-sectional survey. European Journal of Public Health. 2011;**22**:556-561

[83] Cha S, Newman DR, Rahman M, Peterman TA. High rates of repeat chlamydial infections among young women-Louisiana, 2000-2015. Sexually Transmitted Diseases. 2019;**46**:52-57

[84] Söderqvist J, Gullsby K, Stark L, Wikman M, Karlsson R, Herrmann B. Internet-basedself-samplingforchlamydia trachomatis testing: A national evaluation in Sweden. Sexually Transmitted Infections. 2020;**96**:160-165

[85] Huai P, Li F, Chu T, Liu D, Liu J, Zhang F. Prevalence of genital chlamydia trachomatis infection in the general population: A meta-analysis. BMC Infectious Diseases. 2020;**20**:589

[86] ML LF, U.S. Preventive Services Task Force. Screening for chlamydia and gonorrhea: U.S. preventive services task force recommendation statement. Annals of Internal Medicine. 2014;**161**(12):902-910

[87] National Guideline Clearinghouse. Screening for Chlamydial Infection: Recommendation Statement. National Guideline Clearinghouse

[88] Kohlhoff SA, Hammerschlag MR. Treatment of chlamydial infections: 2014 update. Expert Opinion on Pharmacotherapy. 2015;**16**(2):205-212

[89] Huemer M, Shambat SM, Brugger SD, Zinkernagel AS. Antibiotic resistance and persistence—Implications for human health and treatment perspectives. EMBO Reports. 2020;**21**:e51034

[90] Ljubin-Sternak S, Mestrovic T, Vilibic-Cavlek T, Mlinaric-Galinovic G, Sviben M, Markotic A, et al. In vitro susceptibility of urogenital chlamydia trachomatis strains in a country with high azithromycin consumption rate. Folia Microbiologica. 2013;**58**:361-365

[91] Hathorn E, Opie C, Goold P. What is the appropriate treatment for the management of rectal chlamydia trachomatis in men and women? Sexually Transmitted Infections. 2012;**88**:352

[92] Manavi K, Hettiarachchi N, Hodson J. Comparison of doxycycline with azithromycin in treatment of pharyngeal chlamydia infection. International Journal of STD & AIDS. 2016;**27**:1303-1308

[93] Wyrick PB, Knight ST. Pre-exposure of infected human endometrial epithelial cells to penicillin in vitro renders chlamydia trachomatis refractory to azithromycin. The Journal of Antimicrobial Chemotherapy. 2004;**54**:79-85

[94] Shima K, Ledig S, Loeper N, Schiefer A, Pfarr K, Hoerauf A, et al. Effective inhibition of rifampicin-resistant chlamydia trachomatis by the novel DNA-dependent RNA polymerase inhibitor corallopyronin a. International Journal of Antimicrobial Agents. 2018;**52**:523-524

[95] Loeper N, Graspeuntner S, Ledig S, Kaufhold I, Hoellen F, Schiefer A, et al. Elaborations on Corallopyronin a as a novel treatment strategy against genital chlamydial infections. Frontiers in Microbiology. 2019;**10**:943

[96] Yang S, Traore Y, Jimenez C, Ho EA. Autophagy induction and PDGFR-β knockdown by siRNA-encapsulated nanoparticles reduce chlamydia trachomatis infection. Scientific Reports. 2019;**9**:1306

[97] Núñez-Otero C, Bahnan W, Vielfort K, Silver J, Singh P, Elbir H, et al. A 2-Pyridone amide inhibitor of transcriptional activity in chlamydia trachomatis. Antimicrobial Agents and Chemotherapy. 2021;**65**:e01826-e01820

[98] Hamarsheh O, Amro A, Al-Zeer M. In vitro antibacterial activity of selected Palestinian medicinal plants against chlamydia trachomatis. Microbiological Research. 2021;**12**:656-662

[99] Lam HN, Lau T, Lentz A, Sherry J, Cabrera-Cortez A, Hug K, et al. Developing cyclic Peptomers as broad-Spectrum type III secretion system inhibitors in gram-negative bacteria. Antimicrobial Agents and Chemotherapy. 2021;**65**:e01690-e01620

[100] Itoh R, Kurihara Y, Yoshimura M, Hiromatsu K. Bortezomib eliminates persistent chlamydia trachomatis infection through rapid and specific host cell apoptosis. International Journal of Molecular Sciences. 2022;**23**:7434

[101] Barclay L. ACOG recommends expedited partner therapy for STIs. Medscape Medical News. WebMD Inc. May. 2015;**22**:1526-1528

[102] American College of Obstetricians and Gynecologists. Committee opinion no 632: Expedited partner therapy in the management of gonorrhea and chlamydial infection. Obstetrics and Gynecology. 2015;**125**(6):1526-1528

[103] World Health Organization. WHO Guidelines for the Treatment of Chlamydia Trachomatis. Geneva, Switzerland: World Health Organization; 2016

[104] Tsevat DG, Wiesenfeld HC, Parks C, Peipert JF. Sexually transmitted diseases and infertility. American Journal of Obstetrics and Gynecology. 2017;**216**(1):1-9

[105] Linhares IM, Witkin SS. Immunopathogenic consequences of chlamydia trachomatis 60 kDa heat shock protein expression in the female reproductive tract. Cell Stress & Chaperones. 2010;**15**(5):467-473

[106] Meikle S, Zhang X, Marine W, Calonge B, Hamman R, Betz G. Chlamydia trachomatis antibody titers and hysterosalpingography in predicting tubal disease in infertility patients. Fertility and Sterility. 1994;**62**(2):305-312

[107] Coppus S, Land J, Opmeer B, Steures P, Eijkemans M, Hompes P, et al. Chlamydia trachomatis IgG seropositivity is associated with lower natural conception rates in ovulatory subfertile women without visible tubal pathology. Human Reproduction. 2011;**26**(11):3061-3067

[108] Steiner AZ, Diamond MP, Legro RS, Schlaff WD, Barnhart KT, Casson PR, et al. Chlamydia trachomatis immunoglobulin G3 seropositivity is a predictor of reproductive outcomes in infertile women with patent fallopian tubes. Fertility and Sterility. 2015;**104**(6):1522-1526

[109] Stephens AJ, Aubuchon M, Schust DJ. Antichlamydial antibodies, human fertility, and pregnancy wastage. Infectious Diseases in Obstetrics and Gynecology. 2011;**2011**:525182

[110] Passos LG, Terraciano P, et al. The correlation between chlamydia trachomatis and female infertility: A systematic review. Revista Brasileira de Ginecologia e Obstetrícia. 2022;**44**(6):614-620

[111] Menon S, Stansfield SH, Logan B, Hocking JS, Timms P, Rombauts L, et al. Development and evaluation of a multi-antigen peptide ELISA for the diagnosis of chlamydia trachomatis-related infertility in women. Journal of Medical Microbiology. 2016;**65**(09):915-922

[112] den Heijer CDJ, Hoebe CJPA, Driessen JHM, Wolffs P, van den Broek IVF, Hoenderboom BM, et al.

Chlamydia trachomatis and the risk of pelvic inflammatory disease, ectopic pregnancy, and female infertility: A retrospective cohort study among primary care patients. Clinical Infectious Diseases. 2019;**69**(09):1517-1525

[113] Davies B, Turner KME, Frølund M, Ward H, May MT, Rasmussen S. Et al; Danish chlamydia study group. Risk of reproductive complications following chlamydia testing: A population-based retrospective cohort study in Denmark. The Lancet Infectious Diseases. 2016;**16**(09):1057-1064

[114] Ramadhani MY, Mirambo MM, Mbena H, Kihunrwa A, Mshana SE. High prevalence of chlamydia trachomatis infection among infertile women in Mwanza city, Tanzania: A need to introduce screening and treatment programme. Sexually Transmitted Infections. 2017;**93**(2):111

[115] Kayiira A, Zaake D, Lwetabe MW, Sekweyama P. Impact of genital chlamydia trachomatis infection on reproductive outcomes among infertile women undergoing tubal flushing: A retrospective cohort at a fertility Centre in Uganda. Fertility Research and Practice. 2019;**5**:16

[116] Ceccarani C, Foschi C, Parolin C, D'Antuono A, Gaspari V, Consolandi C, et al. Diversity of vaginal microbiome and metabolome during genital infections. Scientific Reports. 2019;**9**(1):14095

[117] Parolin C, Foschi C, Laghi L, Zhu C, Banzola N, Gaspari V, et al. Insights intovaginal bacterial communities andmetabolicprofiles of chlamydia trachomatis infection: Positioning between eubiosis and dysbiosis. Frontiers in Microbiology. 2018;**9**:600

[118] Gazvani R, Coyne L, Anttila T, Saikku P, Paavonen J, Templeton A. Antibodies to chlamydia trachomatis in serum and peritoneal fluid of women with endometriosis. Human Fertility (Cambridge, England). 2011;**14**(01):64-67

Section 5

Pediatric and Adolescent Chlamydial Infection

Chapter 19

Childhood Chlamydia Infections

Hayriye Daloglu

Abstract

Chlamydia pneumoniae and *Chlamydia trachomatis* are significant human pathogens that affect people of all ages worldwide. *Chlamydia psittaci* is a cause of zoonosis, and birds are the reservoirs. All are diseases for which there is no effective vaccine. *C. pneumoniae* is responsible for respiratory tract infections but the majority of recent *C. pneumoniae* research has focused on the persistent infections associated with chronic diseases and has been considered a childhood infection with potential adult consequences. *C. trachomatis* is one of the most common sexually transmitted diseases (STDs), and the prevalence of the infection is particularly high among young people and adolescents. Prepubertal infection of *C. trachomatis* may be a warning sign for probable child sexual abuse (CSA). In addition to its role in genital diseases, trachoma is one of the world's leading preventable causes of blindness. *C. trachomatis* can also cause Lymphogranuloma venereum (LGV), a systemic, sexually transmitted disease characterized by genital ulceration and inguinal lymphadenopathy. This chapter aims to provide an overview of *Chlamydia* infections in childhood and summarize the epidemiology, clinical manifestations, and treatment.

Keywords: *Chlamydia* infections, *Chlamydia pneumonia*, *Chlamydia Trachomatis*, *Chlamydia Psittachi*, Children

1. Introduction

Chlamydia trachomatis and *Chlamydia pneumoniae* are significant human pathogens that affect people of all ages worldwide. *Chlamydia psittaci* is a cause of zoonosis, and birds are the reservoirs. All are diseases for which there is no effective vaccine.

All members of the family share a lipopolysaccharide antigen and use host resources to synthesize chlamydial protein. They also encode the major outer membrane protein (MOMP or OmpA), which is surface-exposed in *C. trachomatis* and *C. psittaci* but not in *C. pneumoniae*. The MOMP is the major determinant of *C. trachomatis* and *C. psittaci* serologic classification [1, 2].

Chlamydiae are obligate intracellular microorganisms that have a distinct developmental cycle. Understanding this life cycle is important because it underlies the potential problems with laboratory diagnosis, persistent infection, and treatment.

1.1 The biology and life cycle

The chlamydial life cycle is biphasic, with two functional and morphological forms that alternate: infectious "elementary bodies" (EBs) and replicative, non-infectious "reticulate bodies" (RB). The metabolically inactive and infectious "Elementary Body" (EB), which is capable of extracellular survival, binds to the surface of host cells via interactions between bacterial ligands and host receptors, resulting in EB endocytosis. The vesicles containing the EBs are referred to as "inclusion." Because multiple EBs can bind to and enter the same host cell, multiple inclusions are formed. EBs differentiate into metabolically active RBs after internalization. RBs are specialized in nutrient acquisition and the expression of proteins required for energy synthesis. RBs replicate by binary fission within inclusion bodies, avoid lysosomes by modifying host cell endocytic pathways by changing or mimicking the inclusion membrane, and transform into EBs with the ability to infect new host cells [3]. Host metabolites are used in this process via interactions with multiple host cell organelles. After 48–72 hours, new EBs are released by cell lysis to infect other cells while leaving the host cell alive. In this one-of-a-kind cycle, RBs, the organism's intracellular form, play a role in disease persistence, while EBs infect new hosts or neighboring host cells [3, 4].

2. *Chlamydia pneumonia*

Chlamydia pneumoniae was first isolated in 1965 in Taiwan from a child's eye in a trachoma vaccine study and named TW-183 because it was the 183rd isolate in the laboratory. It was assumed that the isolate was a *C. trachomatis* serovar, but it was noticed that it did not share any features of *C. trachomatis* previously tested in laboratory or animal studies. After the micro-immunofluorescence (MIF) serologic test for *Chlamydia* was developed in 1972, TW-183 remained untypable [5]. These antibody studies concluded that TW-183 was probably not a cause of eye disease but a very common infection. Meanwhile, TW-183 was shown to be the probable cause of a pneumonitis outbreak in Finland [6]. AR-39 was the name of the isolate cultivated from the 39th student's throat in a university study, with similar characteristics to TW-183 [7]. While "TW-183/AR-39-like organisms" were continuing to be studied in respiratory tract infections, findings suggested that "TWAR" (as a shorthand for typing) strains were most likely a new human *C. psittaci* strain transmitted from human to human without a bird or animal reservoir [5]. They were shown to be responsible for 12% of pneumonia illnesses and 5% of bronchitis in a university outbreak over a 2.5-year period [5].

In 1989, the TWAR organism was officially announced as "*Chlamydia Pneumoniae*" as a new species by Grayston, based on distinct morphology, DNA sequence, and clinical disease spectrum in *Chlamydiae*, 50 years after Joseph E. Smadel first questioned the source of seven "psittacosis cases without known bird contact" [7].

More recently, a new taxonomic classification was proposed after genome sequencing, in which the genus *Chlamydia pneumoniae* would be replaced with a new genus name, *Chlamydophila pneumoniae* [8, 9]. Since the genus *Chlamydophila* would be composed of most veterinary chlamydiae and the proposal was not universally accepted, especially by the clinicians, and since both names are currently in use by different authors, the former, more widely recognized designation (*Chlamydia pneumoniae*), will be used in this review and will refer to *Chlamydophila pneumoniae*, biovar TWAR.

Even though *C. pneumoniae* is a common pathogen responsible for respiratory tract infections, the majority of recent *C. pneumoniae* research has focused on the pathogen's role as a cause of persistent infections in human chronic diseases and is considered a childhood infection with adult consequences. *C. pneumoniae* has been linked to a wide range of diseases, including cardiovascular disease, Alzheimer's disease, arthritis, ischaemic stroke, asthma, and lung cancer [10].

2.1 Pathogenesis

Chlamydia pneumonia appears to enter the human body via the respiratory mucosal epithelium, and it has been shown that, after infecting lung epithelial cells and alveolar macrophages, they can infiltrate different cell types such as monocytes, macrophages, monocyte-derived dendritic cells (DCs), lymphocytes, and neutrophils [10]. When *C. pneumonia* is not eradicated, RBs, keen on hiding from the host immune system within inclusion bodies, can persist intracellularly for long periods of time and cause chronic infection. Chronically infected monocytes can spread all over the body via the lower respiratory tract after intranasal CP inoculation in mice [11].

2.2 Epidemiology

The mode of transmission of the bacteria in children is not well understood, but it is thought to be similar to other respiratory infections, and transmission occurs from human to human through infected respiratory tract secretions.

It is challenging to describe the epidemiology of *C. pneumonia* precisely. The studies published after the initial identification, during the 1990s, defined the organism as being associated with 6–22% of lower respiratory tract infections in children and adults [12–15]. After the consideration of *C. pneumoniae*'s long-term effects, studies continued with an acceleration number in various populations, with different and more sensitive diagnostic methods. Heterogeneity in the serological methods and study population (hospitalized/outpatient, ages, used criteria in the diagnosis) makes it difficult to compare the results.

Serological studies showed that *C. pneumoniae* is common, with a seroprevalence of over 50% among adults, indicating previous infection [16–19]. In addition, prevalence is relatively low in children under five to ten years (7–8%), sharply increases by the age of 20 (%40–55), and continues to increase gradually to rise in the elderly to 70–80% [16, 20].

C. pneumoniae is considered to affect mostly school-aged children, and initial infection time peaks between 5 and 15 years of age; however, with expanding knowledge, this statement may alter as well. Some studies have shown that the prevalence rate of infection in younger children may be similar to that in older ones. A population-based seroepidemiological survey of students from Italy showed that 23% of the first graders had early exposure to *C. pneumoniae* infection in the community [21]. It seems that the age of primary infection due to *C. pneumonia* seems to differ due to the diagnostic test used. Most young children are not able to develop specific antibodies when culture or PCR testing is used. Colonization or possible infection in younger children would also be identified in the absence of a detectable antibody response.

There is no evidence of seasonality. The mean incubation period is 21 days.

2.3 Clinical presentation

Chlamydia pneumoniae infection is frequently asymptomatic or manifests with mild symptoms. *C. pneumonia*, infecting the upper respiratory epithelium in children, can cause or contribute to acute otitis media and sinusitis, as well as protracted cough illnesses and community-acquired pneumonia.

Upper respiratory tract infections caused by *C. pneumoniae* actually do not have a distinctive clinical picture, and patients may be asymptomatic, mildly, or moderately ill, with non-specific respiratory complaints. In general, signs and symptoms of respiratory infections have little value in the diagnosis of *C. pneumoniae*.

Clinical manifestations of the *C. pneumoniae* infection as upper respiratory tract infections were established as pharyngitis, otitis, and sinusitis, with an incidence of 5–10% in the initial studies [7, 22]. Nasopharyngitis (46%) was the most common clinical presentation in school-aged respiratory infections related to *C. pneumoniae*, documented by PCR positivity [23]. In a recent study, *C. pneumoniae* was detected by PCR in 38% of children under 10 years diagnosed with an upper respiratory infection in Brazil [24].

"Sore throat" and "hoarseness" are particular symptoms commonly mentioned in the studies in which either the upper or lower respiratory tract was included [22, 23]. Although fever and related respiratory symptoms can be self-limited, the cough usually follows pharyngitis. The clinical progress can be biphasic and end up in atypical pneumonia. The infection is often associated with a persistent cough when the lower respiratory tract is included. *C. pneumoniae* was isolated in 17% of the infants with prolonged coughing [25]. The mean duration of cough associated with a *C. pneumoniae* infection has been reported as 25–30 days.

Clinical features of *C. pneumoniae* pneumonia are similar to those of other community-acquired pneumonia (CAP), including fever, cough, tachypnea, and shortness of breath. Physical examination may reveal nonexudative pharyngitis, pulmonary rales, and bronchospasm. It is not feasible to distinguish the causative agent according to clinical or routine laboratory tests [26, 27]. Chest radiograph findings generally are nonspecific and include patchy subsegmental infiltration, bilateral infiltrates, segmental and lobar consolidation, and even pleural effusion [27–30].

Data gained from the epidemics painted a clinical picture of mild but long-lasting pneumonia in previously healthy young adults [6]. With our expanding knowledge, it seems that the course of the disease may vary with the patient's age, the presence of co-pathogens, or the existence of comorbidities. Severe and life-threatening infections have been reported [31]. Coinfection with other pathogens is possible and may affect clinical presentation [32].

C. pneumoniae can manifest as severe community-acquired pneumonia in immunocompromised hosts and has been associated with the onset or acute exacerbation of respiratory symptoms in patients with asthma, cystic fibrosis, and acute chest syndrome in children with sickle cell disease; rare cases of meningoencephalitis and myocarditis have also been attributed to the pathogen [33].

2.4 Diagnosis

The micro immunofluorescent (MIF) antibody test is the most sensitive and specific serologic test for acute infections, but it cannot be used to make an instant diagnosis. A fourfold increase in IgG levels in acute and convalescent sera is diagnostic. IgM titers greater than 1:16 are indicative of acute infection. IgM increases 1–2 weeks after the onset of primary infection, but not upon reinfection. It should be considered that early antibiotic treatment may suppress the antibody response.

NAATs, such as real-time polymerase chain reaction (PCR) assays, can detect the organism on nasopharyngeal swabs, bronchoalveolar lavages, and sputum samples with high sensitivity and specificity and are useful for rapid and accurate diagnosis [33]. *C. pneumoniae* can be isolated from swab specimens, sputum, bronchoalveolar lavage, and tissue biopsy specimens, but the organism is relatively hard to culture.

2.5 Treatment

Chlamydia pneumoniae appears sensitive to tetracyclines, macrolides, ketolides, and the majority of fluoroquinolones (e.g., levofloxacin and moxifloxacin but not ciprofloxacin). A total of 70–90% of children with *C. pneumoniae* pneumonia eradicate the organism from the nasopharynx after a 10-day course of erythromycin, clarithromycin, or a 5-day course of azithromycin [26, 34, 35]. When tetracycline or doxycycline is prescribed, typical treatment regimens consist of 14–21 days: 14 days for erythromycin, 7–14 days for fluoroquinolones or clarithromycin, and 5 days for azithromycin.

Clinical improvement occurs in a high proportion of children even if they are untreated or given beta-lactam antibiotics which are thought to be ineffective [36]. On the other hand, despite 10–30 days of appropriate treatment, ongoing isolation of the organism persists in some patients [37].

3. *Chlamydia Trachomatis*

C. trachomatis is the most prevalent sexually transmitted bacterium in the world [38]. It is a significant public health concern [39].

Although chlamydia typically affects sexually active adolescents or adults, this infection can also be transmitted vertically during delivery from their infected mothers.

Prepubertal infection of *C. trachomatis* may be a sign of probable child sexual abuse (CSA), necessitating a multidisciplinary thorough investigation.

In addition to its role in genital diseases and associated perinatal infections, trachoma is one of the world's leading preventable causes of blindness. *C. trachomatis* can also cause Lymphogranuloma venereum (LGV), a systemic, sexually transmitted disease characterized by genital ulceration and inguinal lymphadenopathy.

3.1 Classification

C. trachomatis encodes an abundant surface-exposed protein known as the major outer membrane protein (MOMP or OmpA), which is the primary determinant of serologic classification. Based on antigenic variation in the major OMPs (serovars) and clinical expression, *C. trachomatis* is subdivided into subgroups. Microimmunofluorescence and monoclonal antibody testing have revealed that there are over 18 serovars of *C. trachomatis* classified under three biovars [4].

In developing nations, the trachoma biovar (serovars A–C) is the leading cause of non-congenital blindness, whereas the genital tract biovar (serovars D–K) is the most common sexually transmitted bacterium, each of which is associated with a distinct clinical presentation [1, 3] Serovars A, B, Ba, and C cause trachoma; serovars B, Da, Ga, Ia, and D-K cause oculogenital and neonatal disease; and serovars L1, L2, L2a, and L3 cause lymphogranuloma venereum (LGV).

3.2 Pathogenesis

The major symptoms of *C. trachomatis* infection are not due to direct pathogen activity but rather to the host's immune response to infection. LGV serovars can proliferate in lymph nodes and macrophages, whereas other types of *C. trachomatis* can only replicate in mucosal epithelial cells. After 7–21 days (on average, 10 days), various clinical symptoms manifest due to tissue degradation or the host's inflammatory response. Neutrophil infiltration distinguishes the initial stages of the primary infection. Although lymphocytes and plasma cells contribute to the initial response, they also play a role in the resolution of the infection [40, 41]. Plasma cells predominate in ocular and genital tract infections [42, 43], whereas eosinophils and neutrophils predominate in neonatal pneumonia [44]. Chlamydial infections can be self-limiting and asymptomatic or infections can be persistent for months or years, it is assumed that the host will develop some form of a protective immune response [45–47]. However, natural *C. trachomatis* infection is insufficient to prevent reinfection. Since the majority of chlamydial infections of the genital tract are asymptomatic, the risk of chronic, untreated infections is high.

3.3 Epidemiology

Different strains of *C. trachomatis* infect either the mucosa of the genital tract or the eye. In endemic regions, primarily in Africa and the Middle East, *C. trachomatis* causes trachoma, the leading preventable cause of blindness globally. Approximately 136 million people reside in trachoma-endemic areas in 44 countries [48].

C. trachomatis is the most common bacterial cause of sexually transmitted infections (STIs) worldwide. According to the World Health Organization's (WHO) global surveillance of STIs in 2018, the global estimate of new CT cases in 2016 was 127 million [49]. Genital Chlamydia infections are asymptomatic in 61% of women and 68% of men; consequently, they are frequently misdiagnosed and untreated, resulting in transmission to others.

The most strongly associated sociodemographic factor with chlamydial infection is young age (<20 years). *C. trachomatis* was found in 6.5% of high school students, with rates among girls being more than double those of boys (4.0% versus 9.7%), and rates of infection increased with age [50]. In a study of over 3000 sexually active middle-school-aged female adolescents, 29% of them had at least 1 positive test result, and the highest age-specific prevalence rate (28%) was found in 14-year-old females [51]. The prevalence of CT infection was 11.5% among adolescents and 6.2% among young adult women.

3.4 Clinical presentations of *C. trachomatis* in children

C. trachomatis infects non-ciliated squamocolumnar or transitional epithelial cells that are susceptible (e.g., mucous membranes of the conjunctivae, posterior nasopharynx, urethra, endocervix, and rectum).

3.4.1 Perinatal infection

Typically, a newborn acquires an infection while passing through an infected birth canal, but it is known that transmission via cesarean delivery is possible, whether or not the membranes rupture prematurely. The prevalence of *C. trachomatis* infection in pregnant women varies depending on the population studied, ranging from 2 to 20% [52–54]. As in the general population, young women, particularly adolescents, had the highest prevalence of infection during pregnancy. In a British study of 1216 pregnant women, the overall CT infection prevalence was 2.4%, but it increased to 8.6% under the age of 25 years and 14.3% in the adolescent group [55]. Another study found that 18% of 203 pregnant adolescents had *C. trachomatis* infection in the third trimester of pregnancy [56].

The conclusion of many studies done in the 1980s was that maternal carriage of *C. trachomatis* is associated with a high incidence of clinical illness in infants. Prospective studies of infants born to mothers with chlamydial infection of the cervix have revealed a 50–75% risk of *C. trachomatis* acquisition in at least one anatomic site, including the conjunctiva, nasopharynx, rectum, and vagina [57]. Infants exposed to untreated *C. trachomatis* are estimated to have a 20–50% risk of conjunctivitis and a 5–20% risk of pneumonia [57–59]. In a recent Chinese study, the vertical transmission rate was determined to be 67% after vaginal delivery and 8% after a cesarean section [60]. Symptomatic chlamydia appears in infants mostly between the ages of 4 and 5 weeks, with a range of 2–20 weeks [56, 61].

3.4.1.1 Inclusion conjunctivitis

C. trachomatis has been reported to be the *most prevalent cause* of ophthalmia neonatorum in many countries and neonatal conjunctivitis is the *primary clinical manifestation* of chlamydial infection in neonates [62–64]. The findings of studies conducted in various countries clearly show that the distribution of key etiological agents of newborn conjunctivitis corresponds to the real prevalence of STI infections among pregnant women.

Ocular findings start usually between 5 and 14 days postpartum, although they can occur earlier if a premature membrane rupture is present. Mucopurulent discharge (95%), swelling of the eyelids (73%), and conjunctival erythema (65%) are the defined symptoms [65]. The vast majority of cases resolve spontaneously, but conjunctivitis can be long-lasting and severe; in the condition of severe inflammation, a pseudomembrane formation develops as a result of large exudates adhering to the conjunctivae. Conjunctivae may bleed during the examination or sampling. Corneal ulceration, scarring, and pannus formation are uncommon; and recovery without visual impairment is expected. Bloodstained eye discharge was found to have high specificity and positive predictive value for chlamydial conjunctivitis in a retrospective study of 90 infants from Hong Kong with chlamydial conjunctivitis [66]. At least 50% of infants with chlamydial conjunctivitis also have a nasopharyngeal infection, and 50% of the pneumonia cases have evidence of previous conjunctivitis [56, 67].

Neonatal prophylaxis with antibiotic-containing ointments has no effect on the incidence of chlamydial conjunctivitis or the development of nasopharyngeal carriage and pneumonia [68, 69].

Differential diagnosis of gonococcal and other pyogenic conjunctivitis is not possible based on clinical findings, but ophthalmia neonatorum due to gonococcal infection usually begins earlier (postnatal 3–5 days).

3.4.1.2 Neonatal pneumonia

The importance of *C trachomatis* as a causal pathogen for respiratory illness in young infants is well documented in the literature [62]. *C. trachomatis* seems the etiological agent of 7–30% of the hospitalized pneumonia cases before 6 months of age [70–74].

Clinical manifestations of chlamydial pneumonia typically appear between the ages of 3 and 12 weeks. The majority of the infants are only mildly ill and afebrile. Nasal obstruction and *staccato* cough worsen over one or more weeks. Tachypnea and rallies are found on physical examination, but wheezing is uncommon. An X-ray of the chest will usually show hyper aeration as well as bilateral interstitial infiltration. Peripheral eosinophilia (>400 cells/mm^3) is a distinctive laboratory finding but the total white cell number is usually normal [73, 75]. Concomitant or history of conjunctivitis is present in 30–50% of cases. The absence of fever and significant wheezing may be useful in the differential diagnosis of RSV infection, which is the most common pathogen in this age group.

Infected preterm neonates, may present differently. They can be symptomatic as early as 48 hours after birth, manifesting as idiopathic respiratory distress syndrome, which improved initially but was complicated by apneic spells and feeding difficulties [76]. Severe infections causing respiratory failure are also defined in the literature [77–79].

3.4.1.3 Infections at other sites

It is possible to detect asymptomatic rectal or vaginal *C. trachomatis* in 14% of neonates born to women with chlamydial infection, which can persist for 18 months [80, 81]. The presence of *C. trachomatis* in the genital tract can complicate the evaluation of probable sexual abuse and necessitates a thorough investigation [81].

3.4.2 Infections in older children

No specific clinical syndrome has been associated with *C. trachomatis* in older infants and children. The majority of focus on *C. trachomatis* infection in these children has centered on its association with child sexual abuse. As mentioned previously, perinatal maternal–infant transmission resulting in vaginal and/or rectal infection has been documented with up to three years of prolonged infection.

If *C. trachomatis* established in a prepubertal child from a rectal or genital site, sexual abuse must always be considered and a detailed multidisciplinary assessment of sexual abuse should be performed [82]. There is no evidence in the literature about the transmission of this organism without sexual activity such as via fomites.

3.4.3 Infections in adolescents

3.4.3.1 Oculogenital infections

Half of the approximately 20 million new sexually transmitted infections (STIs) diagnosed annually in the USA affect those aged 15–24 and both male and female STI rates are on the rise, with the majority of this increase occurring among adolescents [83]. It is estimated that one in four sexually active adolescent girls have a sexually transmitted infection, most commonly *C. trachomatis* (CT) and human papillomavirus (HPV) [84].

From a behavioral and biological point of view, adolescents are presumed to engage in high-risk sexual behavior, such as having multiple partners or not using a condom. And due to the biological factors, it is known that adolescent females are susceptible to sexually transmitted diseases due to cervical ectopy, and lower production of cervical mucous. Studies indicate that *C. trachomatis* infection is more prevalent in patients with cervical ectopy, which is more common in adolescents [85, 86]. In addition, most *C. trachomatis* infection is asymptomatic and adolescents are less likely than adults to apply for sexual health services and have STD screening. Healthcare professionals usually do not feel confident about questioning adolescents and young adults about their sexual behaviors, assessing for STI risks, and screening for STIs. These factors contribute to creating an ongoing reservoir for infection and a lower chance of diagnosis and treatment.

Females infected with Chlamydia may develop cervicitis, urethritis, and proctitis, and males may exhibit urethritis, proctitis, and epididymitis as manifestations. In the majority of cases, heterosexual transmission accounts for a high rate. Since the majority of chlamydia infections, including non-genital infections, are asymptomatic, routine screening of at-risk populations is recommended for preventing transmission to sexual partners and preventing complications of untreated infections. A total of 82 Colombian women were followed for five years using serotyping and polymerase chain reaction (PCR) on cervical-scrap samples; it was stated that untreated, approximately 46% of infections were persistent at one year, 18% at two years, and 6% at four years, and manifesting symptoms were dysuria/pyuria syndrome, vaginal discharge, intermittent bleeding, and moderate abdominal pain [47]. Besides, they noticed that *C. trachomatis* can cause vaginitis in adolescence but not in adults; the squamous epithelium of the adult vagina is not vulnerable, and vaginal discharge is generally indicative of endocervical infection.

In women who do not get treatment, an ascending acute urogenital infection can cause severe, long-lasting pelvic inflammation. This can show up as endometritis, salpingitis, PID, chronic pelvic pain, etc., and it can damage the tubes, which can lead to infertility and ectopic pregnancy. The spectrum of PID associated with *C. trachomatis* infection extends from asymptomatic to a severe, acute disease characterized by perihepatitis and ascites (Fitz-Hugh–Curtis syndrome). It has been discovered that chlamydia screening reduces the incidence of PID [87].

In the USA, a national cross-sectional prospective cohort found that 95% of *C. trachomatis*-infected people had no symptoms. The most common symptoms among infected males were urethral discharge (3%) and dysuria (2%), while the most common symptoms among infected females were vaginal discharge (0.3%) and dysuria (4%). And seropositivity was only in 1% of vaginal discharges [88, 89]. A total of 38% of males reporting urethral discharge and 6% of females reporting dysuria were found to be positive for *C. trachomatis*.

Epididymitis, reactive arthritis (including Reiter syndrome), and transmission to females are the primary complications of chlamydial urethritis in men.

Although asymptomatic rectal and nasopharyngeal carriage of *C. trachomatis* can occur in both infants and adults, *C. trachomatis* is also reported as a cause of proctitis [90, 91].

Inclusion conjunctivitis is an extra-genital manifestation of this STD in both sexes that results from oto-inoculation of the eyes with contaminated genital secretion, typically as acute follicular conjunctivitis. The symptoms are usually a sensation of a foreign body in the eye. In most cases, the infection resolves without complications; however, if left untreated, it can persist for months and cause damage.

3.4.3.2 Lymphogranuloma Venereum

LGV is a STI caused by the L1 to L3 *C. trachomatis* serovars.

The bubonic form of the disease is endemic to tropical and subtropical regions. Classically, LGV starts with a small papule or ulcer and days to weeks after the primary lesion resolves spontaneously, unilateral inguinal lymphadenitis, and hemorrhagic proctitis develop. Systemic symptoms may accompany it, including fever, myalgia, and headache. Approximately one-third of inguinal buboes drain, and the rest involute slowly. Due to the persistence of chlamydia in anogenital tissues, a small proportion of patients with LGV develop a chronic inflammatory response with fibrosis, which can lead to chronic genital ulcers or fistulas, rectal strictures, or genital elephantiasis.

3.4.4 Trachoma

Trachoma remains one of the world's primary causes of blindness; approximately 30% of children in a holoendemic region are at risk of blindness due to severe trachoma [47]. Both pannus formation and progressive disease with scarring are thought to be the result of a long-term cycle of active infection and healing over the years.

In areas where trachoma is endemic, infections occur early in life and the disease remains active for several years. Poor hygiene and the presence of eye-seeking insects increase the likelihood of transmission. Inclusion conjunctivitis' characteristic chronic follicular conjunctivitis first appears, then the conjunctivae become more intensely inflamed, and finally, the tarsal conjunctiva fibrosis occurs. Trichiasis (turning of the eyelashes) frequently develops following extensive scarring of the inner surface of the lids. This causes additional corneal ulceration, fibrosis, opacification, and vision loss. Young adolescents with active trachoma can have *C. trachomatis* isolated from conjunctival scrapings and nasopharyngeal cultures.

3.5 Diagnosis

NAATs such as PCR assays are the guideline-recommended method for pathogen identification in acute *urethritis* [92]. First-catch urine or a urethral swab specimen can be used. NAATs also have more sensitivity and specificity than culture in nasopharyngeal and rectal infections both in males and females [93–96]. For *urogenital infections in females*, NAATs are the most sensitive tests as well and are recommended for laboratory diagnosis.

Both cell culture and nonculture assays are sensitive and specific diagnostic techniques such as direct fluorescent antibody tests (DFA) and NAAT, in the diagnosis of *neonatal chlamydial conjunctivitis* [97, 98]. Because eye discharge alone is not sufficient, conjunctival cells are required, and the specimen should be obtained from the everted eyelid using a dacron-tipped swab.

For *chlamydial infant pneumonia*, cell culture is the definitive standard diagnostic test. Specimens collected from the posterior nasopharynx are recommended or tracheal aspirates and lung biopsy specimens if collected. Chlamydia culture in tissue culture is a sensitive and specific method for detecting neonatal chlamydial infections; however, it is time-consuming and costly and has been largely replaced by NAATs. DFA or NAATs can be used in the same specimens but have lower sensitivity and specificity than culture. Microimmunofluorescent (MIF) serum titer of *C trachomatis*-specific immunoglobulin Ig M > 1:32 is diagnostic.

Only molecular testing that is specific to LGV can provide a definitive diagnosis of LGV (for example, PCR-based genotyping).

Trachoma of the eye is typically diagnosed clinically in countries where the disease is endemic.

When concerning possible sexual child abuse, it is preferred the child be referred for complete evaluation and management to an experienced/specialized pediatrician, clinic, or child advocacy center, with a prompt examination for other SDIs as well. If sexual abuse is suspected, appropriate social service and law enforcement agencies must be contacted to evaluate the situation, ensure the child or adolescent's safety, and provide appropriate counseling.

3.6 Treatment

Because the elementary body is metabolically inactive, the treatment should target the intracellular form of the organism and have strong intracellular penetration. And, given CT's 36–48-hour intracellular formation cycle, a long therapeutic duration or a long half-life antibiotic should be chosen to assure appropriate levels of the antibiotic.

To prevent *C. trachomatis* infection-related complications, decrease the risk of transmission to sex partners and newborns in pregnant individuals, resolve the symptoms, eradicate the microorganism, and prevent re-infection, screening and treating adolescents and young people are recommended. After starting doxycycline or azithromycin, clinical improvement is achieved in 83–86% of symptomatic patients with cervicitis and urethritis [98]. By the way, because most of the patients are asymptomatic, microbial eradication should be targeted.

Inclusion conjunctivitis or Pneumonia of infancy: Erythromycin (50 mg/kg/day in 4 doses) for 10–14 days or Azithromycin (10 mg/kg/day) for 5 days [33]. Empiric antibiotic treatment is recommended for neonatal pneumonia till to diagnostic results are available, but not for conjunctivitis [98].

Genital infections in adolescents: CT is shown to be susceptible to tetracyclines, macrolides, and some of fluoroquinolones [99]. Although amoxicillin is effective, penicillins are accused of easing the *in vitro* persistence of the microorganism [100].

If laboratory diagnosis is not possible, symptomatic patients with cervicitis, urethritis, epidydymithis, or acute prostatitis who have had recent known or possible sexual exposure can be offered empiric treatment for CT.

Doxycycline is given as 100 mg twice daily for seven days, or single-dose 1 gram azithromycin is recommended by the CDC in the treatment of genital chlamydia infections [83].

Although doxycycline seems microbiologically more effective than azitromycin, especially in rectal infections [101–103], azitromycin has the advantage of better adherence to treatment with a single dose. Levofloxacin and ofloxacin are the alternative antibiotics recommended.

4. *Chlamydia psittachi* infections

Chlamydophila psittaci can cause systemic infection and pneumonia, often called psittacosis or ornithosis The pathogen *Chlamydophila psittaci* can cause systemic infections and pneumonia, often called psittacosis or ornithosis. Previously, it was classified under the genus of Chlamydia but now it is grouped *with C. pneumoniae* and some other veterinary species in the genus Chlamydophila of the family Chlamydiaceae [4].

4.1 Epidemiology

Psittacosis is responsible for 1% of incident cases of CAP, according to a recent meta-analysis [104]. From 1990 to 2008, the Centers for Disease Control and Prevention (CDC) received 756 reports of psittacosis, of which 9% involved individuals younger than 20 years old [105]. It is not a well-recognized disease by clinicians, there are difficulties in the diagnosis of infection and may be due to underreporting, it is thought that this may not be reflecting the actual number of cases. It is not a well-recognized disease by clinicians, there are difficulties in diagnosing infection, and because of underreporting, this may not reflect the actual number of cases.

C. psittaci is transmitted through the inhalation of aerosols containing respiratory tract secretions, eye secretions, urine, or feces from infected birds. Even limited exposure to infected birds or their droppings can cause illness. Most reported cases of psittacosis have been linked to exposure to domestic birds. Since *C. psittaci* is resistant to drying and can remain infectious for months in the environment, avian exposure may not be reported in some cases.

4.2 Clinical manifestations

Psittacosis classically causes "atypical" pneumonia. Disease presentations can range from minor influenza-like symptoms to severe systemic diseases. The incubation period is typically between 5 and 14 days, but symptoms can appear up to one month after exposure. It is impossible to make a differential diagnosis according to clinical features compared to other pathogens of community-acquired pneumonia [106]. Psittacosis should be considered in any child with pneumonia who has had close contact with birds.

4.3 Diagnosis

Historically, the diagnosis of *C. psittaci* disease was based on clinical presentation and a positive microimmunofluorescence (MIF) with paired sera serologic test results. Despite the fact that the MIF test is generally more sensitive and specific than complement fixation (CF) assays, MIF still exhibits cross-reactivity with other Chlamydia species in some cases. NAATs and PCR tests are currently accessible only in specialized laboratories [107].

4.4 Treatment

Doxycycline, erythromycin, and azithromycin are the drugs recommended for treatment.

Author details

Hayriye Daloglu[1,2]

1 Faculty of Health Sciences Antalya Bilim University, Antalya, Turkey

2 Medicalpark Antalya Hospital, Department of Pediatric Bone Marrow Transplantation Unit, Antalya, Turkey

*Address all correspondence to: hayriye.daloglu@gmail.com

References

[1] Tan M, Bavoil P. Intracellular Pathogens I: Chlamydiales. Washington, DC, USA: American Society for Microbiology Press; 2012

[2] Elwell C, Mirrashidi K, Engel J. Chlamydia cell biology and pathogenesis. Nature Reviews Microbiology. 2016;**14**(6):385-400

[3] Bastidas RJ, Elwell CA, Engel JN, Valdivia RH. Chlamydial intracellular survival strategies. Cold Spring Harbor perspectives in medicine. 2013;**3**(5):a010256

[4] Bachmann NL, Polkinghorne A, Timms P. Chlamydia genomics: Providing novel insights into chlamydial biology. Trends in microbiology. 2014;**22**(8):464-472

[5] Grayston J, Wang S-P. History of Chlamydia pneumoniae (TWAR). *Chlamydia pneumoniae*. The lung and the Heart. Midtown Manhattan, New York City, USA: Springer Publishing; 1999. pp. 1-8

[6] Kleemola M, Saikku P, Visakorpi R, Wang S, Grayston J. Epidemics of pneumonia caused by TWAR, a new chlamydia organism, in military trainees in Finland. Journal of Infectious Diseases. 1988;**157**(2):230-236

[7] Grayston JT, Kuo C-C, Campbell LA, Wang S-P. Chlamydia pneumoniae sp. nov. for chlamydia sp. strain TWAR. International Journal of Systematic and Evolutionary Microbiology. 1989;**39**(1):88-90

[8] Everett KD, Bush RM, Andersen AA. Emended description of the order Chlamydiales, proposal of Parachlamydiaceae fam. Nov. and Simkaniaceae fam. Nov., each containing one monotypic genus, revised taxonomy of the family Chlamydiaceae, including a new genus and five new species, and standards for the identification of organisms. International Journal of Systematic Bacteriology. 1999;**49**(Pt 2):415-440

[9] Schachter J, Stephens RS, Timms P, Kuo C, Bavoil PM, Birkelund S, et al. Radical changes to chlamydial taxonomy are not necessary just yet. International Journal of Systematic and Evolutionary Microbiology. 2001;**51**(Pt 1):249

[10] Porritt RA, Crother TR. Chlamydia pneumoniae infection and inflammatory diseases. Forum on Immunopathological Diseases and Therapeutics. 2016;**7**(3-4):237-254

[11] Yang Z-p, Kuo C-c, Thomas GJ. Systemic dissemination of chlamydia pneumoniae following intranasal inoculation in mice. Journal of Infectious Diseases. 1995;**171**(3):736-738

[12] Grayston JT, Campbell LA, Kuo C-C, Mordhorst CH, Saikku P, Thorn DH, et al. A new respiratory tract pathogen: Chlamydia pneumoniae strain TWAR. Journal of Infectious Diseases. 1990;**161**(4):618-625

[13] Grayston JT. Chlamydia pneumoniae (TWAR) infections in children. The Pediatric infectious disease journal. 1994;**13**(8):675-685

[14] Hammerschlag MR. Chlamydia pneumoniae and the lung. European Respiratory Journal. 2000;**16**(5):1001-1007

[15] Blasi F, Cosentini R, Tarsia P. Chlamydia pneumoniae respiratory

infections. Current Opinion in Infectious Diseases. 2000;**13**(2):161-164

[16] Lin T-M, Kuo C, Chen W, Lin F, Eng H-L. Seroprevalence of chlamydia pneumoniae infection in Taiwan. Journal of Infection. 2004;**48**(1):91-95

[17] Aldous MB, Grayston JT, Wang S-p, Foy HM. Seroepidemiology of chlamydia pneumoniae TWAR infection in Seattle families, 1966-1979. Journal of Infectious Diseases. 1992;**166**(3):646-649

[18] Kanamoto Y, Ouchi K, Mizui M, Ushio M, Usui T. Prevalence of antibody to chlamydia pneumoniae TWAR in Japan. Journal of Clinical Microbiology. 1991;**29**(4):816-818

[19] Montes M, Cilla G, Alcorta M, Pérez-Trallero E. High prevalence of chlamydia pneumoniae infection in children and young adults in Spain. The Pediatric Infectious Disease Journal. 1992;**11**(11):972-973

[20] Chatzidimitriou D, Exidari M, Gioula G, Papakonstantinou P, Melidou A, Gavriilaki E, et al. Seroepidemiology of chlamydia pneumoniae in northern Greece. European Journal of Inflammation. 2009;**7**(3):139-144

[21] Dal Molin G, Longo B, Not T, Poli A, Campello C. A population based seroepidemiological survey of chlamydia pneumoniae infections in schoolchildren. Journal of Clinical Pathology. 2005;**58**(6):617-620

[22] Huovinen P, Riitta L, Thedi Z, Meurman O, Hakkarainen K, Miettinen A, et al. Pharyngitis in adults: The presence and coexistence of viruses and bacterial organisms. Annals of Internal Medicine. 1989;**110**(8):612-616

[23] Norman E, Gnarpe J, Granpe HC. Pneumoniae in children with acute respiratory tract infection. Acta Pediatrics. 1998;**80**:405-409

[24] Alves MS, da Silva CM, dos Santos Ferreira HL, de Abreu S, Silva E, Felipe KKP, et al. High frequency of chlamydia pneumoniae and risk factors in children with acute respiratory infection. Brazilian Journal of Microbiology. 2020;**51**:629-636

[25] Hallander HO, Gnarpe J, Gnarpe H, Olin P. Bordetella pertussis, Bordetella parapertussis, mycoplasma pneumoniae, chlamydia pneumoniae and persistent cough in children. Scandinavian Journal of Infectious Diseases. 1999;**31**(3):281-286

[26] Block S, Hedrick J, Hammerschlag MR, Cassell GH, Craft JC. Mycoplasma pneumoniae and chlamydia pneumoniae in pediatric community-acquired pneumonia: Comparative efficacy and safety of clarithromycin vs. erythromycin ethylsuccinate. The Pediatric infectious disease journal. 1995;**14**(6):471-477

[27] Esposito S, Bosis S, Cavagna R, Faelli N, Begliatti E, Marchisio P, et al. Characteristics of Streptococcus pneumoniae and atypical bacterial infections in children 2-5 years of age with community-acquired pneumonia. Clinical Infectious Diseases. 2002;**35**(11):1345-1352

[28] Puljiz I, Kuzman I, Dakovic-Rode O, Schönwald N, Mise B. Chlamydia pneumoniae and mycoplasma pneumoniae pneumonia: Comparison of clinical, epidemiological characteristics and laboratory profiles. Epidemiology & Infection. 2006;**134**(3):548-555

[29] Chirgwin K, Roblin PM, Gelling M, Hammerschlag MR, Schachter J. Infection

with chlamydia pneumoniae in Brooklyn. Journal of Infectious Diseases. 1991;**163**(4):757-761

[30] Augenbraun MH, Roblin PM, Mandel LJ, Hammerschlag MR, Schachter J. Chlamydia pneumoniae pneumonia with pleural effusion: Diagnosis by culture. The American journal of medicine. 1991;**91**(4):437-438

[31] Tenenbaum T, Heusch A, Henrich B, MacKenzie C, Schmidt K, Schroten H. Acute hemorrhagic pericarditis in a child with pneumonia due to Chlamydophila pneumoniae. Journal of clinical microbiology. 2005;**43**(1):520-522

[32] Miyashita N, Fukano H, Okimoto N, Hara H, Yoshida K, Niki Y, et al. Clinical presentation of community-acquired chlamydia pneumoniae pneumonia in adults. Chest. 2002;**121**(6):1776-1781

[33] Kimberlin DW. Red Book: 2018-2021 Report of the Committee on Infectious Diseases: American Academy of Pediatrics. 2018

[34] Harris J-AS, Kolokathis A, Campbell M, Cassell GH, Hammerschlag MR. Safety and efficacy of azithromycin in the treatment of community-acquired pneumonia in children. The Pediatric infectious disease journal. 1998;**17**(10):865-871

[35] Roblin PM, Hammerschlag MR. Microbiologic efficacy of azithromycin and susceptibilities to azithromycin of isolates of chlamydia pneumoniae from adults and children with community-acquired pneumonia. Antimicrobial Agents and Chemotherapy. 1998;**42**(1):194-196

[36] Esposito S, Bosis S, Faelli N, Begliatti E, Droghetti R, Tremolati E, et al. Role of atypical bacteria and azithromycin therapy for children with recurrent respiratory tract infections. The Pediatric infectious disease journal. 2005;**24**(5):438-444

[37] Hammerschlag MR, Chirgwin K, Roblin PM, Gelling M, Dumornay W, Mandel L, et al. Persistent infection with chlamydia pneumoniae following acute respiratory illness. Clinical Infectious Diseases. 1992;**14**(1):178-182

[38] Sarıer M, Duman I, Göktaş Ş, Demir M, Kukul E. Results of Multiplex Polymerase Chain Reaction Assay to ıdentify Urethritis Pathogens. 2017

[39] Sarier M, Demir M, Turgut H, Hizel A, Emek M, Kukul E, et al. New approach to microscopy of gram-stained urethral smear: The kissing slide method. Sexually Transmitted Diseases. 2020;**47**(10):712-715

[40] Brunham RC, Paavonen J, Stevens CE, Kiviat N, Kuo C-C, Critchlow CW, et al. Mucopurulent cervicitis—The ignored counterpart in women of urethritis in men. New England journal of medicine. 1984;**311**(1):1-6

[41] Rank R, Sanders M. Pathogenesis of endometritis and salpingitis in a Guinea pig model of chlamydial genital infection. The American journal of pathology. 1992;**140**(4):927

[42] Paavonen J, Kiviat N, Brunham RC, Stevens CE, Kuo C-C, Stamm WE, et al. Prevalence and manifestations of endometritis among women with cervicitis. American journal of obstetrics and gynecology. 1985;**152**(3):280-286

[43] Patton D, Taylor H. The histopathology of experimental trachoma: Ultrastructural changes in the conjunctival epithelium. Journal of Infectious Diseases. 1986;**153**(5):870-878

[44] Griffin M, Pushpanathan C, Andrews W. Chlamydia trachomatis pneumonitis: A case study and literature review. Pediatric Pathology. 1990;**10**(5):843-852

[45] McCormack WM, Alpert S, McComb DE, Nichols RL, Semine DZ, Zinner SH. Fifteen-month follow-up study of women infected with chlamydia trachomatis. Obstetrical & Gynecological Survey. 1979;**34**(6):472-477

[46] Bell TA, Stamm WE, Chou Kuo C, Holmes KK, Grayston JT. Chronic chlamydia trachomatis infections in infants. Journal of the American Medical Association. 1992;**267**(3):400-402

[47] Molano M, Meijer CJ, Weiderpass E, Arslan A, Posso H, Franceschi S, et al. The natural course of chlamydia trachomatis infection in asymptomatic Colombian women: A 5-year follow-up study. The Journal of infectious diseases. 2005;**191**(6):907-916

[48] Solomon AW, Burton MJ, Gower EW, Harding-Esch EM, Oldenburg CE, Taylor HR, et al. Trachoma. Nature Reviews Disease Primers. 2022;**8**(1):32

[49] World Health Organization - WHO. Report on global sexually transmitted infection surveillance [Internet]. Geneva: World Health Organization; 2018 [cited 2020 Jun 7]. Available from: https://www.who.int/reproductivehealth/publications/stis-surveillance-2018/en/

[50] Cohen DA, Nsuami M, Etame RB, Tropez-Sims S, Abdalian S, Farley TA, et al. A school-based chlamydia control program using DNA amplification technology. Pediatrics. 1998;**101**(1):E1

[51] Burstein GR, Gaydos CA, Diener-West M, Howell MR, Zenilman JM, Quinn TC. Incident chlamydia trachomatis infections among inner-city adolescent females. Journal of the American Medical Association. 1998;**280**(6):521-526

[52] FitzSimmons J, Callahan C, Shanahan B, Jungkind D. Chlamydial infections in pregnancy. The Journal of Reproductive Medicine. 1986;**31**(1):19-22

[53] Oakeshott P, Hay P, Hay S, Steinke F, Rink E, Kerry S. Association between bacterial vaginosis or chlamydial infection and miscarriage before 16 weeks' gestation: Prospective community based cohort study. BMJ. 2002;**325**(7376):1334

[54] Niccolai LM, Ethier KA, Kershaw TS, Lewis JB, Ickovics JR. Pregnant adolescents at risk: Sexual behaviors and sexually transmitted disease prevalence. American Journal of Obstetrics and Gynecology. 2003;**188**(1):63-70

[55] Much DH, Yeh SY. Prevalence of chlamydia trachomatis infection in pregnant patients. Public Health Reports. 1991;**106**(5):490-493

[56] Hammerschlag MR, Chandler JW, Alexander ER, English M, Koutsky L. Longitudinal studies on chlamydial infections in the first year of life. Pediatric Infectious Disease. 1982;**1**(6):395-401

[57] Hammerschlag MR. Chlamydial and gonococcal infections in infants and children. Clinical Infectious Diseases. 2011;**53**(Suppl. 3):S99-S102

[58] Frommell GT, Rothenberg R, Wang S, McIntosh K. Chlamydial infection of mothers and their infants. The Journal of Pediatrics. 1979;**95**(1):28-32

[59] Hammerschlag MR, Anderka M, Semine DZ, McComb D, McCormack WM. Prospective study of

maternal and infantile infection with chlamydia trachomatis. Pediatrics. 1979;**64**(2):142-148

[60] Yu J, Wu S, Li F, Hu L. Vertical transmission of chlamydia trachomatis in Chongqing China. Current Microbiology. 2009;**58**(4):315-320

[61] Heggie AD, Lumicao GG, Stuart LA, Gyves MT. Chlamydia trachomatis infection in mothers and infants. A prospective study. American Journal of Diseases of Children. 1981;**135**(6):507-511

[62] Darville T, editor. Chlamydia trachomatis Infections in Neonates and Young Children. Seminars in Pediatric Infectious Diseases. Elsevier; 2005;**16**(4):235-244

[63] Zloto O, Gharaibeh A, Mezer E, Stankovic B, Isenberg S, Wygnanski-Jaffe T. Ophthalmia neonatorum treatment and prophylaxis: IPOSC global study. Graefe's Archive for Clinical and Experimental Ophthalmology. 2016;**254**(3):577-582

[64] Zikic A, Schünemann H, Wi T, Lincetto O, Broutet N, Santesso N. Treatment of neonatal chlamydial conjunctivitis: A systematic review and meta-analysis. Journal of the Pediatric Infectious Diseases Society. 2018;**7**(3):e107-ee15

[65] Rours IGIJG, Hammerschlag MR, Ott A, De Faber TJTHN, Verbrugh HA, de Groot R, et al. Chlamydia trachomatis as a cause of neonatal conjunctivitis in Dutch infants. Pediatrics. 2008;**121**(2):e321-e3e6

[66] Mordhorst CH, Dawson C. Sequelae of neonatal inclusion conjunctivitis and associated disease in parents. American Journal of Ophthalmology. 1971;**71**(4):861-867

[67] Tipple MA, Beem MO, Saxon EM. Clinical characteristics of the afebrile pneumonia associated with chlamydia trachomatis infection in infants less than 6 months of age. Pediatrics. 1979;**63**(2):192-197

[68] Hammerschlag MR, Cummings C, Roblin PM, Williams TH, Delke I. Efficacy of neonatal ocular prophylaxis for the prevention of chlamydial and gonococcal conjunctivitis. The New England Journal of Medicine. 1989;**320**(12):769-772

[69] Darling EK, McDonald H. A meta-analysis of the efficacy of ocular prophylactic agents used for the prevention of gonococcal and chlamydial ophthalmia neonatorum. Journal of Midwifery & Women's Health. 2010;**55**(4):319-327

[70] Martinez MA, Millan F, Gonzalez C. Chlamydia trachomatis genotypes associated with pneumonia in Chilean infants. Scandinavian Journal of Infectious Diseases. 2009;**41**(4):313-316

[71] Li Y, Xiong L, Huang Y, Xia Y, Zhou H, Xu F, et al. The clinical characteristics and genotype distribution of chlamydia trachomatis infection in infants less than six months of age hospitalized with pneumonia. Infection, Genetics and Evolution. 2015;**29**:48-52

[72] Rours GI, Hammerschlag MR, Van Doornum GJ, Hop WC, de Groot R, Willemse HF, et al. Chlamydia trachomatis respiratory infection in Dutch infants. Archives of Disease in Childhood. 2009;**94**(9):705-707

[73] Chen CJ, Wu KG, Tang RB, Yuan HC, Soong WJ, Hwang BT. Characteristics of chlamydia trachomatis infection in hospitalized infants with lower respiratory tract infection. Journal

of Microbiology, Immunology, and Infection. 2007;**40**(3):255-259

[74] Balla E, Donders GG, Petrovay F, Urbán E. Seroprevalence of anti-chlamydia trachomatis IgM in neonatal respiratory tract infections in Hungary. Journal of Medical Microbiology. 2017;**66**(8):1114-1117

[75] Attenburrow AA, Barker CM. Chlamydial pneumonia in the low birthweight neonate. Archives of Disease in Childhood. 1985;**60**(12):1169-1172

[76] Long SS, Prober CG, Fischer M. Principles and Practice of Pediatric Infectious Diseases E-Book. Elsevier Health Sciences; 2022. pp.885

[77] Hon KL, Leung AK. Chlamydial pneumonitis: A creepy neonatal disease. Case Reports in Pediatrics. 2013;**2013**:549649

[78] Bellulo S, Bosdure E, David M, Rolain JM, Gorincour G, Dubus JC. Chlamydia trachomatis pneumonia: Two atypical case reports. Archives de Pédiatrie. 2012;**19**(2):142-145

[79] Herieka E, Dhar J. Acute neonatal respiratory failure and chlamydia trachomatis. Sexually Transmitted Infections. 2001;**77**(2):135-136

[80] de Barbeyrac B, Benali L, Clerc M, Garapon S, Bébéar C, Gromb S. Authors reply to: Min Karen lo et al., "a response to: Chlamydia trachomatis infection in children: Do not forget perinatal acquisition." [J forensic legal med 2010;17:450]. Journal of Forensic and Legal Medicine. 2011;**18**(4):187

[81] Hammerschlag MR. Sexually transmitted diseases in sexually abused children: Medical and legal implications. Sexually Transmitted Infections. 1998;**74**(3):167-174

[82] Paediatrics RCo, Health C. The Physical Signs of Child Sexual Abuse: An Updated Evidence-Based Review and Guidance for Best Practice. London, United Kingdom: Royal College of Paediatrics and Child Health; 2015

[83] Workowski KA, Bolan GA. Sexually transmitted diseases treatment guidelines, 2015. MMWR - Recommendations and Reports. 2015;**64**(Rr-03):1, 137

[84] Shannon CL, Klausner JD. The growing epidemic of sexually transmitted infections in adolescents: A neglected population. Current Opinion in Pediatrics. 2018;**30**(1):137-143

[85] Lee V, Foley E, Tobin JM. Relationship of cervical ectopy to chlamydia infection in young women. BMJ Sexual & Reproductive Health. 2006;**32**(2):104-106

[86] Kleppa E, Holmen SD, Lillebø K, Kjetland EF, Gundersen SG, Taylor M, et al. Cervical ectopy: Associations with sexually transmitted infections and HIV. A cross-sectional study of high school students in rural South Africa. Sexually Transmitted Infections. 2015;**91**(2):124-129

[87] Scholes D, Stergachis A, Heidrich FE, Andrilla H, Holmes KK, Stamm WE. Prevention of pelvic inflammatory disease by screening for cervical chlamydial infection. New England Journal of Medicine. 1996;**334**(21):1362-1366

[88] Miller WC, Ford CA, Morris M, Handcock MS, Schmitz JL, Hobbs MM, et al. Prevalence of chlamydial and gonococcal infections among young adults in the United States. Journal of the American Medical Association. 2004;**291**(18):2229-2236

[89] Sarier M, Sepin N, Duman I, Demir M, Hizel A, Göktaş Ş, et al. Microscopy of gram-stained urethral smear in the diagnosis of urethritis: Which threshold value should be selected? Andrologia. 2018;**50**(10):e13143

[90] Quinn TC, Goodell SE, Mkrtichian E, Schuffler MD, Wang SP, Stamm WE, et al. Chlamydia trachomatis proctitis. The New England Journal of Medicine. 1981;**305**(4):195-200

[91] Thompson C, MacAulay A, Smith I. Chlamydia trachomatis infections in the female rectums. Sexually Transmitted Infections. 1989;**65**(4):269-273

[92] Sarier M, Sepin N, Emek M, Germen AT, Hoscan MB, Konuk E, et al. Evaluating the utility of the a.F. genital system test for pathogen diagnosis in acute male urethritis. Andrologia. 2022;**54**(4):e14377

[93] Workowski KA, Bachmann LH, Chan PA, Johnston CM, Muzny CA, Park I, et al. Sexually transmitted infections treatment guidelines, 2021. MMWR - Recommendations and Reports. 2021;**70**(4):1-187

[94] Papp JR, Schachter J, Gaydos CA, Van Der Pol B. Recommendations for the laboratory-based detection of chlamydia trachomatis and Neisseria gonorrhoeae. MMWR -Recommendations and Reports. 2014;**63**(Rr-02):1-19

[95] Meyer T. Diagnostic procedures to detect chlamydia trachomatis infections. Microorganisms. 2016;**4**(3):25

[96] Nwokolo NC, Dragovic B, Patel S, Tong CY, Barker G, Radcliffe K. 2015 UK national guideline for the management of infection with chlamydia trachomatis. International Journal of STD & AIDS. 2016;**27**(4):251-267

[97] Hammerschlag MR, Roblin PM, Gelling M, Tsumura N, Jule JE, Kutlin A. Use of polymerase chain reaction for the detection of chlamydia trachomatis in ocular and nasopharyngeal specimens from infants with conjunctivitis. The Pediatric Infectious Disease Journal. 1997;**16**(3):293-297

[98] Yip PP, Chan WH, Yip KT, Que TL, Kwong NS, Ho CK. The use of polymerase chain reaction assay versus conventional methods in detecting neonatal chlamydial conjunctivitis. Journal of Pediatric Ophthalmology and Strabismus. 2008;**45**(4):234-239

[99] Geisler WM. Diagnosis and Management of Uncomplicated Chlamydia trachomatis infections in adolescents and adults: Summary of evidence reviewed for the 2015 Centers for Disease Control and Prevention sexually transmitted diseases treatment guidelines. Clinical Infectious Diseases. 2015;**61**(Suppl. 8):S774-S784

[100] Wyrick PB. Chlamydia trachomatis persistence in vitro: An overview. The Journal of Infectious Diseases. 2010;**201**(Suppl. 2(Suppl. 2)):S88-S95

[101] Kong FY, Tabrizi SN, Law M, Vodstrcil LA, Chen M, Fairley CK, et al. Azithromycin versus doxycycline for the treatment of genital chlamydia infection: A meta-analysis of randomized controlled trials. Clinical Infectious Diseases. 2014;**59**(2):193-205

[102] Páez-Canro C, Alzate JP, González LM, Rubio-Romero JA, Lethaby A, Gaitán HG. Antibiotics for treating urogenital chlamydia trachomatis infection in men and non-pregnant women. Cochrane Database of Systematic Reviews. 2019;**1**(1):Cd010871

[103] Chandra NL, Broad C, Folkard K, Town K, Harding-Esch EM,

Woodhall SC, et al. Detection of chlamydia trachomatis in rectal specimens in women and its association with anal intercourse: A systematic review and meta-analysis. Sexually Transmitted Infections. 2018;**94**(5):320-326

[104] Hogerwerf L, De Gier B, Baan B, Van Der Hoek W. Chlamydia psittaci (psittacosis) as a cause of community-acquired pneumonia: A systematic review and meta-analysis. Epidemiology & Infection. 2017;**145**(15):3096-3105

[105] McNabb S, Jajosky RA, Hall-Baker PA, Adams DA, Sharp P, Anderson WJ, et al. Summary of notifiable diseases---United States, 2005. MMWR Morbidity and Mortality Weekly Report. 2007;**54**(53):1-92

[106] Beeckman DSA, Vanrompay D. Zoonotic Chlamydophila psittaci infections from a clinical perspective. Clinical microbiology and infection. 2009;**15**(1):11-17

[107] Drob SL. Reading the Red Book: An Interpretive Guide to CG Jung's. Liber Novus: Taylor & Francis; 2023

Chapter 20

Chlamydia pneumoniae and Childhood Asthma

Hayriye Daloglu

Abstract

Asthma is the most common chronic disease in childhood and it is a major global health problem. Asthma is characterized by chronic airway inflammation and the pathogenetic mechanisms leading to asthma are likely to be diverse, and influenced by multiple genetic polymorphisms as well as environmental factors, including respiratory tract infections. *Chlamydia pneumoniae* is a human pathogen belonging to the Chlamydiae family. Since its recognition in 1989, *C. pneumoniae* has been extensively studied for its role as a widespread respiratory pathogen and its potential consequences in both children and adults. Its ability to evade the human immune system, biphasic development cycle, and capacity to spread throughout the host has made it a suspect in many chronic inflammatory diseases, including asthma. Chlamydia pneumonia is of particular interest among the various infections associated with new-onset asthma, asthma severity, and treatment resistance.

Keywords: *Chlamydia pneumoniae*, asthma, childhood asthma, infection-related asthma, severe asthma

1. Introduction

Since its recognition in 1989, *Chlamydia pneumoniae* has been extensively studied for its role as a widespread respiratory pathogen and its potential consequences for both children and adults. Its ability to evade the human immune system, biphasic development cycle, and capacity to spread throughout the host has made it a suspect in many chronic inflammatory diseases, including asthma.

Asthma is the most common chronic disease in childhood [1] and it is a major global health problem, affecting an estimated 300 million people of all ages worldwide [2].

Asthma is characterized by chronic airway inflammation. The pathogenetic mechanisms leading to asthma are likely to be diverse and influenced by multiple genetic polymorphisms as well as environmental factors, including respiratory tract infections. Chlamydia pneumonia is of particular interest among the various infections associated with new-onset asthma, asthma severity, and treatment resistance. This chapter aims to provide an overview of the association between Chlamydia pneumonia and childhood asthma and to summarize the most recent evidence on this topic.

1.1 Asthma

Asthma is an umbrella term for heterogeneous diseases with similar clinical manifestations, but different underlying pathophysiological mechanisms and prognoses. The Global Initiative for Asthma (GINA) defines asthma as "the history of respiratory symptoms such as wheeze, shortness of breath, chest tightness, and cough that vary over time and in intensity, together with variable expiratory airflow limitation" [1]. These symptoms can be triggered by respiratory irritants, exercise, respiratory infections, and exposure to allergens in susceptible individuals.

Asthma symptoms and airflow limitation may resolve with or without treatment, and patients may remain asymptomatic for weeks or months. While many patients with classic asthma symptoms respond well to conventional treatments, some do not. These cases may be related to different underlying mechanisms.

1.2 Asthma phenotypes

Asthma phenotypes define clinically observable characteristics and are classified according to different elements (e.g., the age of onset, triggers, comorbidities, etc.). Besides, asthma endotypes define the underlying biological mechanisms making the clinical characteristics. Detailing the differences in the phenotypes and pathological or molecular characteristics of the content of the inflammation are trying to be explained by genotypes [3–5].

In order to achieve a more personalized medicine, especially for those with severe, treatment-resistant asthma, it seems future research will target classifying phenotypes based on endotypes (pathophysiological mechanisms) and the biomarkers associated with them. Additionally, exploring the etiology and mechanisms of the disease would help to more accurately predict the persistence of childhood asthma and its prognosis.

Several key elements, such as the age of onset, triggering factors, characteristics of symptoms, and biomarkers, have been taken into consideration when determining phenotypes of asthma [6].

Phenotypes by age of onset: This group consists of patients who were diagnosed with asthma at the age of 12 or older, with no definite upper age limit [7]. Typically, this group consists of adults, particularly women, who exhibit asthma that requires high doses of inhaled corticosteroids or is relatively resistant to corticosteroids [8].

Phenotypes by biomarkers: Asthma phenotyping can be conducted on biomarkers found in bronchial biopsy specimens, induced sputum, and peripheral blood, such as eosinophils and neutrophils (and the associated cytokines) that are involved in the Th-2 and non-Th-2 pathways, respectively [5, 9, 10].

A. Type 2 asthma can be further divided into two subtypes: allergic asthma and eosinophilic asthma [11]. (a) Allergic asthma is typically seen in children and is characterized by a history of eczema, allergic rhinitis, or food-drug allergies. This phenotype usually responds well to inhaled corticosteroids. (b) Eosinophilic asthma is identified when a patient's blood eosinophil count is >150/μl, and the eosinophil rate is higher than 2% in the sputum. Features of this phenotype include high eosinophil count, increased asthma severity, late-onset, and steroid resistance.

B. Non-Type 2 asthma refers to a group of patients who do not exhibit biomarkers of type-2 inflammation, such as epidermal prick test-compatible allergic comorbidities or eosinophils in blood/sputum. Their airway inflammation is either neutrophilic or paucigranulocytic (with few inflammatory cells). This non-allergic asthma group does not respond well to inhaled corticosteroid treatment. Neutrophil-derived inflammation, which may be associated with disorganized airway microbiota, appears to be linked to the most severe forms of asthma, typically seen in very young children and teenagers [12].

Asthma severity and asthma control were often used interchangeably. Today, asthma severity is evaluated retrospectively and defined as a condition where high doses and/or multiple medications are required to control the disease. Uncontrolled/difficult asthma is now considered a condition where symptoms persist despite treatment, and patients experience frequent exacerbations or attacks [2, 6, 13, 14].

2. Asthma treatment

The goal of asthma treatment is to achieve daily symptom relief, reduce the risk of future exacerbations, and keep medication use within safe limits in terms of side effects. Asthma treatments fall into three categories: controller drugs (such as inhaled corticosteroids and leukotriene antagonists), symptom-relief/rescue medications (such as fast-acting bronchodilators and inhaled/systemic corticosteroids), and additional therapies (such as long-acting inhaled anticholinergics, low-dose corticosteroids, biologic agents, and immunotherapy) that are utilized when the patient's symptoms remain unchanged despite the use of high-dose controller drugs in settings where the risk factors are controlled [6]. The role of macrolides in the treatment of asthma has been a topic of interest for decades. The use of these medications will be discussed in more detail later in this chapter.

2.1 Childhood asthma

Asthma is the most common chronic disease in children, with a current prevalence ranging from 6–9% [15]. Preschool-aged children are particularly susceptible to symptoms similar to those of asthma, such as acute bronchiolitis and wheezing, making it crucial to predict if they will eventually develop asthma. Follow-up studies have revealed that remission of the disease is possible during adolescence, with rates varying from 15 to 64% [16]. Individuals with a milder onset and lower allergic susceptibility have a higher probability of remission [6].

Allergic asthma is the most common phenotype in childhood and is characterized by a history of atopic dermatitis, allergic rhinitis, food allergies, and IgE mediation. Eosinophilic infiltration marks airway inflammation in these patients. Nonallergic asthma is the second most common phenotype, which is marked by neutrophilic inflammation and lacks an atopic component [17].

Research suggests that multiple genetic and environmental factors interact to influence clinical manifestation, bronchial hyperresponsiveness, and the presence of atopy. It is now acknowledged that asthma has an integral relationship with the immune system. Atopy and asthma are related, although it is not a direct correlation since not all atopic people develop asthma, and not all asthmatics have detectable allergic sensitivity. Increased levels of IgE, the release of allergens from mast cells, the growth of eosinophils in the lungs, inflammation in the airways, and an imbalance of Th1 and Th2 responses indicate that a dysregulated immune system contributes to the development of asthma.

2.2 Asthma and hygiene hypothesis

Epidemiological studies have provided evidence for a rise in asthma and allergic illnesses in industrialized countries over recent decades, leading to the development of the "hygiene hypothesis." This hypothesis proposes that a lack of early childhood exposure to infectious agents, symbiotic microorganisms (e.g., probiotics), and parasites increases susceptibility to allergic diseases by altering the immune system. Evidence suggests that populations with greater exposure to infectious agents, such as in developing countries or families with more children, have a lower prevalence of allergic diseases. It is thought that decreased exposure to the microbial environment in more developed countries results in an immune system that is more likely to elicit allergic responses, rather than the protective immune responses that exposure to these organisms could elicit.

However, recent studies have suggested that the hygiene hypothesis may not be applicable to asthma, but instead, asthma may be connected to infections experienced during the life cycle [18–20]. The immune response generated from these infections is dependent on the route, duration, dose, and a person's genetic makeup [21].

2.3 The microbiome of the airway

Recent studies have suggested that the "microbiome of the respiratory tract" may play a role in the development of asthma [22]. This is supported by two studies that revealed notable variations between the quantity and variety of microbial populations in healthy individuals and asthmatics [23, 24]. Microbiomes, also known as microbial flora, are generally not considered to be a threat to human health since they are usually present in the lungs and other small environments in the body. However, as our understanding of these organisms and their effects on diseases such as atopy and asthma increases, their impact should be taken into account.

Research into the microbiome of the gut has established that the airways also contain a typical flora, with varying numbers, diversity, and distribution of prokaryotic species. Early research into this new field has suggested that various types of bacteria that are present in increased numbers in asthmatic airways may be contributing to the chronic airway inflammation and hyperreactivity that characterize asthma. A study with a relatively small sample size found that treatment with clarithromycin improved patients with increased bacterial populations and diversity [23].

Moreover, the microbial populations of the gastrointestinal tract are also being studied, and early antibiotic exposure has been linked to the development of atopy and asthma by altering the gastrointestinal tract flora [25–27]. The significance of these differences is yet to be fully determined.

2.4 Asthma and infection

For more than 20 years, researchers have been investigating whether asthma is an infectious disease, but a definitive answer has yet to be found [28]. Investigating the origins of asthma is challenging because it is difficult to collect samples from the lungs of children. It is now believed that a combination of genetic mutations and environmental conditions is responsible for the various pathways of asthma, making it a syndrome with a typical clinical presentation but with a myriad of potential pathogenic mechanisms.

Recent research suggests that the prolonged presence of certain microorganisms in the bronchi may be linked to the development of asthma. Acute viral infections are well-known triggers of asthma exacerbations in both adults and children. In contrast, little is known about the role of chronic infections in the pathogenesis of the disease itself.

Asthma can be caused by a variety of factors, including atopy, respiratory infections, genetic predisposition, and a Th2-biased immune response. Polymorphisms in host defense genes can also influence the host's innate immune response. The effect of infectious agents on asthma can vary depending on the type of asthma, such as childhood- or adult-onset, atopic or nonatopic, and neutrophilic, eosinophilic, or paucigranulocytic leukocyte airway predominance.

Numerous studies suggest that early-life lower respiratory tract infections, especially those caused by viruses such as Rhinoviruses (RV) and Respiratory Syncytial Virus (RSV), are linked to an increased risk of school-age asthma [29]. Additionally, atypical bacteria, such as *Mycoplasma pneumoniae* and *C. pneumoniae*, may also contribute to persistent infections and be involved in the development of asthma [30–33]. Of particular interest is the role of *C. pneumoniae*, an obligate intracellular respiratory pathogen, in both asthma severity and treatment resistance [34].

3. *C. pneumoniae*: a pathogen causing more than pneumoniae

C. pneumoniae is a widespread cause of infection, with an estimated seroprevalence of over 50% among adults in many countries [35–37]. However, the prevalence is relatively low in children under 5 to 10 years old (7–8%), but it sharply increases to 40–55% in those aged 20 and continues to increase gradually, reaching 70–80% in the elderly [38, 39].

In 1989, Grayston identified *C. pneumoniae* as a novel species based on its distinct morphology, DNA sequence, and associated clinical disease spectrum within the Chlamydiae family [40]. Subsequently, *C. pneumoniae* has been linked to 6–22% of upper and lower respiratory tract infections, including pharyngitis, laryngitis, sinusitis, bronchitis, and pneumonia, in both children and adults [41–43]. This obligatory intracellular pathogen has been associated with an extensive range of conditions, such as cardiovascular disease, Alzheimer's disease, arthritis, lung cancer, diabetes, and asthma [44].

3.1 Biology and developmental cycle

C. pneumoniae is a human pathogen belonging to the Chlamydiae family. Its developmental cycle is complex and involves alternating between an infectious, extracellular elementary body, and a noninfectious, intracellular reticulate body. These two forms exist in a membrane-bound compartment called an inclusion, located inside a mucosal cell. After multiple replications, the reticulate body returns to the elementary body form and is released from the host cell, enabling it to infect nearby cells. This life cycle plays a crucial role in the molecular pathogenesis of chronic chlamydial infections.

To inject effector molecules into host cells, Chlamydia spp. utilizes a type III secretion system (T3SS). This T3SS produces a unique family of proteins known as inclusion membrane proteins (Incs). Incs are essential for the intracellular survival of Chlamydia spp. as they recruit host proteins to the inclusion, hijack the endocytic-lysosomal pathway, and help maintain the structural integrity of the inclusion. Additionally, Incs can enhance virulence by interfering with host antimicrobial pathways, promoting resistance to apoptosis, or constructing novel complexes with unique functions [45, 46].

Although studies of *C. trachomatis* have contributed significantly to our understanding of chlamydial infection and metabolism in humans, not all of these findings apply to *C. pneumoniae*. Significant differences in transcription, metabolism, and morphology exist between *C. pneumoniae* and other chlamydial species.

Research has shown that *C. pneumoniae* can modulate host cell apoptosis to evade detection by the host's immune system by interfering with tumor necrosis factor-alpha (TNF-alpha) and various signaling pathways [47]. This trait of the microorganism suggests that if the host cell can survive after the expulsion of extracellular vesicles, it could enable further reinfection and the maintenance of chronic, asymptomatic disease. The ability of *C. pneumoniae* to spread from the lungs to distant body parts and persist in those tissues for an extended period is essential to the development of the infection [48].

Persistence of Chlamydia Infection: Chlamydia infection is caused by the direct effects of chlamydial proteins, as well as mechanisms that utilize the host cell's machinery. When exposed to stressful conditions, Chlamydiae cease production of infectious extracellular bodies (EBs) and instead form viable but noninfectious forms characterized by a continued synthesis of unprocessed 16S rRNA and genomic replication [47]. These persistent forms can remain in the host for a prolonged period and are often associated with enlarged and malformed RBs, which can return to the normal developmental cycle when the inducing factor is removed [44]. *In vitro*, experiments have shown that several factors, including exposure to interferon-gamma (IFN) or antibiotics (such as penicillin and amoxicillin) and nutrient deprivation, can trigger the formation of persistent forms.

4. Asthma and *C. pneumoniae*

In the early 1990s, Hahn and colleagues were the first to suggest a possible link between *C. pneumoniae* and asthma when they observed a connection between Ig levels, wheezing, and adult-onset asthma [49]. To further investigate this association, they followed 10 patients who had acute C. pneumonia infection and *de novo* wheezing for 10 years, collecting clinical and microbiological data [50]. Among the 10 patients, one had pneumonia, while the other nine had bronchitis. Of the nine with bronchitis, four improved without treatment, while the remaining five developed chronic asthma during follow-up.

The investigation of the association between *C. pneumoniae* and asthma is impeded by the lack of standardized, sensitive, and specific detection methods for the pathogen. Nucleic acid amplification tests (NAATs), such as real-time PCR assays, offer accurate and efficient means of diagnosing acute *C. pneumoniae* infections [51]. However, the microimmunofluorescent antibody test is the most sensitive and specific serologic test for acute infection [40], despite its technical challenges and subjective interpretation. *C. pneumoniae* culturing is difficult and should be performed in cell culture. Additionally, there are practical and ethical obstacles to sampling the lower respiratory tract in representative populations of asthma patients and control subjects. Clinical research serological testing methods are limited by the high prevalence of antibodies to *C. pneumoniae* in the general population and the short duration of the initial antibody response (3–5 years), indicating that chronic infection and reinfection are common [52]. Serological methods cannot distinguish between acute, chronic, or reactivated prior infections. Therefore, new molecular diagnostic methods, such as PCR, have been developed to detect the pathogen's DNA. Although PCR testing can detect uncultivable organisms, it cannot differentiate between viable and nonviable organisms when used in antibiotic treatment studies [53]. However, reverse transcriptase-PCR can identify metabolic activity by detecting messenger RNA and may overcome this limitation [54].

Several studies using serological diagnostic techniques have linked C. pneumoniae to stable asthma in both adults and children. The studies used heat-shock proteins (HSPs) of *C. pneumoniae*, which are overproduced in persistent infections and associated with hypersensitivity and immunopathology [55]. Significant differences in the prevalence of antibodies to these HSPs were observed [56–58]. Falck et al. found that persistently increased levels of *C. pneumoniae* IgA antibodies were associated with pronounced symptoms of chronic respiratory tract disease [56]. A recent study concluded that asthmatics with IgA and IgG against *C. pneumoniae* have more severe disease with increased airway obstruction, higher doses of ICS, more signs of air trapping, and less type-2 inflammation [59].

A dose-response relationship between *C. pneumoniae* HSP60 IgA antibodies and pulmonary function has also been observed, with an inverse association seen between IgG antibodies to *C. pneumoniae* and percent-predicted FEV1 in asthmatics with elevated IgG and/or IgA levels. These elevated levels of IgA antibodies have also been associated with a higher daytime asthma symptom score and the need for high-dose inhaled corticosteroids. In general, higher *C. pneumoniae* antibody titers appear to be linked to several asthma severity markers [60].

A study involving 332 asthmatic patients discovered a significant correlation between asthma and elevated levels of IgG antibodies to *C. pneumoniae*, with the strongest correlation being observed in non-atopic longstanding asthma [58]. However, a population-based study conducted in Italy found a significant correlation between *C. pneumoniae* seropositivity and atopy among young adults [59].

Regarding children with reactive airway disease, Emre et al. discovered a correlation between *C. pneumoniae* infection and wheezing, with 85.7% of the 14 wheezing asthmatic patients testing positive for *C. pneumoniae* [61]. Immunoblotting detected anti-*C. pneumoniae* IgE, while anti-*C. pneumoniae* IgG and IgM were not detected by microimmunofluorescence. This suggests that the production of specific IgE may be a mechanism underlying reactive airway disease in some patients with *C. pneumoniae* infection. A subsequent study of asthmatic children found *C. pneumoniae*-specific IgE antibodies even in the absence of acute airway infection (negative PCR), suggesting that *C. pneumoniae* can stimulate allergic responses [61].

Studies comparing the T helper responses in *C. pneumoniae*-infected peripheral blood mononuclear cells (PBMC) of asthmatic patients to those of non-asthmatic control subjects revealed that *C. pneumoniae* infection can induce allergic responses in asthmatic PBMC, as indicated by an increase in the production of Th2-type cytokines (such as IL-4) and induction of IgE responses [62]. Recent studies with similar findings have suggested that *C. pneumoniae* infection may trigger IgE-specific responses in both asthmatic children and adult asthma patients [63, 64].

Research has indicated that *C. pneumoniae* infections can lead to the development of organism-specific IgE chemical mediators, which can cause airway inflammation and consequent wheezing. Furthermore, CP-specific IgE has been linked to severe persistent asthma, indicating that persistent infection may be causing asthma symptoms. Therefore, treating the underlying *C. pneumoniae* infection may help to lessen or even abolish symptoms [65].

Teig et al. conducted a study involving 38 children with stable chronic lung disease and 42 healthy controls. They found that 24% of the children with lung disease tested positive for *C. pneumoniae* using PCR, while none of the controls tested positive [66]. In a similar study, Cunningham et al. detected *C. pneumoniae* DNA in nasal specimens from

28% of stable asthmatic children, and the PCR result remained positive for a few months [67]. Biscione et al. utilized reverse transcriptase PCR to detect RNA of the major outer membrane protein (MOMP) from *C. pneumoniae*, which is only created during productive infection. This method was found to distinguish colonization from productive infection. They reported an increase in the detection of this organism in asthmatic patients compared to nonatopic spouses of asthmatic patients who served as controls [68].

There is evidence that C. pneumoniae infection may be related to asthma exacerbations. Acute asthma exacerbations are a common cause of hospitalization and visits to the Emergency Department (ED) in children, and they account for a significant proportion of asthma-related issues. Respiratory infections have been strongly linked to exacerbations, making them potential targets for treatment. Evidence suggests that *C. pneumoniae* is associated with asthma attacks, particularly in cases of severe attacks in children [69, 70]. Furthermore, atypical bacterial infections have been shown to cause attacks that are associated with persistent symptoms and a slower rate of recovery after 3 weeks [71].

Mounting evidence suggests that C. pneumoniae could play a role in the pathogenesis of asthma. Components of *C. pneumoniae*, such as transcription factors, have been found to activate components in bronchial tissue, leading to increased cytokine release and airway remodeling [72]. Furthermore, studies have shown that patients with *C. pneumoniae*-specific antibodies are more likely to experience severe airway inflammation than those without [73]. These findings suggest that *C. pneumoniae* reactivation could be a potential trigger for neutrophilic airway inflammation in people with asthma.

C. pneumonia infections might be worsening asthma. Webley found that 33% of asthma patients had C. pneumonia present in their bronchoalveolar lavage (BAL) samples by culture, and 67% were PCR-positive [74]. In a study of a heterogeneous group of children with asthma and recurrent bronchial obstructions, Schmidt et al. reported a 52% PCR-positivity rate for *C. pneumonia* in bronchoalveolar lavage specimens [75]. This suggests that C. pneumonia infections are more common in asthmatic patients than previously thought. It is worth considering whether *C. pneumonia* infection or colonization has a worsening effect on chronic respiratory diseases, as these invasive procedures such as bronchoscopy are only performed in treatment-resistant patients.

C. pneumoniae infection has been linked to an increase in the number and longevity of immune and inflammatory cells, which can lead to a reduced response to steroid treatment and increase the likelihood of treatment resistance [76].

A subpopulation of 5–25% of asthmatics, typically those with more severe disease and uncontrolled symptoms despite high doses of steroids, are labeled as having severe, steroid-resistant asthma. Respiratory infections are being implicated in the pathogenesis of severe, steroid-resistant asthma, and neutrophil-dominated endotypes of disease. Neutrophilic asthma is found to be associated with increased bacterial burden and interleukin 8 levels [34]. It has been suggested that neutrophilic asthma is less responsive than eosinophilic asthma to anti-inflammatory therapies, including corticosteroids. A study of children with asthma found that those who were PCR-positive for *C. pneumoniae* had higher concentrations of IL-8 and neutrophils in their bronchoalveolar lavage fluid than those who were PCR-positive for *C. trachomatis* or mycoplasma organisms but PCR-negative for *C. pneumoniae* [34]. This suggests that undiagnosed *C. pneumoniae* infections in children may contribute to inadequately controlled asthma by inducing IL-8.

Several studies have suggested that chronic *C. pneumoniae* infection is associated with a decline in respiratory function and more severe disease in both children and adults [68, 77, 78], and these associations are supported by biologically plausible mechanisms [79]. Cigarette smoke exposure is a known risk factor for steroid resistance in asthma [80]. Similarly, *C. pneumoniae* (CP) is known to induce ciliostasis of the pulmonary bronchial epithelium [81] and can infect alveolar macrophages and lung monocytes, resulting in increased production of TNF-, IL-1, IL-6, and IL-8, as well as human bronchial smooth muscle cells, leading to the production of IL-6 and basic fibroblast growth factor (with potential effects on bronchial hyperreactivity and lung remodeling) and chronic infection exposes tissues to cHSP60 and LPS, which have been linked to increased inflammation and asthma [82].

Numerous clinical studies have found associations between C. pneumoniae infection and the onset of childhood asthma. However, the relationship between *C. pneumoniae* infection and late-onset asthma in adult studies has yielded contradictory findings. A cross-sectional study conducted on patients with severe, late-onset, nonatopic asthma showed intriguing results suggesting a possible link between *C. pneumoniae* infection and fixed airway obstruction in adults [83].

A case-control study conducted in Italy found that children aged 2–14 years who presented to the pediatric emergency department with an acute episode of wheezing had a significantly higher incidence (15.5%) of acute *C. pneumoniae* infection compared to healthy controls [83]. Follow-up revealed that those who were not treated with antibiotics were more likely to experience recurrent wheezing than those without the infection. A study conducted in Japan also demonstrated similar findings, with higher CP-IgM levels present in hospitalized wheezing infants than in controls and a higher incidence of asthma in those with *C. pneumoniae* infection than in those without [84]. A larger follow-up study conducted 2 years later revealed that *C. pneumoniae* infection, a family history of allergic diseases, the number of eosinophils, and the serum IgE concentration at the initial examination were risk factors for asthma progression [85].

The use of mouse models has enabled researchers to determine the mechanisms by which Chlamydia respiratory infections in early life may be associated with the emergence and increased severity of allergic airway disease (AAD) later in life. Infections at all ages (neonatal, infant, and adult) were found to induce inflammation. However, it was observed that chlamydial infection during early life, but not in adulthood, was associated with the development of asthmatic characteristics in allergen-induced AAD. In particular, neonatal and infant infections were found to result in mixed type 1/type 2 immunity with increased levels of interleukin-13 (IL-13) and interferon (IFN), which, in turn, was associated with increased mucus-secreting cells and airway hyperreactivity (AHR) in AAD later in life, when compared to age-matched uninfected controls [86, 87]. Jupelli et al. later confirmed the effects of infant infection on the structure and function of the respiratory system [88]. Interestingly, it was found that infant infection increased the number of airway eosinophils [84, 85, 89]. Further investigation revealed that inflammation and AHR can lead to steroid resistance [75].

5. Macrolides in asthma treatment

Macrolides, such as clarithromycin and azithromycin, have been extensively studied for decades as a potential treatment for asthma. Although the results of clinical trials have been controversial, they are now included in severe adult asthma treatment guidelines as an additive agent due to their antibacterial, antiviral, anti-inflammatory, and immunomodulatory features [90–92]. The anti-inflammatory effects of macrolides may be particularly beneficial for patients with type 2 inflammation, while the antibiotic and antiviral effects may prevent respiratory infections in patients with neutrophilic inflammation [93].

Macrolides have been found to be effective in treating both eosinophilic and non-eosinophilic asthma phenotypes as adjunctive therapy in severe asthma [91, 94].

It is well-known that severe asthma can present with different phenotypes, such as increased concentrations of eosinophils or neutrophils and IL-8 in the airways. Patients with neutrophilic asthma have been shown to respond better to macrolide therapy and this type of asthma is thought to be more associated with bacterial pathogens and IL-8 [95]. Infection-mediated asthma is particularly related to neutrophilic, steroid-resistant asthma, leading many studies to focus on atypical bacterial infections in asthma and the effectiveness of macrolide treatment [96].

Two randomized, double-blind, placebo-controlled studies have reported contrasting results. Kraft and colleagues reported that clarithromycin treatment substantially increased FEV1 in asthmatic patients with PCR evidence of *C. pneumoniae* or *M. pneumoniae* infection in upper or lower airway samples [97]. However, the study conducted by Sutherland and colleagues did not support these findings [98]. The contrasting results can be attributed to the difficulty of accurately diagnosing atypical bacterial infections, as reported in a related meta-analysis [99].

6. Conclusion

Asthma is a heterogeneous disease that presents with similar clinical manifestations, is characterized by airway inflammation, and is likely to have different mechanisms of pathogenesis. Research suggests that multiple genetic and environmental factors, including respiratory pathogens and airway microbiome, interact to influence clinical manifestation, bronchial hyperresponsiveness, and the presence of atopy.

In addition to the role of viral infections in early life, many clinical and animal studies support the role of Chlamydia related respiratory infections in the development of asthma. Furthermore, *Chlamydia pneumonia* has been linked to severe and steroid-resistant asthma.

Author details

Hayriye Daloglu[1,2]

1 Faculty of Health Sciences, Antalya Bilim University, Turkey

2 Department of Pediatric Bone Marrow Transplantation Unit, Medicalpark Antalya Hospital, Turkey

*Address all correspondence to: hayriye.daloglu@gmail.com

References

[1] Chronic Respiratory Disease Collaborators Global, regional, and national deaths, prevalence, disability-adjusted life years, and years lived with disability for chronic obstructive pulmonary disease and asthma, 1990-2015: A systematic analysis for the global burden of disease study 2015. Lancet Respiratory Medicine. 2017;**5**(9):691-706

[2] Masoli M, Fabian D, Holt S, Beasley R. The global burden of asthma: Executive summary of the GINA dissemination committee report. Allergy. 2004;**59**(5):469-478

[3] Anderson GP. Endotyping asthma: New insights into key pathogenic mechanisms in a complex, heterogeneous disease. Lancet. 2008;**372**(9643):1107-1119

[4] Moore WC, Meyers DA, Wenzel SE, Teague WG, Li H, Li X, et al. Identification of asthma phenotypes using cluster analysis in the severe asthma research program. American Journal of Respiratory and Critical Care Medicine. 2010;**181**(4):315-323

[5] Wenzel SE. Asthma phenotypes: The evolution from clinical to molecular approaches. Nature Medicine. 2012;**18**(5):716-725

[6] Çelik G, Soyer Ö, Aydın Ö. Astım Tanı ve Tedavi Rehberi 2020 Güncellemesi. Türk Toraks Derneği. 2020;**1**(1):187-232

[7] Miranda C, Busacker A, Balzar S, Trudeau J, Wenzel SE. Distinguishing severe asthma phenotypes: Role of age at onset and eosinophilic inflammation. The Journal of Allergy and Clinical Immunology. 2004;**113**(1):101-108

[8] Derneği TT. ASTIM. Official Journal of the Turkish Thoracic Society. 2016;**17**:72

[9] Wenzel SE. Asthma: Defining of the persistent adult phenotypes. Lancet. 2006;**368**(9537):804-813

[10] Wenzel SE, Schwartz LB, Langmack EL, Halliday JL, Trudeau JB, Gibbs RL, et al. Evidence that severe asthma can be divided pathologically into two inflammatory subtypes with distinct physiologic and clinical characteristics. American Journal of Respiratory and Critical Care Medicine. 1999;**160**(3):1001-1008

[11] Hekking PP, Bel EH. Developing and emerging clinical asthma phenotypes. The Journal of Allergy and Clinical Immunology. In Practice. 2014;**2**(6): 671-680

[12] Brooks CR, Van Dalen CJ, Harding E, Hermans IF, Douwes J. Effects of treatment changes on asthma phenotype prevalence and airway neutrophil function. BMC Pulmonary Medicine. 2017;**17**(1):169

[13] Chung KF, Wenzel SE, Brozek JL, Bush A, Castro M, Sterk PJ, et al. International ERS/ATS guidelines on definition, evaluation and treatment of severe asthma. The European Respiratory Journal. 2014;**43**(2):343-373

[14] Taylor DR, Bateman ED, Boulet LP, Boushey HA, Busse WW, Casale TB, et al. A new perspective on concepts of asthma severity and control. The European Respiratory Journal. 2008;**32**(3):545-554

[15] Toskala E, Kennedy DW. Asthma risk factors. The International Forum of Allergy & Rhinology. 2015;**5** (Suppl. 1):S11-S16

[16] Tai A, Tran H, Roberts M, Clarke N, Gibson AM, Vidmar S, et al. Outcomes of childhood asthma to the age of 50 years. The Journal of Allergy and Clinical Immunology. 2014;**133**(6):1572-8.e3

[17] Deliu M, Yavuz TS, Sperrin M, Belgrave D, Sahiner UM, Sackesen C, et al. Features of asthma which provide meaningful insights for understanding the disease heterogeneity. Clinical and Experimental Allergy. 2018;**48**(1):39-47

[18] Strachan DP. Hay fever, hygiene, and household size. BMJ. 1989;**299**(6710):1259-1260

[19] Strachan DP. Family size, infection and atopy: The first decade of the "hygiene hypothesis". Thorax. 2000;**55**(Suppl. 1):S2-S10

[20] Brooks C, Pearce N, Douwes J. The hygiene hypothesis in allergy and asthma: An update. Current Opinion in Allergy and Clinical Immunology. 2013;**13**(1):70-77

[21] Prokopakis E, Vardouniotis A, Kawauchi H, Scadding G, Georgalas C, Hellings P, et al. The pathophysiology of the hygiene hypothesis. International Journal of Pediatric Otorhinolaryngology. 2013;**77**(7):1065-1071

[22] Huang YJ, Boushey HA. The microbiome in asthma. The Journal of Allergy and Clinical Immunology. 2015;**135**(1):25-30

[23] Huang YJ, Nelson CE, Brodie EL, Desantis TZ, Baek MS, Liu J, et al. Airway microbiota and bronchial hyperresponsiveness in patients with suboptimally controlled asthma. The Journal of Allergy and Clinical Immunology. 2011;**127**(2):372-81.e1-3

[24] Hilty M, Burke C, Pedro H, Cardenas P, Bush A, Bossley C, et al. Disordered microbial communities in asthmatic airways. PLoS One. 2010;**5**(1):e8578

[25] Penders J, Thijs C, van den Brandt PA, Kummeling I, Snijders B, Stelma F, et al. Gut microbiota composition and development of atopic manifestations in infancy: The KOALA birth cohort study. Gut. 2007;**56**(5):661-667

[26] Kozyrskyj AL, Ernst P, Becker AB. Increased risk of childhood asthma from antibiotic use in early life. Chest. 2007;**131**(6):1753-1759

[27] Droste JH, Wieringa MH, Weyler JJ, Nelen VJ, Vermeire PA, Van Bever HP. Does the use of antibiotics in early childhood increase the risk of asthma and allergic disease? Clinical and Experimental Allergy. 2000;**30**(11):1547-1553

[28] Lemanske RF Jr. Is asthma an infectious disease?: Thomas A Neff lecture. Chest. 2003;**123**(Suppl. 3): 385s-390s

[29] van Meel ER, Mensink-Bout SM, den Dekker HT, Ahluwalia TS, Annesi-Maesano I, Arshad SH, et al. Early-life respiratory tract infections and the risk of school-age lower lung function and asthma: A meta-analysis of 150,000 European children. The European Respiratory Journal. 2022;**60**(4). DOI: 10.1183/13993003.02395-2021

[30] Holt PG, Sly PD. Viral infections and atopy in asthma pathogenesis: New rationales for asthma prevention and treatment. Nature Medicine. 2012;**18**(5):726-735

[31] Atkinson TP. Is asthma an infectious disease? New evidence. Current Allergy and Asthma Reports. 2013;**13**(6):702-709

[32] Metz G, Kraft M. Effects of atypical infections with mycoplasma and chlamydia on asthma. Immunology and Allergy Clinics of North America. 2010;**30**(4):575-585 vii-viii

[33] Edwards MR, Bartlett NW, Hussell T, Openshaw P, Johnston SL. The microbiology of asthma. Nature Reviews. Microbiology. 2012;**10**(7):459-471

[34] Hansbro PM, Kim RY, Starkey MR, Donovan C, Dua K, Mayall JR, et al. Mechanisms and treatments for severe, steroid-resistant allergic airway disease and asthma. Immunological Reviews. 2017;**278**(1):41-62

[35] Kanamoto Y, Ouchi K, Mizui M, Ushio M, Usui T. Prevalence of antibody to *Chlamydia pneumoniae* TWAR in Japan. Journal of Clinical Microbiology. 1991;**29**(4):816-818

[36] Montes M, Cilla G, Alcorta M, Pérez-Trallero E. High prevalence of *Chlamydia pneumoniae* infection in children and young adults in Spain. The Pediatric Infectious Disease Journal. 1992;**11**(11):972-973

[37] Aldous MB, Grayston JT, Wang SP, Foy HM. Seroepidemiology of *Chlamydia pneumoniae* TWAR infection in Seattle families, 1966-1979. The Journal of Infectious Diseases. 1992;**166**(3):646-649

[38] Lin TM, Kuo CC, Chen WJ, Lin FJ, Eng HL. Seroprevalence of *Chlamydia pneumoniae* infection in Taiwan. The Journal of Infection. 2004;**48**(1):91-95

[39] Chatzidimitriou D, Exidari M, Gioula G, Papakonstantinou P, Melidou A, Gavriilaki E, et al. Seroepidemiology of *Chlamydia pneumoniae* in northern Greece. European Journal of Inflammation. 2009;7(3):139-144

[40] Grayston JT, Kuo C-C, Campbell LA, Wang S-P. *Chlamydia pneumoniae* sp. nov. for chlamydia sp. strain TWAR. International Journal of Systematic and Evolutionary Microbiology. 1989;**39**(1):88-90

[41] Hammerschlag MR. *Chlamydia pneumoniae* and the lung. The European Respiratory Journal. 2000;**16**(5):1001-1007

[42] Blasi F, Cosentini R, Tarsia P. *Chlamydia pneumoniae* respiratory infections. Current Opinion in Infectious Diseases. 2000;**13**(2):161-164

[43] Grayston JT. Infections caused by *Chlamydia pneumoniae* strain TWAR. Clinical Infectious Diseases. 1992;**15**(5):757-761

[44] Roulis E, Polkinghorne A, Timms P. *Chlamydia pneumoniae*: Modern insights into an ancient pathogen. Trends in Microbiology. 2013;**21**(3):120-128

[45] Bastidas RJ, Elwell CA, Engel JN, Valdivia RH. Chlamydial intracellular survival strategies. Cold Spring Harbor Perspectives in Medicine. 2013;**3**(5):a010256

[46] Elwell C, Mirrashidi K, Engel J. Chlamydia cell biology and pathogenesis. Nature Reviews. Microbiology. 2016;**14**(6):385-400

[47] Schoborg RV. Chlamydia persistence -- a tool to dissect chlamydia--host interactions. Microbes and Infection. 2011;**13**(7):649-662

[48] Witte L, Droemann D, Dalhoff K, Rupp J. *Chlamydia pneumoniae* is frequently detected in the blood after acute lung infection. The European Respiratory Journal. 2011;**37**(3):712-714

[49] Hahn DL, Dodge RW, Golubjatnikov R. Association of *Chlamydia pneumoniae* (strain TWAR) infection with wheezing, asthmatic bronchitis, and adult-onset asthma. Journal of the American Medical Association. 1991;**266**(2):225-230

[50] Hahn DL, McDonald R. Can acute chlamydia pneumoniae respiratory tract infection initiate chronic asthma? Annals of Allergy, Asthma & Immunology. 1998;**81**(4):339-344

[51] Kimberlin DW. Red Book: 2018-2021 Report of the Committee on Infectious Diseases. Elk Grove Village, USA: American Academy of Pediatrics; 2018

[52] Kuo CC, Jackson LA, Campbell LA, Grayston JT. Chlamydia pneumoniae (TWAR). Clinical Microbiology Reviews. 1995;**8**(4):451-461

[53] Gencay M, Roth M. *Chlamydia pneumoniae* infections in asthma: Clinical implications. American Journal of Respiratory Medicine. 2003;**2**(1):31-38

[54] Khan MA, Potter CW, Sharrard RM. A reverse transcriptase-PCR based assay for in-vitro antibiotic susceptibility testing of *Chlamydia pneumoniae*. The Journal of Antimicrobial Chemotherapy. 1996;**37**(4):677-685

[55] Kinnunen A, Paavonen J, Surcel HM. Heat shock protein 60 specific T-cell response in chlamydial infections. Scandinavian Journal of Immunology. 2001;**54**(1-2):76-81

[56] Falck G, Gnarpe J, Hansson LO, Svärdsudd K, Gnarpe H. Comparison of individuals with and without specific IgA antibodies to *Chlamydia pneumoniae*: Respiratory morbidity and the metabolic syndrome. Chest. 2002;**122**(5):1587-1593

[57] Huittinen T, Hahn D, Anttila T, Wahlström E, Saikku P, Leinonen M. Host immune response to *Chlamydia pneumoniae* heat shock protein 60 is associated with asthma. The European Respiratory Journal. 2001;**17**(6):1078-1082

[58] Sävykoski T, Harju T, Paldanius M, Kuitunen H, Bloigu A, Wahlström E, et al. *Chlamydia pneumoniae* infection and inflammation in adults with asthma. Respiration. 2004;**71**(2):120-125

[59] Calmes D, Huynen P, Paulus V, Henket M, Guissard F, Moermans C, et al. Chronic infection with *chlamydia pneumoniae* in asthma: A type-2 low infection related phenotype. Respiratory Research. 2021;**22**(1):72

[60] Black PN, Scicchitano R, Jenkins CR, Blasi F, Allegra L, Wlodarczyk J, et al. Serological evidence of infection with *chlamydia pneumoniae* is related to the severity of asthma. The European Respiratory Journal. 2000;**15**(2):254-259

[61] Emre U, Sokolovskaya N, Roblin PM, Schachter J, Hammerschlag MR. Detection of anti-chlamydia pneumoniae IgE in children with reactive airway disease. The Journal of Infectious Diseases. 1995;**172**(1):265-267

[62] Shulman A, Kohlhoff S, Estrella E, Kalra K, Smith-Norowitz T, Durkin H, et al. IgE responses to *Chlamydia pneumoniae* (Cpn) in allergic asthma. Journal of Allergy and Clinical Immunology. 2010;**125**(2), Supplement 1:AB48. DOI: 10.1016/j.jaci.2009.12.224

[63] Smith-Norowitz TA, Chotikanatis K, Erstein DP, Perlman J, Norowitz YM, Joks R, et al. *Chlamydia pneumoniae* enhances the Th2 profile of stimulated peripheral blood mononuclear cells from asthmatic patients. Human Immunology. 2016;**77**(5):382-388

[64] Smith-Norowitz TA, Loeffler J, Huang Y, Klein E, Norowitz YM, Hammerschlag MR, et al. *Chlamydia pneumoniae* immunoglobulin E antibody levels in patients with asthma compared with non-asthma. Heliyon. 2020;**6**(2):e03512

[65] Hahn DL, Schure A, Patel K, Childs T, Drizik E, Webley W. *Chlamydia pneumoniae*-specific IgE is prevalent in asthma and is associated with disease severity. PLoS One. 2012;**7**(4):e35945

[66] Teig N, Anders A, Schmidt C, Rieger C, Gatermann S. *Chlamydophila pneumoniae* and *Mycoplasma pneumoniae* in respiratory specimens of children with chronic lung diseases. Thorax. 2005;**60**(11):962-966

[67] Cunningham AF, Johnston SL, Julious SA, Lampe FC, Ward ME. Chronic *Chlamydia pneumoniae* infection and asthma exacerbations in children. The European Respiratory Journal. 1998;**11**(2):345-349

[68] Biscione GL, Corne J, Chauhan AJ, Johnston SL. Increased frequency of detection of *Chlamydophila pneumoniae* in asthma. The European Respiratory Journal. 2004;**24**(5):745-749

[69] Iramain R, De Jesús R, Spitters C, Jara A, Jimenez J, Bogado N, et al. *Chlamydia pneumoniae*, and *Mycoplasma pneumoniae*: Are they related to severe asthma in childhood? The Journal of Asthma. 2016;**53**(6):618-621

[70] Freymuth F, Vabret A, Brouard J, Toutain F, Verdon R, Petitjean J, et al. Detection of viral, *Chlamydia pneumoniae* and *Mycoplasma pneumoniae* infections in exacerbations of asthma in children. Journal of Clinical Virology. 1999;**13**(3):131-139

[71] Thumerelle C, Deschildre A, Bouquillon C, Santos C, Sardet A, Scalbert M, et al. Role of viruses and atypical bacteria in exacerbations of asthma in hospitalized children: A prospective study in the Nord-pas de Calais region (France). Pediatric Pulmonology. 2003;**35**(2):75-82

[72] KrüllM,BockstallerP,WuppermannFN, Klucken AC, Mühling J, Schmeck B, et al. Mechanisms of *Chlamydophila pneumoniae*-mediated GM-CSF release in human bronchial epithelial cells. American Journal of Respiratory Cell and Molecular Biology. 2006;**34**(3):375-382

[73] Wark PA, Johnston SL, Simpson JL, Hensley MJ, Gibson PG. *Chlamydia pneumoniae* immunoglobulin a reactivation and airway inflammation in acute asthma. The European Respiratory Journal. 2002;**20**(4):834-840

[74] Webley WC, Salva PS, Andrzejewski C, Cirino F, West CA, Tilahun Y, et al. The bronchial lavage of pediatric patients with asthma contains infectious Chlamydia. American Journal of Respiratory and Critical Care Medicine. 2005;**171**(10):1083-1088

[75] Schmidt SM, Müller CE, Bruns R, Wiersbitzky SK. Bronchial *Chlamydia pneumoniae* infection, markers of allergic inflammation and lung function in children. Pediatric Allergy and Immunology. 2001;**12**(5):257-265

[76] Beagley KW, Huston WM, Hansbro PM, Timms P. Chlamydial infection of immune cells: Altered function and implications for disease. Critical Reviews in Immunology. 2009;**29**(4):275-305

[77] Hahn DL, Bukstein D, Luskin A, Zeitz H. Evidence for *Chlamydia pneumoniae* infection in steroid-dependent asthma. Annals of

Allergy, Asthma & Immunology. 1998;**80**(1):45-49

[78] von HL. Role of persistent infection in the control and severity of asthma: Focus on chlamydia pneumoniae. The European Respiratory Journal. 2002;**19**(3):546-556

[79] Cho YS, Kim TB, Lee TH, Moon KA, Lee J, Kim YK, et al. *Chlamydia pneumoniae* infection enhances cellular proliferation and reduces steroid responsiveness of human peripheral blood mononuclear cells via a tumor necrosis factor-alpha-dependent pathway. Clinical and Experimental Allergy. 2005;**35**(12):1625-1631

[80] Thomson NC, Chaudhuri R, Livingston E. Asthma and cigarette smoking. The European Respiratory Journal. 2004;**24**(5):822-833

[81] Shemer-Avni Y, Lieberman D. *Chlamydia pneumoniae*-induced ciliostasis in ciliated bronchial epithelial cells. The Journal of Infectious Diseases. 1995;**171**(5):1274-1278

[82] Webley WC, Hahn DL. Infection-mediated asthma: Etiology, mechanisms and treatment options, with focus on chlamydia pneumoniae and macrolides. Respiratory research. 2017;**18**(1):1-12

[83] ten Brinke A, van Dissel JT, Sterk PJ, Zwinderman AH, Rabe KF, Bel EH. Persistent airflow limitation in adult-onset nonatopic asthma is associated with serologic evidence of *Chlamydia pneumoniae* infection. The Journal of Allergy and Clinical Immunology. 2001;**107**(3):449-454

[84] Zaitsu M. The development of asthma in wheezing infants with *Chlamydia pneumoniae* infection. The Journal of Asthma. 2007;**44**(7):565-568

[85] Zaitsu M. Does *Chlamydia pneumoniae* infection trigger to development of asthma in wheezy infants? The Journal of Asthma. 2009;**46**(9):967-968

[86] Horvat JC, Starkey MR, Kim RY, Phipps S, Gibson PG, Beagley KW, et al. Early-life chlamydial lung infection enhances allergic airways disease through age-dependent differences in immunopathology. The Journal of Allergy and Clinical Immunology. 2010;**125**(3):617-625

[87] Starkey MR, Nguyen DH, Brown AC, Essilfie AT, Kim RY, Yagita H, et al. Programmed death ligand 1 promotes early-life chlamydia respiratory infection-induced severe allergic airway disease. American Journal of Respiratory Cell and Molecular Biology. 2016;**54**(4):493-503

[88] Jupelli M, Murthy AK, Chaganty BK, Guentzel MN, Selby DM, Vasquez MM, et al. Neonatal *Chlamydial pneumonia* induces altered respiratory structure and function lasting into adult life. Laboratory Investigation. 2011;**91**(10):1530-1539

[89] Esposito S, Blasi F, Arosio C, Fioravanti L, Fagetti L, Droghetti R, et al. Importance of acute *Mycoplasma pneumoniae* and chlamydia pneumoniae infections in children with wheezing. The European Respiratory Journal. 2000;**16**(6):1142-1146

[90] Paçaci G. Astımda uzun süreli makrolid tedavisi. Tüberküloz ve Toraks. 2021;**69**(4):520-534

[91] Boulet LP, Reddel HK, Bateman E, Pedersen S, FitzGerald JM, O'Byrne PM. The global initiative for asthma (GINA): 25 years later. The European Respiratory Journal. 2019;**54**(2). DOI: 10.1183/13993003.00598-2019

[92] Holguin F, Cardet JC, Chung KF, Diver S, Ferreira DS, Fitzpatrick A, et al. Management of severe asthma: A European Respiratory Society/American Thoracic Society guideline. The European Respiratory Journal. 2020;**55**(1). DOI: 10.1183/13993003.00588-2019

[93] Hiles SA, McDonald VM, Guilhermino M, Brusselle GG, Gibson PG. Does maintenance azithromycin reduce asthma exacerbations? An individual participant data meta-analysis. The European Respiratory Journal. 2019;**54**(5). DOI: 10.1183/13993003.01381-2019

[94] Altenburg J, de Graaff CS, van der Werf TS, Boersma WG. Immunomodulatory effects of macrolide antibiotics - part 2: Advantages and disadvantages of long-term, low-dose macrolide therapy. Respiration. 2011;**81**(1):75-87

[95] Brusselle GG, Joos G. Is there a role for macrolides in severe asthma? Current Opinion in Pulmonary Medicine. 2014;**20**(1):95-102

[96] Wood LG, Simpson JL, Hansbro PM, Gibson PG. Potentially pathogenic bacteria cultured from the sputum of stable asthmatics are associated with increased 8-isoprostane and airway neutrophilia. Free Radical Research. 2010;**44**(2):146-154

[97] Kraft M, Cassell GH, Pak J, Martin RJ. *Mycoplasma pneumoniae* and *Chlamydia pneumoniae* in asthma: Effect of clarithromycin. Chest. 2002;**121**(6):1782-1788

[98] Sutherland ER, King TS, Icitovic N, Ameredes BT, Bleecker E, Boushey HA, et al. A trial of clarithromycin for the treatment of suboptimally controlled asthma. The Journal of Allergy and Clinical Immunology. 2010;**126**(4):747-753

[99] Wong EH, Porter JD, Edwards MR, Johnston SL. The role of macrolides in asthma: Current evidence and future directions. The Lancet Respiratory Medicine. 2014;**2**(8):657-670

Chapter 21

Adolescents' World: Know One Tell One against Unsafe Sexual Behaviours, Teenage Pregnancies and Sexually Transmitted Infections Including Chlamydia

Walter C. Millanzi

Abstract

Addressing adolescents' sexual and reproductive health (SRH) matters using multidisciplinary pedagogical innovations may assure the proper development and well-being of adolescents so that they reach the adulthood stage healthy and strong enough to produce for their future investment. This is in response to sustainable development goal number 3, target 3.7, and SDG4, target 4.7 in particular emphasizes the universal availability and accessibility of sexual information and education among people and knowledge and skills for gender equality, human rights and sustainable lifestyles by 2030, respectively. Yet, the innovative strategies may respond to a call stated by SGD5 (gender equality), target 5.3 which advocates the elimination of child, early, and forced marriages, and target 5.6 which focuses on ensuring universal access to SRH and rights to all by 2030.

Keywords: adolescents, chlamydia infection, sexual behaviours, sexual and reproductive health, sexually transmitted infections, teenage pregnancies, young people

1. Introduction

This chapter has been informed and validated by several published reports, literature, relevant international organizational publications, country-based materials, and ongoing initiatives (between 2017 and 2022 years). The reviewed documents included those related to young people's sexual and reproductive health against sexually transmitted infections (STIs) including human immunodeficiency virus (HIV), chlamydia, and teenage pregnancies among adolescents around the globe. Search engines for published research articles, reports, web pages, books, and or conferences preceding included google, google scholar, WBMED, and/or PUBMED. The criteria for the articles were set at not <2017 year of publications, and or only articles that addressed issues around STIs among young people. The review started by analysing the concept of adolescents, the global trend of unsafe sexual behaviours

IntechOpen

among young people, followed by the global trend of STIs/HIV, chlamydia, teenage pregnancies, factors linked with unsafe sexual behaviours, and the global trend of various strategies against STIs among adolescents.

2. Findings

2.1 The global trend of adolescents

Addressing adolescents' sexual and reproductive health (SRH) matters using multidisciplinary pedagogical innovations may assure the proper development and well-being of adolescents so that they reach the adulthood stage healthy and strong enough to produce for their future investment [1, 2]. This is in response to sustainable development goal number 3, target 3.7, and SDG4, target 4.7 in particular emphasizes the universal availability and accessibility of sexual information and education among people and knowledge and skills for gender equality, human rights and sustainable lifestyles by 2030, respectively [3]. Yet, the innovative strategies may respond to a call stated by SGD5 (gender equality), target 5.3 which advocates the elimination of child, early, and forced marriages, and target 5.6 which focuses on ensuring universal access to SRH and rights to all by 2030.

From the point of view of human life history theory, adolescence marks the beginning of a young individual's journey into sexual development, which can be an exciting, worrying, and/or difficult period. Adolescence is a stage of socio-sexual maturation and the construction of social and economic skills, which may increase reproductive success during later life. It is acknowledged through global statistics that adolescents determines a huge opportunity to transform the social and economic fortunes of any nation if they are formed properly during the early years of their lives [4, 5]. The proper formation here means developing adolescents with safe, good, and age-appropriate personal characters, identities, and social responsibilities for healthy adulthood [6].

Reports have defined adolescence as a transition period from childhood to adulthood [7]. The adolescence stage has been categorized into three stages including early adolescents (10–12 years), middle adolescents (13–16 years), and late adolescents (17–19 years) [8]. All stages are reported to be characterized by a tremendous amount of changes including biological, pubertal, and neuro-behavioural changes [9]. The term 'biological changes' here means physical growth and intellectual maturity milestone from childish to adulthood behaviours; while 'pubertal change' is a series of significant releases of sex hormones that influence physical maturity and emotional fluctuation [10]. Neuro-behavioural changes are deliberated to encompass all adolescent-related characteristics including an increase in risk-taking, attention-seeking, trial and error, violence, and or injuries [11].

Scholars have defined adolescence as a period whereby adolescents experience changes in social responsibilities that need close parental guidance, monitoring, and social support toward their life potential [12, 13]. Social responsibilities are defined here as a person's concern for self, others' welfare, sense of duty, avoidance of destructive behaviours, civil involvement, and responsible attitudes towards others [14]. Timely and age-appropriate sexual and reproductive health (SRH) information and education among adolescents are closely linked with healthy adolescence stages. As described by Denno et al. [15], the adolescence stage is always considered to be a healthy period when nurtured in ethical standards and acceptable socio-cultural norms. It is impressive to note that the number of adolescents keeps on increasing around the globe, which is perceived as a result of good parenthood demonstrated by parents, relatives, and other people.

The 2010 data shows that about 55% of the total global adolescents live in Asia and the Pacific with 29% in South Asia and India, 26% in East Asia, and the Pacific including China. Contrariwise, adolescents in Sub-Saharan Africa account for 16% of the world's total adolescent population with equal distribution between Eastern, Western, Southern, and Central Africa. Referring to the UNFPA [16] report, the adolescent population distribution is predicted to decline by 18% in Asia and the Pacific while in Sub-Saharan Africa, adolescents aged 10–17 years old will significantly rise to about 23% by 2030. Data indicate that the largest national increase in adolescent girls will mostly happen in the Sub-Saharan African countries including Tanzania which encompasses about 90%, the highest being Zambia (99%) followed by Malawi (93%).

Adolescents aged 10–19 years are of school age which is authoritatively well-defined at the country level for secondary and tertiary education [16, 17]. Updated data on adolescents by [18] estimates that of the 7.2 (higher than that reported in 2010) billion world population, 42% (over 3 billion) are younger than 25 years, while 18% (1.2 billion) are adolescents aged 10–19 years. About 88% of adolescents live in developing countries whereby Sub-Saharan Africa (SSA) constitutes 18%. It is also projected that between 2010 and 2030 the adolescent population in Sub-Saharan Africa will increase to 1.3 billion [19]. Tanzanian adolescents aged between 10- and 19 years account for 11,858,193 (23%) of the country's population (N = 51,557,365). Early adolescents (10–14 years) make up 13%, while late adolescents (15–19 years) make up 10% of the total population, respectively [20–22].

The global view holds the belief that, if adolescents are nurtured well, and the rearing process, parental control, and social scaffolding are assured to them they will one day be young professionals, entrepreneurs, farmers, teachers, social workers, engineers, nurses, doctors, technicians, politicians, designers, good parents, and new brave thinkers [23, 24]. However, adolescents at the adolescence stage may feel that they are old enough to start sexual activities, which need future-oriented parenting styles to assure proper character, good social responsibilities, and future investments [10, 25].

Although their sexual freedom and activity patterns differ markedly according to geographical, cultural, and religious backgrounds, it is acknowledged that they need continuous parental and academic guidance to reach their adulthood with good health and strong enough to produce to contribute to the socio-economic prosperity of their nations [26, 27]. Effective support, particularly on sexual education interventions for adolescents who are about to begin their sexual lives appears to have potential and long-lasting effects in enhancing their academic and behavioural outcomes.

2.2 The global trend of unsafe sexual behaviours among adolescents

A healthy adolescence stage is argued to determine strong and healthy adulthood, which is associated with increased job market opportunities that are believed to increase productivity rates in reproductive health and economic aspects, respectively [28]. Increased productivity rates are argued by scholars to have the potential of promoting economic growth and prosperity at individual, family, and national levels in response to the sustainable development goal number 1 (SDG1) of no poverty in the world [29, 30]. However, the literature argues that most adolescents are not developed appropriately in their characters, identity, and social responsibilities to contribute to economic opportunities [31].

Aristotle [32] notes that adolescents often live out of their control with a sense that they are always right to their desires and acts, regardless of how beneficial or hazardous they are to live. Literature has demonstrated that adolescents in their early years of life are driven by a sense that they are mature enough, and thus, they are obsessed with impulses to interact with diverse people and the largest social networks that constantly require them to be socially competent [33, 34]. Sometimes they demonstrate attention-seeking and reckless behaviours including disputes with their parents, peers, teachers at schools, and other people in society, and unsafe sexual behaviours that expose them to sexual exploitation [35].

Unsafe sexual behaviours among adolescents aged between 10 and 19 years, for example, have become the most prevailing problem around the globe [36–38]. Unsafe sexual behaviours include such manners as; early initiation, unsafe sexual behaviours, incorrect and inconsistent usage of contraceptive methods, having multiple sexual partners, frequent sexual intercourse, drug abuse before, or while having sexual activity, and or engaging in sexual intercourses for money or materials gain [36, 39]. Early initiation of unsafe sexual behaviours among adolescents is considered a problem as it is often associated with early and unintended teenage pregnancies and or new sexually transmitted infections (STIs) such as syphilis, gonorrhoea, chlamydia, and/or human immunodeficiency virus (HIV) just to mention a few [40, 41].

Reports such as that by UNICEF [42] indicate that 11 and 6% of girls and boys, respectively claim to have had sex before the age of 15 years. They reported early sexual debut, being involved in a sexual partnership with older men, and having unprotected sexual intercourse in their lives. Almost 57% of young women and 48% of young men across the world report having had sexual intercourse by the age of 18 years [43]. An estimate of unsafe sexual behaviours among young people in Tanzania shows that approximately 57 and 48% of young women and men, respectively, report having had sex by the age of 18 years [20]. These pieces of data show that unsafe sexual behaviours among adolescents are still a public concern around the globe.

Available data may indicate that despite the effect of the existing strategies, there might be a need to rethink, adapt and test other pedagogies that aim at empowering young people with soft skills against unsafe sexual behaviour. Participatory and collaborative sexual education pedagogies among teachers and health workers that involve adolescents in the first position may become a sustainable solution in addressing unsafe sexual behaviours among adolescents. Addressing unsafe sexual behaviours among them may promise a fruitful fight against STIs/HIV, teenage pregnancies, and school dropouts among adolescents.

Unintended pregnancies in the adolescence stage for example are also linked with several adverse health outcomes associated with childbearing such as obstetric complications before, during, and after delivery including eclampsia, post-partum haemorrhage, fistula, and or premature deaths [37, 44]. Children born from an adolescent girl are at risk of higher potential deaths, and low birth weights [45]. Unintended teenage pregnancies from unsafe sexual behaviours are more often associated with educational outcomes such as interrupting schooling leading to school dropouts [46, 47]. Early and unintended teenage pregnancies are linked with social and economic outcomes including endangering their future economic opportunities such as reduced job market opportunities that would contribute to the economic growth and prosperity at an individual, family, and national level at large [15].

Although sexual behaviours may be seen as emotional involvement, for some adolescents it may start as a commercial endeavour that may lead to emotional (or vice versa) and health, educational and socioeconomic consequences [48]. Adolescents who are empowered with sexual and reproductive health (SRH) knowledge, and soft skills (self-esteem, and assertiveness skills) are believed to be able to demonstrate self-control over the urges to engage in sexual relationships, marry young, and or have children at young ages [49]. However, different reports on sexual education in developing countries claim that adolescents are not well empowered with the necessary soft skills for safe sexual behavioural change [50, 51].

Needless to say, scholars such as Envuladu et al. [39] and Kaale et al. [37] disclose that unsafe sexual behaviours among adolescents are very obvious with misinformation about SRH matters and poor self-regulation of sexual emotions and behaviour at an early age, something that may need to be addressed accordingly. Tallying with a belief of the current study, poor self-regulation among adolescents is reported to be proximal to sexual risk-taking and might have more sexual partners later in their lives [45, 52].

The majority of adolescents tend to fail to make informed and reasoned decisions about sexual activities early in their lives when they encounter sexual pressures, dilemmas, and or temptations from peers, adults, or strangers [53]. Mlyakado [54, 55] exposes that most adolescents have less negotiating power over sexual pressures and coercions on safer sexual behaviour. To embark on the situation, Chilisa et al. [56] argue that by improving their SRH knowledge and soft skills, adolescents may be able to abstain from sexual intercourses and hence decide to delay sexually aroused relationships, intend to reduce the number of sexual partners if any and or negotiate for consistent and accurate use of condoms for safe sexual activities.

2.3 A global trend of STIs/HIV among adolescents

Reports have provided pieces of evidence, which demonstrate that sexually transmitted infections have increased to >1 million newly infected people on daily basis. An estimate made by the World Health Organization [57] indicates that about 376 million people were newly infected with chlamydia (127 million), gonorrhoea (87 million), syphilis (6 million), and trichomoniasis (150 million) while 500 million people were infected with genital herpes, respectively. Being at young ages, many adolescents engage in unsafe sexual behaviours, which are commonly associated with incidences of sexually related infections [37].

Adolescents' health problems, for example, have been connected to the prevalence of sexually transmitted infections (STIs) and human immunodeficiency virus (HIV) infections which account for 60 and 69% of global and Sub-Saharan Africa, respectively [58]. STIs such as gonorrhoea, syphilis, trichomoniasis, HIV, chlamydia, and/or genital herpes among the cohort of adolescents are prevailing at the global, regional, and national levels [59, 60]. The HIV report by UNAIDS [61], for example, has informed that although trends of new global HIV infections have continued to decline from 3.4 million in 1996 to 1.8 million in 2017, the UNAIDS report published online in 2021 has reported 38,000,000 people are living with HIV, up from 30.7 million in 2010.

Approximately 690,000 died of AIDS-related causes in 2019, a decrease (37%) from 1.1 million in 2010; of which, an estimated 600,000 deaths occurred among adults and 95,000 deaths among children <15 years [62]. Available reports uncover that about 76 million people have been infected with HIV since the beginning of the HIV epidemic [63]. However, the current UNAIDS report has exposed that there were still 1.7 million new HIV infections in 2019, which is equivalent to about 5000 new HIV infections per day [62]. Sums of 1.5 million people are adults while 150,000 are adolescents. Approximately, 250,000 young people of school age were newly HIV-infected whereby about 182,599 (73%) of them were residing in Sub-Saharan [64].

The overall global HIV decline progress rate (including that of young people) has been counted in the report to be slower than the requirement to reach a decline to 500,000 new infections by 2020. Needless to say, like other developing countries,

Tanzania has 4.8% of people living with HIV of which there has been a remarkable increase in the prevalence from 1.3 million in 2010 to 1.7 million in 2019 [65]. However, it is worth noting that deaths associated with acquired immunodeficiency syndrome (AIDS) have decreased from 52,000 people in 2010 to 27,000 in 2019. The same decline in the trend of HIV/AIDS has been reported in Zanzibar whereas, the prevalence is low with only 6990 people living with HIV while the number of new HIV infections has decreased from 82,000 in 2018 to 77,000 in 2019.

Despite the decrease in HIV prevalence among adolescents and adults (15–49 years) from 5.1% in 2014 to 4.8% in 2019 in Tanzania, 5.8% (N = 104,400) of the adolescents who are living with HIV in the globe (N = 1,800,000), are in Tanzania [65]. Almost 8600 new HIV infections occur among children between the ages of zero and the middle adolescent stage (0–14 years); whereas 93,000 children of the same age range live with HIV. Out of the 27,000 estimated AIDS-related deaths in the country, 5900 deaths occur among children (0–14 years).

Approximately, 99,000 adolescents aged between 10 and 19 years are living with HIV; of whom about 57,000 are adolescent girls. It is estimated that out of the 77,000 new HIV infections occurring in the country, 10,000 are adolescents aged between 10 and 19 years. Despite some improvements in reducing the rate of new STIs/HIV among adolescents, the reported trend may imply that the existing strategies are either not sustainable, not reaching a large and appropriate age group of adolescents, or something is missing, be it in their design, implementation, or evaluation.

2.4 A global trend of chlamydia infections among adolescents

By considering its significance not only in this book but also in the promotion of sexual and reproductive health among young people, reports have uncovered that chlamydia infections among others have become to be the most diagnosed STI with an incidence of 1.6 million in 2020, which is equivalent to 481 per 100,000 population regardless the existing strategies to lower down its burden [66, 67]. Nevertheless, the report has demonstrated that of the infected individuals with STIs, 53% were young people between 15 and 24 years adolescents inclusive. It may feel upsetting to find that 62% of STIs were incidences of chlamydia among adolescents in the year 2020.

Such a piece of data may imply that despite all good and positive initiatives against STIs at the global, regional and national levels, it appears that the trend of chlamydia infections among you people including adolescents is critical and may need to be prioritized by engaging them in the front line against it. Although the uptake of chlamydia screening is keeping in a high race, an international organization such as the Centers for Disease Control and Prevention (CDC) has demonstrated the intent to boost it to 77% by 2030 [66].

Sometimes STIs may be counted to be less fatal in peoples' health but, chlamydia can result in reproductive tract morbidities including but not limited to ectopic pregnancies (to females), infertility, pelvic inflammatory diseases particularly in women of reproductive age, and new-borns morbidity and mortality health outcomes [68, 69]. Additionally, the health burden of chlamydia infection may be linked with someone feeling shame after acquiring it, being faced with different forms of maltreatment from stigma, the reluctance of young people to talk about SRH matters, exposure to active sexual relationships and or engage in the productive activities [70].

The increasing trend of chlamydia infection among young people including adolescents may be used as an alert to the respective authorities for special collaborative efforts to be given appropriate weight to reach them [71]. Tallying to the existing initiatives against chlamydia infections among young people, mounting the scope of SRH preventive interventions such as screening programs, and education programs may be crucial to the proper development of the young generation towards a healthy adulthood [72].

A strong and healthy generation is believed to have the appropriate social responsibilities and fuel economic fortunes for the prosperity of regions and nations around the globe [28, 44]. Needless to say, the trend compels the need for increased collaborative initiatives that will focus on reaching and bringing out the forgotten and hidden young cohort so they to be provided with rehabilitative services such as timely and right health treatments, counselling, and extra-curricular activities [73]. It appears to be timely for the higher authorities such as policymakers and ministry, schools, health facilities, religious facilities, parents/caregivers, and other stakeholders to unite and advocate for young people against chlamydia.

2.5 A global trend of teenage pregnancies among adolescents

Apart from the trend of STIs/HIV among adolescents, adolescents aged between 15 and 19 years face the challenge of getting unplanned pregnancies [74]. Although WHO [75] estimated a high (16 million) number of girls aged 15–19 years give birth each year, the number declined to 12 million girls in 2019 [76]. WHO [76] has reported a decline in the adolescent fertility rate from 56 births per 1000 adolescent women in 2000 to 45 births in 2015 and 44 births in 2019.

Despite the decline of the fertility rate in the globe, the level has remained high (19.3%) in Sub-Saharan Africa whereby, adolescent fertility accounts for 101 births per 1000 adolescent women. Owing to the high adolescent fertility rate, an estimated 21 million girls (15–19 years) become pregnant every year, while 12 million of them give birth and approximately 2.5 million (12%) of them become mothers by the age of 16 years. The prevalence appears to be high in East Africa (21.5%) and low (9.2%) in Northern Africa [33, 52].

Reports about teenage pregnancies in East African regions show that the highest percentage exists in Uganda (23.8%) and Tanzania (22.8%). Rwanda (7.3%) and Ethiopia (12.4%) have the lowest rate as compared to other African regions. Currently, the adolescent fertility rate in Tanzania, in particular, has reached 128 pregnancies per 1000 women against the target of fewer than 100 pregnancies per 1000 women by 2020 [20]. MoHCDGEC [77] reports that 27% of adolescents in Tanzania get underage pregnancies. Adolescents are always blamed for the current trend as their fault as perceived by parents and the community at large [78].

The trend of teenage pregnancies among adolescents is perceived by what has commonly been reported to be due to poor parenting, and sexual masculinities which are linked to sociocultural norms, migrations, social media, drug abuse, peer pressure, poverty, and or the existence of sugar daddy and sugar mommy [79]. The trend is also linked to inadequate implementation and evaluation of health policy and co-related health strategic plans and lack of health-seeking behaviour (to access the available SRH services) among adolescents [74]. However, the most forgotten aspect, which, if addressed to its maximum, might change the current trend of teenage pregnancies, would be soft skills, which are believed to enhance informed and reasoned decisions over an act among people.

2.6 Factors associated with trends of unsafe sexual behaviours among adolescents

Scholars such as Wolinsky [80] have argued that nothing under the earth occurs without a cause. **Figure 1** shows the bioecological concepts that root in the ecological

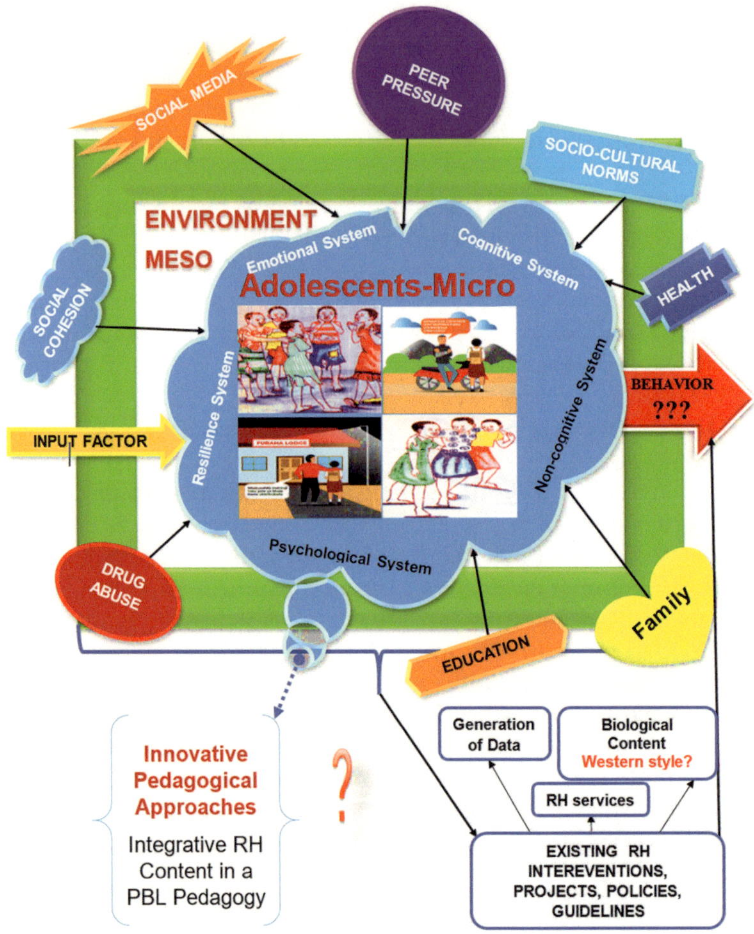

Figure 1.
Bioecological correlates of adolescents' sexual behaviours. Source: Dr. Walter C. Millanzi (PhD).

system of human life, which demonstrate factors that potential in determining adolescents' SRH [81]. The theory believes that an individual's behaviour is shaped by several factors ranging from biological, social, cultural, and technological to politics. The theory stipulates that the environment where a child is put affects the shaping of a child's behaviour, and thus, needs to be structured into layers or systems as important building blocks to their development.

The five recommended systems by the theory include microsystem (child's proximal interaction with family, school, neighbourhood, or childcare environment); and mesosystem (indirect child's interaction with the microsystem structures such as child's teacher and parents, and parents with neighbours). Other systems consist of the exosystem (child's distal interaction with society to feel positive or negative outcomes to the microsystem such as parents' work schedules or community-based resources). "A child interacts outside of his/her system via the macro-system" (the outermost layer of a child including cultural values, customs, and laws that can also influence the mesosystem and exosystem).

On the other hand, the review of existing documents, interventions, projects, policies, and guidelines revealed that the RH content focuses more on biological contents

DOI: http://dx.doi.org/10.5772/intechopen.109048

such as definitions of concepts, biological changes in human beings' health, diseases and their causes, effects of the disease on health, and the preventive measures of diseases. However, issues around the emotional and psychological aspects (soft skills: critical thinking and reasoned judgment, resilience, self-esteem, assertiveness skills, and negotiation skills) were less addressed in the RH contents for adolescents.

Most programs, and or projects have been reported to depend on external funding to work [82]. Depending on external funding from program donors may open new avenues for Non-governmental Organizations (NGOs) to decide and prioritize what, why, when, and how to facilitate SRH learning among adolescents. The content scenarios, problems, stories, and examples in the existing SRH lesson materials, for example, appear to be more of western styles than African situations. Adopting and implementing western styles for facilitating SRH learning among African countries' adolescents without considering the input factor to adolescents' behaviours predicts the permanent mismatch between what is supposed to be provided, the right dosage, timing, and frequency among them, and the real-life events in low-resource countries.

The review of the existing documents exposed that despite the RH lesson materials borrowing western styles, conventional pedagogies are commonly used to facilitate SRH learning in adolescents. If the RH lesson materials and its associated pedagogical knowledge mismatch continue, adolescents will not only continue to be formed in a conventional style but also lack soft skills to solve social and economic problems in their real-life phenomena. With this brief review, this chapter disseminates a need to address the gap by adopting ecological systems of human life theory to help shape the materials by considering important factors to be addressed too during the development and implementation of integrated RH lesson materials in PBP. **Figure 1** illustrates the concept.

Literature [10, 52, 83–85] claims that factors such as age, sex, religious influence, and unsafe sexual behaviours among adolescents contribute greatly to teenage pregnancies amongst adolescents. Furthermore, limited education and employment, drug abuse, exposure to media, low self-esteem, and inability to refuse sexual temptations catalyse the trend of unsafe sexual behaviour among adolescents resulting in STIs/HIV, teenage pregnancies, and school dropouts [86, 87]. Factors such as socio-cultural, economic, and environmental factors including peer influence, coerced sexual relations, and sexual intercourse with adults have been linked to the early onset of adolescents' unsafe sexual behaviour [36, 88].

Similarly, unequal gender power relations, the pressure to marry and bear children early, poverty, lack of parental counselling and guidance, and inadequate comprehensive sexuality education have been mentioned as contributing to the persistence of the trend [89]. Still, health services related to factors such as inadequate and unskilled health workers, lack of youth-friendly comprehensive sexuality education at health facilities, costs of contraceptives, and long waiting times at clinics have been associated with adolescents' unsafe sexual behaviour [28]. The detailed trend of STIs/HIV, teenage pregnancies, and school dropouts among adolescents with co-related factors presented above, for example, has been linked closely with the early onset of unsafe sexual behaviours [90]. This may be the case because, as argued by previous studies, sexual emotions and abilities to make reasoned and informed decisions develop gradually at young ages [91].

Sexual emotions here include the desire for intimacy, friendship, and belonging, which at this age translate into temptations to sexual acts at an age when they have little understanding of their consequences [92]. Indeed, suggested data from Schiller [93] on neuroscience is that changes in affective processing during adolescence may be critical to understanding unsafe behaviour in this age period. Christopher et al. [94] unfold that adolescents with poor self-regulation of sexual emotion and behaviour at an early age are more prone to sexual risk-taking and might have more sexual partners later in their lives. In that regard, it appears that although sexual behaviour may be seen as emotional involvement, for some adolescents it may start as a commercial endeavour that may lead to emotional (or vice versa) and health, educational and socio-economic consequences.

2.7 Global response to adolescents' SRH

The reviewed reports and literature indicate a remarkable need to rethink innovative, sustainable, and multidisciplinary pedagogical strategies to enhance the proper formation of the right personality and character leading to social responsibility among adolescents [95]. Initiatives have been in place to develop adolescents with good personalities and characters for social responsibilities and their future investment through multidisciplinary strategies to enhance their sexual selves [96]. The initiatives are rooted in the sustainable development goals 3 (SDGs3) target 3.7 (universal accessibility of sexual information and education among people by 2030) and SDG4 target number 4.7 (knowledge and skills for gender equality, human rights and sustainable lifestyles by 2030) [30].

Various health policies and SRH guidelines have been developed to be adopted and implemented across the world including low and middle-income countries Tanzania inclusive [97]. The policies and guidelines seem to work better in ensuring that sexual and reproductive health rights and associated services (such as menstrual hygiene education and pads, and contraceptives) are available and accessible among adolescents in health facilities and schools. Owing to the presence of political and health policies in middle and low-income countries, whereby, for example, adolescents are advocated against sexual abuses and exploitations towards preventing teenage pregnancies, STIs/HIV, and school dropouts that are linked with teenage pregnancies [98, 99].

Several interventions include, but are not limited to, building boarding schools, enrolment of students to stay at school hostels, policy and legislation reinforcement by the government, sexual education clubs, large-scale reproductive and family planning methods campaigns, projects, and sexual health education training among teachers are being implemented to address unsafe sexual behaviour among adolescents [20, 100]. The National School Health Program provides adolescents with many healthcare services such as SRH information and its associated services and counselling support to address their SRH challenges [20].

Although the SRH content varies widely across nations and schools, the Ministry of Education and Vocational Training has tried to integrate sexual education and STIs/HIV education into the national school curriculum [101–104]. Scholars' works [105, 106] reveal that parents, teachers, and or health workers have a positive attitude towards STI screening and the implementation of school-based sexual educational syllabi among adolescents. However, they claim to experience trouble when they try teaching the social and physiological parts of it by using conventional pedagogies such as lectures, discussions, demonstrations, and storytelling, and or initiating communication with adolescents about SRH matters.

However, the outcry among stakeholders links the permanent use of conventional pedagogies with the permanence facilitation of biological than psychological SRH contents among adolescents [107, 108]. Topics such as the human reproductive system and sexual health behaviour are taught in the classrooms with great care and respect; taking into consideration the prevailing socio-cultural sensitive issues. School teachers and health workers who are invited to facilitate SRH learning among adolescents in schools, tend to make their own decisions regarding what, how, and when to implement it, which is commonly facilitated by using didactic pedagogies [100].

The SRH lesson materials are claimed to adopt more western lifestyle contents, problems, and scenarios, which hardly reflect the existing contexts of adolescents [109]. The noted SRH pedagogical situation may indicate that there is no formal guideline with pedagogical prescriptions to guide teachers, health workers, and other facilitators in facilitating SRH learning among adolescents [82, 110]. Furthermore, as it has been exposed by literature the existing guidelines seem to lack robust prescriptions about the coverage, dosage, timing, frequency, and associated pedagogies to facilitate comprehensive and age-appropriate SRH lesson materials among adolescents [111].

Findings by Bilinga and Mabula [100], for example, have noted that teachers and or health workers implement the existing curriculum materials using conventional teaching and assessment approaches as pedagogical bases in facilitating SRH learning among adolescents. Pressures on schools to demonstrate the effective inclusion of comprehensive SRH issues alongside innovative pedagogical approaches open new avenues for educators to decide what, why, when, and how to facilitate SRH learning among adolescents [82]. The permanent use of conventional pedagogies in school curricula, project, interventions, and other programs is argued here to lead to pedagogical inadequacies when facilitating SRH learning among adolescents [111].

To continue implementing SRH education programs via conventional pedagogies may imply that teachers, health workers, and or other facilitators might continue experiencing challenges in assisting adolescents to develop self-control over sexual temptations, harassment, and peer/parental sexual pressure when they resort to using didactic pedagogies [112]. Developing adolescents under conventional pedagogies may imply that they will grow up misinformed about comprehensive SRH information, and its consequences will remain common [109]. To facilitate the empowerment of adolescents on their SRH matters, information about sex, pubertal development, teenage pregnancy, STIs/HIV, and contraception; multidisciplinary strategies, which advocate participatory, collaborative, and age-appropriate pedagogies are proclaimed [113].

Scholars and practitioners [114–119] encourage basic education to adopt and implement participatory and collaborative pedagogies in facilitating sexual and reproductive health learning among adolescents. The implementation of collaborative and participatory pedagogies has also been supported by some literature to be timely as they enhance, not only inquiry learning but also active engagement in learning and the development of hands-on skills in solving real-life problems among adolescents [6, 45, 83, 120]. Moreover, most projects advocate extra-curricular activities among adolescents such as farming, gardening, games, and or entrepreneurship works. Extra-curricular activities are believed to promote adolescents' hard skills more than soft skills, which they need to make informed, conscious, reasoned, and responsible decisions over sexual behaviours.

Yet, scholars [2, 13] have argued that if comprehensive sexual and reproductive health education is facilitated by using participatory and collaborative pedagogies, the interaction and communication about sensitive SRH topics among teachers, healthcare workers, and other facilitators become very easy. Amidst the existing efforts, most of the existing strategies focus more on adolescents' empowerment in life skills than the pedagogical issues prescribed in school curricula. The projects are argued to not advocate multidisciplinary strategies in facilitating SRH learning to adolescents including education and health fields [121]. Some projects are claimed to be unsustainable because they largely depend on external funding along with the prescribed curricula, which are more of a conventional style and have adopted western styles that do not blend with the African context [122, 123].

2.8 Sexual information and education versus sexual behaviours among adolescents

Adolescents' behaviours have been described by medical, psychosocial, and educational scientists as being malleable owing to internal and external stressors [120, 124, 125]. Owing to globalization, changes in social roles and responsibilities, and migrations, the current situation has plenty of sources of sexual information and education among adolescents including schools, healthcare professionals, parents, religious facilities, media, and peers [6, 83, 126]. These sources are expected to enhance the sexual well-being of adolescents by developing them with good SRH knowledge, and soft skills and thus, shape their safe sexual behaviours. However, literature has critiqued some of the sources to be not valid enough to provide accurate and age-appropriate SRH information and education among adolescents such as media and peer groups [121].

Most social media including television, radio, online music, movies, cinema, and peer groups, just to mention a few, are currently disseminating SRH health information and education without considering the sociocultural, age, and gender differences contexts of the consumers. Sources, including parents, healthcare professionals, and religious facilities are reported to be rarely available to sit and educate their children about SRH [23, 46]. The duty of providing accurate and age-appropriate SRH information and education among adolescents seems to fall on schools [127]. However, the identification of factors that determine adolescents' biological changes, neurobehavioral changes, and social maturation to pursue their roles and responsibilities in society needs to be given priority during the development of SRH lesson materials [5]. Based on this context scholar appear in the frontline in advocating innovative interventional researches to address the informative contextual gap observed in this chapter for the well-being of young people to contribute to the socio-economic prosperity of nations, regions and the globe at large [128].

3. Conclusion

Although the uptake of chlamydia screening and treatment is keeping in the high race, its incidence among young people remains high. With this regard to the knowledge disseminated in this chapter, there seems to be a need for establishing a multidisciplinary pedagogical guideline for teachers, health workers, and or other facilitators of SRH learning for adolescents, especially in middle and low-income countries.

Author details

Walter C. Millanzi
Department of Nursing Management and Education, School of Nursing and Public Health, The University of Dodoma, Dodoma, Tanzania

*Address all correspondence to: wcleo87@gmail.com; walter.millanzi@udom.ac.tz

References

[1] Millanzi WC, Kibusi SM, Osaki KM. Effect of integrated reproductive health lesson materials in a problem-based pedagogy on soft skills for safe sexual behaviour among adolescents: A school-based randomized controlled trial in Tanzania. Zhou M, editor. PLoS One [Internet]. 22 February 2022;**17**(2):e0263431. Available from: https://dx.plos.org/10.1371/journal.pone.0263431 [Cited: 23 February 2022]

[2] Millanzi WC. The Effectiveness of Integrated Reproductive Health Lesson Materials in a Problem-Based Pedagogy on Knowledge, Soft Skills, and Sexual Behaviours among Adolescents in Tanzania [Internet]. University of Dodoma Institutional Repository; 2021. Available from: http://repository.udom.ac.tz

[3] Osborn D, Cutter A, Ullah F. Universal sustainable development goals: Understanding the transformational challenge for developed countries. Universal Sustainable Development Goals [Internet]. 2015. pp. 1-24. Available from: https://sustainabledevelopment.un.org/index.php?page=view&type=400&nr=1684&menu=35

[4] UNFPA. Strategic Plan 2018-2021. 2018. Available from: https://www.unfpa.org/sites/default/files/pub-pdf/18-044_UNFPA-SP2018-EN_2018-03-12-1244_0.pdf

[5] Millanzi WC, Osaki KM, Kibusi SM. Non-cognitive skills for safe sexual behavior: An exploration of baseline abstinence skills, condom use negotiation, self-esteem, and assertiveness skills from a controlled problem-based learning intervention among adolescents in Tanzania. Global Journal of Medical Research [Internet]. 2020;**20**(10):1-18. Available from: https://medicalresearchjournal.org/index.php/GJMR/article/view/2215/2104

[6] Zulu JM, Blystad A, Haaland MES, Michelo C, Haukanes H, Moland KM. Why teach sex education in school? Teacher discretion in implementing comprehensive sexuality education in rural Zambia. International Journal for Equity in Health [Internet]. 2019;**18**(1):1-10. Available from: https://doi.org/10.1186/s12939-019-1023-1

[7] UNICEF. Experiences and Accounts of Pregnancy amongst Adolescents [Internet]. Panamá: UNFPA; 2014. p. 82. Available from: www.unicef.org/lac

[8] WHO. Adolescent Pregnancy: Issues in Adolescent Health and Development [Internet]. Geneva, Switzerland: WHO Library Cataloguing-in-Publication Data; 2007. pp. 1-86. Available from: https://www.who.int/news-room/fact-sheets/detail/adolescent-pregnancy [Cited: 14 October 2019]

[9] WHO. Adolescent Pregnancy Fact Sheet [Internet]. 2014. pp. 1-4. Available from: http://apps.who.int/iris/bitstream/10665/112320/1/WHO_RHR_14.08_eng.pdf%0Awww.who.int/reproductivehealth

[10] Mbachu CO, Agu IC, Eze I, Agu C, Ezenwaka U, Ezumah N, et al. Exploring issues in caregivers and parent communication of sexual and reproductive health matters with adolescents in Ebonyi State, Nigeria. BMC Public Health [Internet]. 17 January 2020;**20**(1):1-77. Available from: https://doi.org/10.1186/s12889-019-8058-5

[11] Doremus-Fitzwater TL, Barreto M, Spear LP. Age-related differences in impulsivity among adolescent

and adult Sprague-Dawley rats. Behavioral Neuroscience [Internet]. 2012;**126**(5):735-41. Available from: https://doi.org/10.1037/a0029697

[12] Wendy B, Sherry K. Teacher-student perspectives of invisible pedagogy: New directions in online problem-based learning environments. Electronic Journal of e-Learning [Internet]. 2016;**14**(4):235-43. Available from: http://search.ebscohost.com/login.aspx?direct=true&db=eue&AN=119642364&amp%5Cnlang=ko&site=ehost-live

[13] Millanzi WC, Osaki KM, Kibusi SM. The effect of educational intervention on shaping safe sexual behavior based on the problem-based pedagogy in the field of sex education and reproductive health: Clinical trial among adolescents in Tanzania. Health Psychology and Behavioral Medicine [Internet]. 2022;**10**(1):262-90. Available from: https://doi.org/10.1080/21642850.2022.2046474

[14] Scales PC, Blyth DA, Berkas TH, Kielsmeier JC. The effects of service-learning on middle school students' social responsibility and academic success. Journal of Early Adolescence [Internet]. 26 July 2000;**20**(3):332-58. Available from: https://journals.sagepub.com/doi/10.1177/0272431600020003004 [Cited: 3 June 2021]

[15] Denno DM, Hoopes AJ, Chandra-Mouli V. Effective strategies to provide adolescent sexual and reproductive health services and to increase demand and community support. Journal of Adolescent Health [Internet]. 2015;**56**(1):S22-41. Available from: http://dx.doi.org/10.1016/j.jadohealth.2014.09.012

[16] UNFPA. Adolescent Pregnancy: A Review of the Evidence. UNFPA [Internet]. 2013. pp. 1-58. Available from: https://www.unfpa.org

[17] UNFPA. A review of 23 countries in harmonizing the legal environment for adolescent sexual and reproductive health and rights 2 [Internet]. 2017. pp. 1-24. Available from: https://esaro.unfpa.org/sites/default/files/pub-pdf/2017-08-Laws and Policies-Digital_0.pdf

[18] WHO. World health statistics 2018: Monitoring health for the SDGs, sustainable development goals. In: CC BY-NC-SA 3.0 IGO. Vol. 10. 2018. Available from: https://creativecommons.org/licenses/by-nc-sa/3.0/igo

[19] WHO. Adolescent pregnancy. The Medical Journal of Australia. 2019;**142**(8):490. Available from: DOI: 10.5694/j.1326-5377.1985.tb113469.x

[20] MoHCDGEC. National Adolescent Health and Development Strategy 2018-2022. 2018;**2057**:1-41. Available from: https://tciurbanhealth.org/wp-content/uploads/2017/12/020518_Adolescent-and-Development-Strategy-Tanzania_vF.pdf

[21] Ministry of Finance and Planning. Available from: https://nbs.go.tz

[22] NBS. Tanzania Hiv Impact Survey (This) 2016-2017. (December 2017), 2016-2017. 2018. Available from: http://www.nbs.go.tz/nbs/takwimu/this2016-17/Tanzania_SummarySheet_English

[23] Maly C, Mcclendon KA, Baumgartner JN, Nakyanjo N, Ddaaki WG, Serwadda D, et al. Perceptions of adolescent pregnancy among teenage girls in Rakai, Uganda. Global Qualitative Nursing Research [Internet]. 2017;**4**(1):12. Available from: http://www.creativecommons.org/licenses/by-nc/4.0/

[24] Doyle AM, Ross DA, Maganja K, Baisley K, Masesa C, Andreasen A, et al. Long-term biological and behavioural

impact of an adolescent sexual health intervention in Tanzania: Follow-up survey of the community-based Mema kwa vijana trial. PLoS Medicine. 2010;**7**(6):1-14

[25] Decat P, De Meyer S, Jaruseviciene L, Orozco M, Ibarra M, Segura Z, et al. Sexual onset and contraceptive use among adolescents from poor neighborhoods in Managua, Nicaragua. The European Journal of Contraception & Reproductive Health Care [Internet]. 2015;**20**(2):88-100. Available from: https://doi.org/10.3109/13625187.2014.955846

[26] Mpondo F, Ruiter AC, Schaafsma D, van den Borne B, Reddy PS. Understanding the role played by parents, culture, and the school curriculum in socializing young women on sexual health issues in rural South African communities. SAHARA-J. 2018;**15**(1):42-49

[27] Muhwezi WW, Katahoire AR, Banura C, Mugooda H, Kwesiga D, Bastien S, et al. Perceptions and experiences of adolescents, parents and school administrators regarding adolescent-parent communication on sexual and reproductive health issues in urban and rural Uganda Adolescent Health. Reproductive Health [Internet]. 2015;**12**(1):1-16. Available from: http://dx.doi.org/10.1186/s12978-015-0099-3

[28] Wado YD, Sully EA, Mumah JN. Pregnancy and early motherhood among adolescents in five East African countries: A multi-level analysis of risk and protective factors. BMC Pregnancy and Childbirth. 2019;**19**(1):1-11

[29] Tadjer H, Lafifi Y, Seridi-Bouchelaghem H, Gülseçen S. Improving soft skills based on students' traces in problem-based learning environments. Interactive Learning Environments [Internet]. 2020. Available from: https://doi.org/10.1080/10494820.2020.1753215 [Cited: 12 June 2021]

[30] United Nations. The sustainable development goals [Internet]. Jensen L, editor. Design for Global Challenges and Goals. New York: United Nations publication issued by the Department of Economic and Social Affairs; 2021. pp. 12-25. Available from: https://unstats.un.org/sdgs

[31] Lanari D, Mangiavacchi L, Pasqualini M. Adolescent sexual behaviour and academic performance of Italian students. Genus [Internet]. 2020;**76**(1). Available from: https://doi.org/10.1186/s41118-020-00093-4

[32] Aristotle. The young are heated by nature as drunken men by wine [Internet]. The Rhetoric of Aristotle. 1886. Available from: https://www.quotenova.net/authors/aristotle/q4w3px [Cited: 11 May 2021]

[33] Kassa GM, Arowojolu AO, Odukogbe AA, Yalew AW. Prevalence and determinants of adolescent pregnancy in Africa: A systematic review and Meta-analysis 11 Medical and Health Sciences 1117 Public Health and Health Services. BMC Reproductive Health [Internet]. 2018;**15**(1):1-17. Available from: https://doi.org/10.1186/s12978-018-0640-2

[34] Barry CT, Sidoti CL, Briggs SM, Reiter SR, Lindsey RA. Adolescent social media use and mental health from adolescent and parent perspectives. Journal of Adolescence. 2017;**61**:1-11

[35] Ivanova O, Rai M, Mlahagwa W, Tumuhairwe J, Bakuli A, Nyakato VN, et al. A cross-sectional mixed-methods study of sexual and reproductive health knowledge, experiences and access to services among refugee adolescent girls in the Nakivale refugee settlement,

Uganda. Reproductive Health [Internet]. 2019;**16**(1):1-11. Available from: https://doi.org/10.1186/s12978-019-0698-5

[36] Nkata H, Teixeira R, Barros H. A scoping review on sexual and reproductive health behaviors among Tanzanian adolescents. Public Health Reviews [Internet]. 2019;**40**(1):1-15. Available from: https://doi.org/10.1186/s40985-019-0114-2

[37] Kaale G, Muhanga M. Sexual health knowledge among secondary school students in Morogoro, Tanzania: Half full or full empty? International Journal of Health. 2017;**5**(2):120

[38] Keto T, Tilahun A, Mamo A. Knowledge, attitude and practice towards risky sexual behaviors among secondary and preparatory students of Metu town, Southwestern Ethiopia. BMC Public Health [Internet]. 2020;**20**(1):1-8. Available from: https://doi.org/10.1186/s12889-020-09371-4

[39] Envuladu EA, De Kwaak Anke V, Zwanikken P, Zoakah AI. Sexual and reproductive health challenges of adolescent males and females in some Communities of Plateau State Nigeria. International Journal of Psychology and Behavioral Sciences [Internet]. 2017;**7**(2):55-60. Available from: file:///C:/Users/jboss/Downloads/10.5923.j.ijpbs.20170702.02.pdf

[40] United Nations. World Fertility and Family Planning 2020: Highlights [Internet]. 2020. p. 42. Available from: https://www.un.org/development/desa/pd/sites/www.un.org.development.desa.pd/files/files/documents/2020/Jan/un_2020_worldfertilityfamilyplanning_highlights.pdf

[41] De Castro F, Rojas-martı R, Uribe-zu P. Sexual and reproductive health outcomes are positively associated with comprehensive sexual education exposure in Mexican high-school students. PLoS One [Internet]. 2018;**13**(3):1-15. Available from: https://doi.org/10.1371/journal. pone.0193780

[42] United Nations Children's Fund. The State of the World's Children: Adolescence an Age of Opportunity. 2011. p. 134

[43] Izugbara CO, Wekesah FM, Tilahun T, Amo-Adjei J, Tsala Dimbuene ZT. Family Planning in East Africa: Trends and Dynamics [Internet]. African Population and Health Research Center (APHRC); 2018. Available from: info@aphrc.org

[44] Panjaitan AA. Model of prevention of adolescent unwanted pregnancy in Indonesia: Review article. International Journal of Research in Law, Economic and Social Sciences [Internet]. 2019;1(2):**60**-73. Available from: https://doi.org/10.32501/injuriless.v1i2.125

[45] Chavula MP, Svanemyr J, Zulu JM, Sandøy IF. Experiences of teachers and community health workers implementing sexuality and life skills education in youth clubs in Zambia. Global Public Health [Internet]. 4 March 2021;**20**(2):1-15. Available from: https://doi.org/10.1080/17441692.2021.1893371 [Cited: 31 May 2021]

[46] Alabi OT, Oni IO. Teenage pregnancy in Nigeria: Causes, effect, and control. International Journal of Academic Research in Business and Social Sciences [Internet]. 2017;**7**(2):17-32. Available from: http://dx.doi.org/10.6007/IJARBSS/v7-i2/2610abstract

[47] Ndibalema P. Making sense of basic education statistics in Tanzania: Emerging issues and implications for future practice. International Journal of Elementary Education. 2019;**8**(1):26

[48] Yi S, Tuot S, Yung K, Kim S, Chhea C, Saphonn V. Factors associated with risky sexual behavior among unmarried most-at-risk young people in Cambodia. American Journal of Public Health Research. 2014;**2**(5):211-220

[49] Landry M, Turner M, Vyas A, Wood S. Social media and sexual behavior among adolescents: Is there a link? JMIR Public Health and Surveillance [Internet]. 2017;**3**(2):e28. Available from: http://publichealth.jmir.org/2017/2/e28/

[50] Human Rights Watch. "I had a dream to finish school": Barriers to secondary education in Tanzania [Internet]. 2017. pp. 1-108. Available from: http://www.hrw.org

[51] Kalolo A, Kibusi SM. The influence of perceived behaviour control, attitude, and empowerment on reported condom use and intention to use condoms among adolescents in rural Tanzania. Reproductive Health [Internet]. 2015;**12**(1):1-9. Available from: https://doi.org/10.1186/s12978-015-0097-5

[52] Yakubu I. Determinants of adolescent pregnancy in sub-Saharan Africa: A systematic review. Reproductive Health [Internet]. 2018;**15**(15):1-11. Available from: https://doi.org/10.1186/s12978-018-0460-4

[53] Ambrosia M, Eckstrand KL, Morgan JK, Allen NB, Jones NP, Sheeber L, et al. Temptations of friends: Adolescents' neural and behavioral responses to best friends predict risky behavior. Social Cognitive and Affective Neuroscience [Internet]. 2018;**13**(5):483-91. Available from: https://doi.org/10.1093/scan/nsy028

[54] Mlyakado BP. Schoolgirls' knowledge of, and efforts against risky sexual activity: The needs for sex education in schools. International Journal of Education [Internet]. 2013;**5**(1):69-80. Available from: http://dx.doi.org/10.5296/ije.v5i1.2825

[55] Petro Mlyakado B, Timothy N. Effects of students' sexual relationship on academic performance among secondary school students in Tanzania. Academic Research International [Internet]. 2014;**5**(4):278-86. Available from: www.savap.org.pk%5Cnwww.journals.savap.org.pk

[56] Chilisa R, Tlhabano K, Vista C, Pheko M, Losike N, Mosime S, Mpeta K, Balogun SK. Self-efficacy, self-esteem and the intention to practice safe sex among Batswana adolescents. IOSR Journal of Humanities and Social Science [Internet]. 2013;**9**(2):87-95. Available from: www.iosrjournals.org

[57] WHO. Sexually Transmitted Infections (STIs) [Internet]. WHO Publications; 2022. Available from: https://www.who.int/en/news-room/fact-sheets/detail/sexually-transmitted-infections-(STIS) [Cited: 7 November 2022]

[58] UNAIDS. Global Aids Monitoring 2018 [Internet]. Global AIDS Monitoring 2018: Indicators for Monitoring the 2016 United Nations Political Declaration on Ending AIDS. 2018. Available from: http://www.unaids.org/sites/default/files/media_asset/global-aids-monitoring_en.pdf

[59] Jamison CD, Coleman JS, Mmeje O. Improving women's health and combatting sexually transmitted infections through expedited partner therapy. Obstetrics & Gynecology [Internet]. 1 March 2019;**133**(3):416. Available from: https://www.ncbi.nlm.nih.gov/pmc/articles/PMC7136014/ [Cited: 7 November 2022]

[60] Kularatne RS, Niit R, Rowley J, Kufa-Chakezha T, Peters RPH, Taylor MM, et al. Adult gonorrhea,

chlamydia and syphilis prevalence, incidence, treatment and syndromic case reporting in South Africa: Estimates using the spectrum-STI model, 1990-2017. PLoS One [Internet]. 1 October 2018;**13**(10):e0205863. Available from: https://journals.plos.org/plosone/article?id=10.1371/journal.pone.0205863 [Cited: 7 November 2022]

[61] UNAIDS. 2017 Global HIV Statistics. 2018. p. 5. Available from: http://www.unaids.org/sites/default/files/media_asset/UNAIDS_FactSheet_en.pdf

[62] Global Health Policy. The Global HIV/AIDS Epidemic | KFF [Internet]. The Global HIV/AIDS Epidemic. 2021. Available from: https://www.kff.org/global-health-policy/fact-sheet/the-global-hivaids-epidemic/ [Cited: 8 May 2021]

[63] UNAIDS. July 2020 Core Epidemiology Slides | UNAIDS [Internet]. UNAIDS; 2020. Available from: https://www.unaids.org/en/resources/documents/2020/core-epidemiology-slides [Cited: 8 May 2021]

[64] UNAIDS. Young people, HIV and AIDS young people at school. 2017. Available from: https://www.avert.org/professionals/hiv-social-issues/key-affected-populations/young-people

[65] UNICEF. AIDS HIV and AIDS [Internet]. Dar es Salaam, Tanzania; 2020. Available from: https://www.unicef.org/tanzania/media/2436/file/HIVProgrammeFactSheet.pdf

[66] The Lancet Child & Adolescent Health. Youth STIs: An epidemic fuelled by shame. Lancet Child & Adolescent Health [Internet]. 1 June 2022;**6**(6):353. Available from: http://www.thelancet.com/article/S2352464222001286/fulltext [Cited: 7 November 2022]

[67] Aguirrebengoa OA, Garcia MV, Sanchez MR, D'Elia G, Méndez BC, Arrancudiaga MA, et al. Risk factors associated with sexually transmitted infections and HIV among adolescents in a reference clinic in Madrid. PLoS One [Internet]. 2020;**15**(3):e0228998. Available from: https://journals.plos.org/plosone/article?id=10.1371/journal.pone.0228998 [Cited: 7 November 2022]

[68] Unemo M, Bradshaw CS, Hocking JS, de Vries HJC, Francis SC, Mabey D, et al. Sexually transmitted infections: Challenges ahead. The Lancet Infectious Diseases. 2017;**17**(8):e235-e279

[69] Fernández-Huerta M, Espasa M. *Mycoplasma genitalium* co-infection with *Chlamydia trachomatis* and *Neisseria gonorrhoeae* among asymptomatic patients: The silent wick for macrolide resistance spread. Sexually Transmitted Infections. 2019;**95**(5):391

[70] Morales A, Garcia-Montaño E, Barrios-Ortega C, Niebles-Charris J, Garcia-Roncallo P, Abello-Luque D, et al. Adaptation of an effective school-based sexual health promotion program for youth in Colombia. Social Science & Medicine [Internet]. 2019;**222**(June 2018):207-15. Available from: https://doi.org/10.1016/j.socscimed.2019.01.011

[71] Gabster A, Mayaud P, Ortiz A, Castillo J, Castillero O, Martínez A, et al. Prevalence and determinants of genital *Chlamydia trachomatis* among school-going, sexually experienced adolescents in urban and rural indigenous regions of Panama. Sexually Transmitted Infections [Internet]. 1 June 2021;**97**(4):304-11. Available from: https://sti.bmj.com/content/97/4/304 [Cited: 7 November 2022]

[72] Yuh T, Micheni M, Selke S, Oluoch L, Kiptinness C, Magaret A, et al. Sexually transmitted infections among Kenyan adolescent girls and young women with limited sexual experience. Frontiers in Public Health. 2020;**8**:303

[73] Wangu Z, Burstein GR. Adolescent sexuality: Updates to the sexually transmitted infection guidelines. Pediatric Clinics of North America. 2017;**64**(2):389-411

[74] Uromi SM. Schoolgirl pregnancies as a most critical and rapidly growing challenge in Tanzania. International Journal of Innovation Science and Research [Internet]. 2014;**10**(1):191-4. Available from: http://www.ijisr.issr-journals.org/

[75] WHO. World Health Organization: Adolescent Pregnancy Fact Sheet No. 364 [Internet]. 2018. Available from: https://www.who.int/en/news-room/fact-sheets/detail/adolescent-pregnancy [Cited: 7 November 2019]

[76] WHO. Adolescent pregnancy. Medical Journal of Australia [Internet]. 2019;**142**(8):490. Available from: www.who.int/reproductivehealth

[77] MoHCDGEC. Child Marriage in Tanzania. 2017. DOI: 10.1016/S0140-6736(00)94317-4

[78] USAID. Sexual and reproductive health in early and later adolescence: DHS data on youth age 10-19. DHS Comp Reports [Internet]. 2017;**45**:1-112. Available from: https://www.dhsprogram.com/pubs/pdf/CR45/CR45.pdf

[79] Weldemariam KT, Gezae KE, Abebe HT. Reasons and multilevel factors associated with unscheduled contraceptive use discontinuation in Ethiopia: Evidence from Ethiopian demographic and health survey 2016. BMC Public Health. 2019;**19**(1):1-15

[80] Wolinsky S. Nothing Comes From Nothing: The Complete One Hundred Most Frequently Asked Questions [Internet]. eBook; 2016. Available from: http://toolbook.site/go/read.php?id=B01CRKAJ4C [Cited: 12 February 2021]

[81] Paquette D, Ryan J. Bronfenbrenner's Ecological Systems Theory [Internet]. ReserachGate; 2001. Available from: https://www.researchgate.net/publication/265485344_Bronfenbrenner's_Ecological_Systems_Theory [Cited: 4 June 2021]

[82] Cardoso JC, Mwolo MP. Assessment of non-formal sexual education strategies for adolescent girls: The case of Tanzania. Ensaio [Internet]. 2017;**25**(95):527-47. Available from: https://10.0.6.54/S0104-40362017002501111527

[83] Kamangu AA, John MR, Nyakoki SJ. Barriers to parent-child communication on sexual and reproductive health issues in East Africa: A review of qualitative research in four countries. Journal of African Studies and Development [Internet]. 2017;**9**(4):45-50. Available from: http://www.academicjournlas.org/JASD

[84] El Kazdouh H, El-Ammari A, Bouftini S, El Fakir S, El Achhab Y. Perceptions and intervention preferences of Moroccan adolescents, parents, and teachers regarding risks and protective factors for risky sexual behaviors leading to sexually transmitted infections in adolescents: qualitative findings. Reproductive Health [Internet]. 2019;**16**(138):1-17. Available from: https://doi.org/10.1186/s12978-019-0801-y

[85] Watsi L, Tarkang EE. Demographic determinants of risky sexual behaviours among senior high school students in the Hohoe Municipality, Ghana. The Pan African Medical Journal [Internet]. 2020;**2797**:1-12. Available from: https://www.clinical-medicine.panafrican-med-journal.com/content/article/2/81/full%0A

[86] De-Sousa C, dos Santos RS, Santana KC, Souzas R, Leite ÁJM, de Medeiros DS. Sexual behavior

and associated factors in rural adolescents. Revista de Saúde Pública [Internet]. 2018;**52**(39):1-11. Available from: https://doi.org/10.11606/S1518-8787.2018052006988

[87] Waktole ZD. Sexual behaviors and associated factors among youths in Nekemte town, East Wollega, Oromia, Ethiopia: A cross-sectional study. PLoS One [Internet]. 2019;**14**(7):1-10. Available from: https://doi.org/10.1371/journal.pone.0220235

[88] Do HN, Nguyen DN, Nguyen HQT, Nguyen AT, Nguyen HD, Bui TP, et al. Patterns of risky sexual behaviors and associated factors among youths and adolescents in Vietnam. International Journal of Environmental Research and Public Health [Internet]. 2020;**17**(6): 1-14. Available from: https://doi.org/10.3390/ijerph17061903

[89] UNFPA. Marrying Too Young: End Child Marriage [Internet]. New York, NY, USA; 2012. pp. 1-76. Available from: https://www.unfpa.org/webdav/site/global/shared/documents/publications/2012/MarryingTooYoung.pdf

[90] Pradhan R, Wynter K, Fisher J. Factors associated with pregnancy among married adolescents in Nepal: Secondary analysis of the national demographic and health surveys from 2001 to 2011. International Journal of Environmental Research and Public Health. 2018;**15**(2):1-12

[91] Busi S. Barriers of discussion concerning sexual and reproductive health issues among adolescents and parents, Hawassa, SNNPR, Ethiopia. Biomedical Journal of Scientific & Technical Research. 2017;**1**(7):1-7

[92] Mutanana N, Mutara G. Factors contributing to teenage pregnancies in a rural community of Zimbabwe. Journal of Biology, Agriculture and Healthcare [Internet]. 2015;**5**(14):29-34. Available from: www.iiste.org

[93] Schiller P. Seven Skills for School Success [Internet]. Images.Gryphonhouse.Com. 2009. Available from: https://images.gryphonhouse.com/content/SevenSkillsForSchoolSuccess PDIHANDOUT.pdf

[94] Christopher M. Relationships of parental monitoring and emotion regulation with early adolescents' sexual behaviors. Physiology & Behavior [Internet]. 2016;**176**(1):100-106. Available from: https://doi.org/10.1016/j.gde.2016.03.011

[95] Visser M. Rethinking HIV prevention for school-going young people based on current behaviour patterns. SAHARA-J: Journal of Social Aspects of HIV/AIDS [Internet]. 2017;**14**(1):64-76. Available from: https://doi.org/10.1080/17290376.2017.1376704

[96] Osorio A, Lopez-del Burgo C, Ruiz-Canela M, Carlos S, de Irala J. Safe-sex belief and sexual risk behaviours among adolescents from three developing countries: A cross-sectional study. BMJ Open. 2015;**5**(4):e007826

[97] Savage-Oyekunle OA, Nienaber A. Adolescent girls' access to contraceptive information and services: An analysis of legislation and policies, and their realization, in Nigeria and South Africa. African Human Rights Law Journal [Internet]. 2015;**15**(2):433-48. Available from: https://doi.org/10.17159/1996-2096/2015/v15n2a10

[98] Svanemyr J, Amin A, Robles OJ, Greene ME. Creating an enabling environment for adolescent sexual and reproductive health: A framework and promising approaches. Journal of Adolescent Health [Internet]. 2015;**56**(1):S7-14. Available

from: http://dx.doi.org/10.1016/j.jadohealth.2014.09.011

[99] Human Rights Watch. Tanzania: Q & A on Ban on Pregnant Girls and World Bank Education Loan | Human Rights Watch [Internet]. Human Rights Watch; 2020. Available from: https://www.hrw.org/news/2020/04/24/tanzania-q-ban-pregnant-girls-and-world-bank-education-loan [Cited: 8 May 2021]

[100] Bilinga M, Mabula N. Teaching sexuality education in primary schools in Tanzania: Challenges and implications. Journal of Education and Practice [Internet]. 2014;**5**(27):21-31. Available from: http://www.iste.org/journals/

[101] MoEST. Basic Education Curriculum Standard III–VI. World Police & Paramilitary Forces; 2016. p. 199

[102] MoEVT. Science Syllabus for Primary Schools: Class I–VII. 2nd ed. Tanzania Institute of Education, editor. Dar es Salaam, Tanzania: Tanzania Institute of Education; 2005. pp. 1-199

[103] MoEVT. Biology Syllabus for Ordinary Secondary Education: Form I–IV [Internet]. 2nd ed. Tanzania Institute of Education, editor. Dar es Salaam, Tanzania: Tanzania Institute of Education; 2005. pp. 1-220. Available from: https://www.moevt.org.tz

[104] TIE. Curriculum for ordinally level secondary education in Tanzania [Internet]. 2007. Available from: www.tie.go.tz

[105] Wanje G, Masese L, Avuvika E, Baghazal A, Omoni G, Mcclelland RS. Parents' and teachers' views on sexual health education and screening for sexually transmitted infections among in-school adolescent girls in Kenya: A qualitative study. Reproductive Health [Internet]. 2017;**14**(95):1-11. Available from: http://creativecommons.org/licenses/by/4.0/

[106] Baku EA, Agbemafle I, Kotoh AM, Adanu RMK. Parents' experiences and sexual topics discussed with adolescents in the Accra Metropolis, Ghana: A qualitative study. Hindawi Advances in Public Health [Internet]. 2018;**2018**:12. Available from: https://doi.org/10.1155/2018/5784902

[107] Boti N, Hussein S, Shegaze M, Shibru S, Shibiru T, Zerihun E, et al. Effects of comprehensive sexuality education on the comprehensive knowledge and attitude to condom use among first-year students in Arba Minch University: A quasi-experimental study. BMC Research Notes [Internet]. 2019. pp. 1-7. Available from: https://doi.org/10.1186/s13104-019-4746-6

[108] Kemigisha E, Bruce K, Ivanova O, Leye E, Coene G, Ruzaaza GN, et al. Evaluation of a school-based comprehensive sexuality education program among very young adolescents in rural Uganda. BMC Public Health [Internet]. 28 October 2019;**19**(1). Available from: https://doi.org/10.1186/s12889-019-7805-y

[109] Boonstra HD. Advancing sexuality education in developing countries: Evidence and implications. Evidence-Based Approaches to Sex Education [Internet]. 2021;**14**(3):370-80. Available from: https://doi.org/10.4324/9781315755250-33

[110] Doubova SV, Martinez-Vega IP, Infante-Castaeda C, Prez-Cuevas R. Effects of an internet-based educational intervention to prevent high-risk sexual behavior in Mexican adolescents. Health Education Research [Internet]. 2017;**32**(6):487-98. Available from: https://doi.org/10.1093/her/cyx074

[111] Haruna H, Hu X, Wah Chu SK. Adolescent school-based sexual health education and training: A literature review

on teaching and learning strategies. Global Journal of Health Sciences [Internet]. 2018;**10**(3):172. Available from: https://doi.org/10.5539/gjhs.v10n3p172

[112] Celiker HD. Development of metacognitive skills: Designing problem-based experiments with prospective science teachers in a biology laboratory. Educational Research and Reviews - Academic Journals [Internet]. 2015;**10**(11):1487-95. Available from: http://www.academicjournals.org/ERR

[113] Daliana N, Farid N, Rus SC, Dahlui M, Al-Sadat N, Aziz NA. Predictors of sexual risk behaviour among adolescents from welfare institutions in Malaysia: A cross-sectional study. BMC Public Health [Internet]. 2014;**14**(Suppl. 3):1-8. Available from: http://www.biomedcentral.com/1471-2458/14/S3/S9

[114] Amoako-Sakyi D, Amonoo-Kuofi H. Problem-based learning in resource-poor settings: Lessons from a medical school in Ghana. BMC Medical Education. 2015;**15**(1):1-8

[115] Zabit MNM. Problem-based learning on students critical thinking skills in teaching business education in Malaysia: A literature review. American Journal of Business Education [Internet]. 2010;**3**(6):19-32. Available from: https://www.researchgate.net/publication/288880295

[116] Masek A, Yamin S. A comparative study of the effect of problem-based learning and traditional learning approaches on students' knowledge acquisition BT—Current trends in nanotechnology education. International Journal of Engineering Education [Internet]. 2012;**28**(5):1161-7. Available from: https://aliasmasek@uthm.edu.my

[117] Keziah A. A comparative study of problem-based and lecture-based learning in secondary school students' motivation to learn science. International Journal of Scientific and Technological Research [Internet]. 2010;**1**(November):126-31. Available from: http://www.academicjournals.org/IJSTER

[118] Millanzi WC, Kibusi SM. Exploring the effect of problem-based facilitatory teaching approach on metacognition in nursing education: A quasi-experimental study of nurse students in Tanzania. Nursing Open [Internet]. 2020;**2020**(February):1-15. Available from: https://doi.org/10.1002/nop2.514

[119] Caswell CA. Design and facilitation of problem-based learning in graduate teacher education: An MA TESOL case. Interdisciplinary Journal of Problem-Based Learning [Internet]. 2017;**11**(1). Available from: https://doi.org/10.7771/1541-5015.1623

[120] Laddunuri MMP. The sexual behaviour of secondary school adolescent students in Tanzania: Patterns and trends. International Journal of Caring Sciences [Internet]. 2013;**6**(3):472-84. Available from: https://search.proquest.com/docview/1445366569?accountid=169732

[121] Pozo KC, Chandra-Mouli V, Decat P, Nelson E, De Meyer S, Jaruseviciene L, et al. Improving adolescent sexual and reproductive health in Latin America: Reflections from an International Congress. Reproductive Health [Internet]. 2015;**12**(1). Available from: http://www.reproductive-health-journal.com/content/12/1/11

[122] Kemigisha E, Ivanova O, Ruzaaza GN, Ninsiima AB, Kaziga R, Bruce K, et al. Process evaluation of a comprehensive sexuality education intervention in primary schools in South Western Uganda. Sexual & Reproductive Healthcare [Internet]. 2019;**21**(June):

51-9. Available from: https://doi.org/10.1016/j.srhc.2019.06.006

[123] Ahmed N, Flisher AJ, Mathews C, Mukoma W, Jansen S. HIV education in South African schools: The dilemma and conflicts of educators. Scandinavian Journal of Public Health. 2009; **37**(Suppl. 2):48-54

[124] Unique IB, Adogu PO, Nwabueze AS, Adinma ED, Ubajaka CF, Onwasigwe C. Factors influencing sexual behavior among female adolescents in Onitsha, Nigeria. Open Journal of Obstetrics and Gynecology [Internet]. 2014;(December):987-95. Available from: http://dx.doi.org/10.4236/ojog.2014.416139

[125] Iordanescu E, Iordanescu C, Draghici A. Time and gender influence in sexual behavior of Romanian adolescents. Procedia Social and Behavioral Sciences [Internet]. 2015;**187**:757-61. Available from: http://dx.doi.org/10.1016/j.sbspro.2015.03.160

[126] Landry M, Turner M, Vyas A, Wood S. Social Media and Sexual Behavior among Adolescents: Is there a link? 2017;3.

[127] Baker-Henningham H. The role of early childhood education programs in the promotion of child and adolescent mental health in low- and middle-income countries. International Journal of Epidemiology. 2014;**43**(2):407-433

[128] USAID. Key Soft Skills for Cross-Key Soft Skills for Cross-Sectoral Youth Outcomes [Internet]. Washington, DC: USAID's YouthPower: Implementation, YouthPower Action; 2016. Report No.: AID-OAA-TO-15-00003. Available from: http://documents.worldbank.org/curated/en/569931468331784110/pdf/816730BRI0AGI00Box0379842B00PUBLIC0.pdf